theclinics.com

NEUROLOGIC CLINICS

Stroke

GUEST EDITORS
Sean D. Ruland, DO
Philip B. Gorelick, MD, MPH, FACP

CONSULTING EDITOR
Randolph W. Evans, MD

November 2008 • Volume 26 • Number 4

SAUNDERS
An Imprint of Elsevier, Inc.
PHILADELPHIA LONDON TORONTO MONTREAL SYDNEY TOKYO

W.B. SAUNDERS COMPANY
A Division of Elsevier Inc.

1600 John F. Kennedy Blvd., Suite 1800, Philadelphia, PA 19103-2899

http://www.theclinics.com

NEUROLOGIC CLINICS
November 2008
Editor: Donald Mumford

Volume 26, Number 4
ISSN 0733-8619
ISBN-13: 978-1-4160-6322-3
ISBN-10: 1-4160-6322-6

Neurologic Clinics (ISSN 0733-8619) is published quarterly by Elsevier Inc., 360 Park Avenue South, New York, NY 10010–171. Months of issue are February, May, August, and November. Business and editorial offices: 1600 John F. Kennedy Blvd., Suite 1800, Philadelphia, PA 19103-2899. Customer Service Office: 11830 Westline Industrial Drive, St. Louis, MO 63146. Accounting and circulation offices: 11830 Westline Industrial Drive, St. Louis, MO 63146. Periodicals postage paid at New York, NY, and additional mailing offices. Subscription prices are $235.00 per year for US individuals, $378.00 per year for US institutions, $118.00 per year for US students, $295.00 per year for Canadian individuals, $454.00 per year for Canadian institutions, $328.00 per year for international individuals, $454.00 per year for international institutions, and $167.00 for Canadian and foreign students/residents. To receive student/resident rate, orders must be accompanied by name of affiliated institution, date of term, and the *signature* of program/residency coordinator on institution letterhead. Orders will be billed at individual rate until proof of status is received. Foreign air speed delivery is included in all *Clinics* subscription prices. All prices are subject to change without notice. POSTMASTER: Send address changes to *Neurologic Clinics*, Elsevier Periodicals Customer Service, 11830 Westline Industrial Drive, St. Louis, MO 63146. **Customer Service: 1-800-654-2452 (US). From outside of the US, call 314-453-7041. Fax: 314-453-5170. E-mail: JournalsCustomerService-usa@elsevier.com (for print support); JournalsOnlineSupport-usa@elsevier.com (for online support).**

Reprints. For copies of 100 or more of articles in this publication, please contact the Commercial Reprints Department, Elsevier Inc., 360 Park Avenue South, New York, New York, 10010-1710; Tel.: (+1) 212-633-3812; Fax: (+1) 212-462-1935, and E-mail: reprints@elsevier.com.

Neurologic Clinics is also published in Spanish by Nueva Editorial Interamericana S.A., Mexico City, Mexico.

Neurologic Clinics is covered in *Current Contents/Clinical Medicine, MEDLINE/PubMed (Index Medicus), EMBASE/Excerpta Medica*, and *PsycINFO*, and *ISI/BIOMED.*

Printed in the United States of America.

CONSULTING EDITOR

RANDOLPH W. EVANS, MD, Clinical Professor of Neurology, Baylor College of Medicine, Houston, Texas

GUEST EDITORS

SEAN D. RULAND, DO, Department of Neurology and Rehabilitation, Department of Neurosurgery, University of Illinois College of Medicine at Chicago, Chicago, Illinois

PHILIP B. GORELICK, MD, MPH, FACP, John S. Garvin Professor and Head, Director, Center for Stroke Research, Department of Neurology and Rehabilitation, University of Illinois College of Medicine at Chicago, University of Illinois Medical Center, Chicago, Illinois

CONTRIBUTORS

HAROLD P. ADAMS, Jr, MD, Professor of Neurology; Director, Division of Cerebrovascular Diseases; and Director, University of Iowa Stroke Center, Division of Cerebrovascular Diseases, Department of Neurology, Carver College of Medicine, University of Iowa, Iowa City, Iowa

MARIA I. AGUILAR, MD, Assistant Professor, Department of Neurology, Mayo Clinic, Phoenix, Arizona

VENKATESH AIYAGARI, MBBS, DM, Co-Director, Neurocritical Care, Department of Neurology and Rehabilitation, Section of Cerebrovascular Disease and Neurological Critical Care, University of Illinois College of Medicine at Chicago, Chicago, Illinois

VICTOR ALETICH, MD, Section Chief, Neuroendovascular Division, Department of Neurosurgery, University of Illinois at Chicago, Chicago, Illinois

SEPIDEH AMIN-HANJANI, MD, Assistant Professor; and Co-Director, Neurovascular Surgery, Department of Neurosurgery, University of Illinois at Chicago, Chicago, Illinois

WILLIAM W. ASHLEY, Jr, MD, PhD, MBA, Department of Neurosurgery, University of Illinois at Chicago, Chicago, Illinois

AAMIR BADRUDDIN, MD, Cerebrovascular and Neurological Critical Care Section, Department of Neurology and Rehabilitation, University of Illinois at Chicago, Chicago, Illinois

QASIM BASHIR, MD, Neuroendovascular Division, Department of Neurosurgery, University of Illinois at Chicago, Chicago, Illinois

CHERYL D. BUSHNELL, MD, MHS, Associate Professor, Department of Neurology, Wake Forest University Health Sciences, Winston-Salem, North Carolina

R. CHARLES CALLISON, MD, Fellow in Vascular Neurology, Division of Cerebrovascular Diseases, Department of Neurology, Carver College of Medicine, University of Iowa, Iowa City, Iowa

FADY T. CHARBEL, MD, Professor and Head; and Director, Neurovascular Surgery, Department of Neurosurgery, University of Illinois at Chicago, Chicago, Illinois

WENDE FEDDER, RN, MBA, Director Stroke Center, Alexian Brothers Hospital Network, Neuroscience Institute Stroke Center, Elk Grove Village, Illinois

WILLIAM D. FREEMAN, MD, Assistant Professor, Departments of Neurology and Critical Care, Mayo Clinic, Jacksonville, Florida

ALISSA R. GORELICK, DO, Emergency Medicine Residency Program, Department of Emergency Medicine, University of Illinois College of Medicine at Chicago, University of Illinois Medical Center, Chicago, Illinois

PHILIP B. GORELICK, MD, MPH, FACP, John S. Garvin Professor and Head, Director, Center for Stroke Research, Department of Neurology and Rehabilitation, University of Illinois College of Medicine at Chicago, University of Illinois Medical Center, Chicago, Illinois

REBBECA A. GRYSIEWICZ, DO, Chief Resident, Department of Neurology and Rehabilitation, University of Illinois at Chicago, Chicago, Illinois

ASLAM M. KHAJA, MD, Assistant Professor of Neurology, Department of Neurology Rehabilitation, University of Illinois at Chicago, Chicago, Illinois

LEWIS B. MORGENSTERN, MD, Director of the Stroke Program; Professor of Neurology, Epidemiology, Emergency Medicine and Neurosurgery, The University of Michigan Health System Cardiovascular Center, Ann Arbor, Michigan

DILIP K. PANDEY, MD, PhD, Associate Professor, Department of Neurology and Rehabilitation, University of Illinois at Chicago, Chicago, Illinois

PETER M. ROTHWELL, MD, PhD, FRCP, FMedSci, Professor of Clinical Neurology, University of Oxford, Stroke Prevention Research Unit, University Department of Clinical Neurology, John Radcliffe Hospital, Headington, United Kingdom

TATJANA RUNDEK, MD, PhD, Associate Professor of Neurology, Department of Neurology, Miller School of Medicine, University of Miami, Miami, Florida

RALPH L. SACCO, MD, MS, FAHA, FAAN, Miller Professor of Neurology, Epidemiology and Human Genetics, Department of Neurology, Miller School of Medicine, University of Miami, Miami, Florida

EDWARD P. SLOAN, MD, MPH, FACEP, Professor of Emergency Medicine; Director, Research Development, Department of Emergency Medicine, University of Illinois College of Medicine at Chicago, Chicago, Illinois

FERNANDO D. TESTAI, MD, PhD, Vascular Neurology Fellow, Department of Neurology and Rehabilitation, Section of Cerebrovascular Disease and Neurological Critical Care, University of Illinois College of Medicine at Chicago, Chicago, Illinois

KURIAN THOMAS, MD, Clinical Instructor, Department of Neurology, Jesse Brown Veteran's Administration Medical Center, Chicago, Illinois

KEITH R. THULBORN, MD, PhD, Professor of Radiology, Physiology and Biophysics; Director, Center for Magnetic Resonance Research, University of Illinois Medical Center at Chicago, Chicago, Illinois

BRIAN TRIMBLE, MD, Assistant Professor of Neurology, University of Washington, Seattle, Washington; and Neurologist, Alaska Native Medical Center, Anchorage, Alaska

CONTENTS

FORTHCOMING ISSUES

February 2009

Neuroimaging
Laszlo Mechtler, MD, *Guest Editor*

May 2009

Primary Headache
Randolph W. Evans, MD, *Guest Editor*

August 2009

Movement Disorders
Joseph Jankovic, MD, *Guest Editor*

RECENT ISSUES

August 2008

Current Issues in Clinical Neurovirology: Pathogenesis, Diagnosis and Treatment
Christopher Power, MD and Richard T. Johnson, MD, *Guest Editors*

May 2008

Neurologic Critical Care
Romergryko G. Geocadin, MD and Robert D. Stevens, MD, *Guest Editors*

February 2008

Sports Neurology
Cory Toth, MD, FRCPC, *Guest Editor*

ELSEVIER
SAUNDERS

NEUROLOGIC CLINICS

Neurol Clin 26 (2008) xiii–xiv

Preface

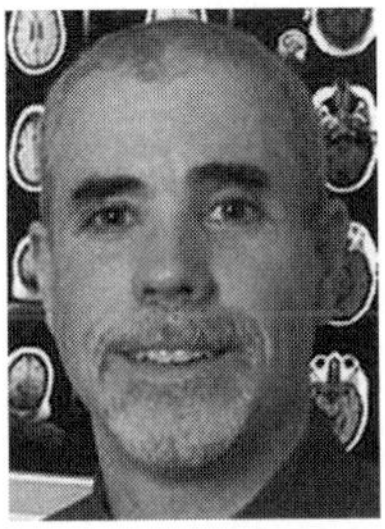

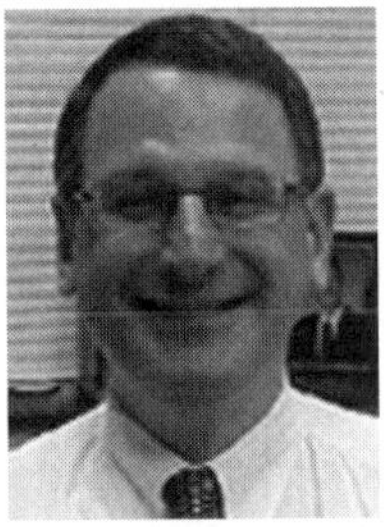

Sean D. Ruland, DO   Philip B. Gorelick, MD, MPH, FACP
Guest Editors

Over the past 2 decades there has been an explosion of information regarding stroke, including enhanced insight into the epidemiology, novel risk factors, preventive strategies, acute management, and surgical and endovascular management techniques. This information has transformed cerebrovascular disease from a previously considered futile entity to one of enthusiasm and optimism. Newer subspecialties such as vascular neurology, neurovascular surgery, and neuroendovascular intervention have evolved and a substantial amount of randomized clinical trial data has expanded the therapeutic armamentarium for stroke prevention and acute treatment. These have come none-too-soon considering the magnitude of the global burden of cerebrovascular disease.

In this issue of *Neurologic Clinics* we have solicited contributions from authors who have a great diversity of expertise and experience and can provide the reader with an overview focusing on new lessons learned and future directions of the evolving field of stroke. The first section features new insights in stroke epidemiology including an expansive discussion of the epidemiology of intracerebral hemorrhage. Then, there is an article about novel uses of neuroimaging techniques for assessing hemodynamic effects of cerebrovascular disease, risk stratification, and clinical course. The second section is devoted to the acute management of stroke. The importance of coordinated emergency department care leads off this portion of the issue. Subsequently, the current and future of thrombolysis and neuroprotectants, and general management principles for acute ischemic stroke are covered.

0733-8619/08/$ - see front matter
doi:10.1016/j.ncl.2008.09.016

The next two articles review the management and controversies surrounding medical and surgical treatments of hemorrhagic stroke. The third section focuses on stroke prevention strategies and begins with an article on risk factor control, including statin use and blood pressure lowering. New randomized clinical trial information regarding appropriate antithrombotic use, new insights from the carotid endarterectomy studies, and a discussion of cardioembolic stroke follow. This section closes with a provocative article on the evolution of endovascular interventions for prevention of ischemic and hemorrhagic stroke. Next, we focus on special at-risk populations including minorities and women. The final article is an historic overview of quality improvement initiatives in stroke care. This includes lessons learned from studies of organized stroke care, and proposed legislation to bridge existing gaps in the quality of care. This timely information helps to highlight the momentum gained by stroke center certification processes in the United States and worldwide.

Although the quantity of new information on stroke prevention, diagnosis and treatment could easily fill a multi-volume text, we emphasize new advances, highlights and hot-button topics in the field, and provide evidence-based guides to treatment and prevention. We extend our gratitude to the authors for their outstanding contributions; the publishing editor, Donald Mumford and the Elsevier staff for their guidance, tireless work and enduring patience to keep the project on a timely schedule for publication; and our families for their endless support.

Sean D. Ruland, DO
Department of Neurology and Rehabilitation
Department of Neurosurgery
The University of Illinois College of Medicine at Chicago
912 S. Wood Street Room 855N (mailcode 796)
Chicago, IL 60612, USA

E-mail address: sruland@uic.edu

Philip B. Gorelick, MD, MPH, FACP
Department of Neurology and Rehabilitation
The University of Illinois College of Medicine at Chicago
912 S. Wood Street Room 855N (mailcode 796)
Chicago, IL 60612, USA

E-mail address: pgorelic@uic.edu

Section I

Understanding the Antecedents of Stroke, Stroke Subtypes, Stroke Causality and Neuroimaging in Stroke

ELSEVIER
SAUNDERS

Neurol Clin 26 (2008) 871–895

NEUROLOGIC
CLINICS

Epidemiology of Ischemic and Hemorrhagic Stroke: Incidence, Prevalence, Mortality, and Risk Factors

Rebbeca A. Grysiewicz, DO[a], Kurian Thomas, MD[b], Dilip K. Pandey, MD, PhD[a,*]

[a]*Department of Neurology and Rehabilitation, University of Illinois at Chicago, Chicago, IL 60612, USA*

[b]*Department of Neurology, Jesse Brown Veteran's Administration Medical Center, 820 South Damen, Chicago, IL 60612, USA*

Annually, 15 million people worldwide suffer a stroke. Of these, 5 million die and another 5 million are left permanently disabled, placing immense burdens on family and community. The World Health Organization (WHO) estimates that a stroke occurs every 5 seconds [1]. In 2002, stroke-related disability was the sixth most common cause of reduced disability-adjusted life-years (DALYs). DALYs are the sum of life-years lost as a result of premature death and years lived with disability adjusted for severity. It is estimated that by 2030 stroke-related disability in western societies will be ranked as the fourth most important cause of DALYs [2]. In 2005, it accounted for approximately 10% of all deaths worldwide. Globally, stroke is the second leading cause of death [3].

In the United States, a stroke occurs approximately every 40 seconds; that translates into 2160 strokes per day. About 780,000 Americans have a new or recurrent stroke each year. Stroke is the primary cause of profound long-term disability in the United States with an estimated 5.8 million stroke survivors in 2008. The societal burden of stroke, including the cost of health care, is considerable. Despite the difficulties in the evaluation of indirect costs, the total cost of stroke has been estimated at $65.5 billion in 2008. Mortality from stroke extends beyond 150,000 people annually, making it the third leading cause of death in the United States. Almost 1 out of every 16 Americans will die as a consequence of stroke [4].

* Corresponding author.
E-mail address: dpandey@uic.edu (D.K. Pandey).

doi:10.1016/j.ncl.2008.07.003 **neurologic.theclinics.com**

Definitions

Stroke is the rapid development of a focal neurologic deficit caused by a disruption of blood supply to the corresponding area of brain. Transient ischemic attack (TIA), by convention, is a focal neurologic deficit lasting less than 24 hours. Recent definitions of TIA describe focal symptoms that last less than 1 hour and do not reveal evidence of infarction [5]. The relevant concept is that TIA is a predictor of stroke [6]. The risk for stroke is greatest in the first 90 days after TIA (between 8%–10%), with practically half of those occurring within the first 7 days [7,8]. Within 5 years, studies report that nearly 30% of people who had TIAs suffer a stroke [8].

Classification of stroke

Strokes can either be ischemic (an occlusion of a blood vessel) or hemorrhagic (a rupture of a blood vessel). Hemorrhagic strokes include intracerebral hemorrhage (ICH, bleeding within the brain) and subarachnoid hemorrhage (SAH, bleeding between the inner and outer layers of tissue covering the brain within the subarachnoid space).

Most strokes in the United States, approximately 87%, are ischemic [4]. Ischemic strokes have been further categorized into subtypes according to the mechanism of injury. These subtypes include large-artery atherosclerosis, cardiogenic embolism, small vessel occlusive disease, stroke of other determined cause, and stroke of undetermined cause [9]. The majority, approximately 60%, of all new ischemic strokes are classified as large-artery atherosclerosis, cardioembolic, or small vessel diseases [10].

ICH and SAH account for approximately 10% and 3% of all strokes, respectively [4]. About 36% to 69% of ICH is deep in location, 15% to 32% is lobar, 7% to 11% is cerebellar, and 4% to 9% is in the brain stem [11].

Incidence, prevalence, and recurrence of stroke

Worldwide, stroke incidence ranges from 240 per 100,000 in Dijon, France (standardized to the European population aged 45–84 years), to about 600 per 100,000 in Novosibirsk, Russia [2]. Data from the Framingham Heart Study (FHS) indicate that the age-adjusted incidence of clinical stroke and atherothrombotic brain infarction per 1000 person-years in 1950 to 1977, 1978 to 1989, and 1990 to 2004 was 7.6, 6.2, and 5.3 in men and 6.2, 5.8, and 5.1 in women, respectively. Clinical stroke in FHS excludes TIA, silent cerebral infarcts, or hemorrhage detected solely by imaging [12].

Estimates of ICH incidence around the world vary, but have generally ranged from 10 to 20 per 100,000 per year [13]. The age-, race-, and sex-adjusted annual incidence of ICH in the Greater Cincinnati–Northern Kentucky Stroke Study (GCNKSS) was 2.9 per 100,000 [11].

The age- and sex-adjusted annual incidence of SAH in the Northern Manhattan Stroke Study (NOMASS) was 9.7 per 100,000 [14].

Prevalence of stroke varies by race/ethnicity in the United States. According to the 2005 Centers for Disease Control and Prevention Behavioral Risk Factor Surveillance System survey the prevalence of stroke was 6.0% among American Indian/Alaska Natives, 4.0% among blacks, 2.6% among Hispanics, 2.3% among whites, and 1.6% among Asians [4].

The risk for recurrent ischemic stroke is 2% at 7 days, 4% at 30 days, 12% at 1 year, and 29% at 5 years after initial cerebral ischemia [15]. The risk for recurrent stroke at 30 days on the basis of stroke subtype is 18.5% for large-artery cervical or intracranial atherosclerosis with stenosis, 5.3% for cardioembolism, 1.4% for lacunar infarction, and 3.3% for infarct of uncertain cause [16]. The risk for recurrence of cerebral hemorrhage is low, partly because of high 30-day mortality following the event. In 19 studies from 15 countries the crude cumulative recurrence rate of ICH varied from 0 to 24% [17]. In a recent study in New Zealand, the risk for recurrence of ICH was 2.1 per 100 in the first year [17].

Case fatality and mortality

The overall mortality for stroke in the United States in 2004 was 50 per 100,000. About 70% to 80% of all stroke deaths are ischemic [18]. Hemorrhagic strokes are less prevalent but more likely to be fatal. The proportion of hemorrhagic stroke deaths varies among race/ethnic group. The percentage of hemorrhagic stroke of all stroke deaths among people aged 35 years or older in 1991 to 1998 was 38% for Asian and Pacific Islanders, 32% for Hispanics, 26% for American Indians and Alaskan Natives, 24% for blacks, and 18% for whites [19].

Globally, the average 30-day case fatality following first ischemic stroke is about 22.9% with the exception of Japan (17%) and Italy (33%) [20]. The 30-day case fatality among people 45 to 64 years of age in the Atherosclerosis Risk in Communities study (ARIC) was 8% to 12% for ischemic stroke and 37% to 38% for hemorrhagic stroke [18]. According to the Rochester Epidemiologic Project, the risk for death after first ischemic stroke was 7% at 7 days, 14% at 30 days, 27% at 1 year, and 53% at 5 years [15]. The most common causes of death after ischemic stroke in the United States are cardiovascular events (22%), respiratory infection (21%), and initial stroke complications (14%) [15]. Long-term mortality following ischemic stroke varies according to stroke subtype. The 5-year mortality following each type of ischemic stroke in the Rochester Epidemiologic Project was: large-artery cervical or intracranial atherosclerosis with stenosis, 32.2%; cardioembolism, 80.4%; lacunar infarction, 35.1%; and infarct of uncertain cause, 48.6% [16].

The 30-day case fatality rate of ICH ranges from 37.6% in GCNKSS to 52% in Oxfordshire Community Stroke Project [21,22]. Volume of the ICH as measured on CT scan and the Glasgow Coma Scale on admission are predictors of mortality in the first 30 days. Death at 1 year for ICH varies by location of ICH: 51% for deep, 57% for lobar, 42% for cerebellar, and 65% for brain stem hemorrhages. Of those that survive the hospitalization, only 20% are functionally independent at 6 months [23]. In population-based studies, the 30-day case fatality rate in a patient who had SAH varied from 26% to 46% [14,21].

Risk factors for ischemic stroke

Epidemiologic studies have established myriad stroke risk factors. Some of these are not modifiable, such as hereditary factors, but are pivotal in correctly identifying those at high risk (Table 1). Factors relating to lifestyle and environment (Tables 2 and 3) may typically be modified or controlled by proven strategies based on randomized clinical trials.

Age

For each consecutive decade after 55 years of age, the risk for stroke approximately doubles [8]. Atherosclerosis increases with age, subsequently increasing the risk for ischemic stroke and myocardial infarction. The prevalence of stroke for individuals older than 80 years of age is approximately 27%, compared with 13% for individuals 60 to 79 years of age [4].

Race

The annual incidence of age-adjusted initial ischemic strokes per 100,000 in people 20 years of age or older in NOMASS was 88 in whites, 191 in blacks, and 149 in Hispanics [24]. According to ARIC study data, the age-adjusted incidence of stroke per 100,000 population in people 45 to 84 years of age is 360 in white males, 230 in white females, 660 in black males, and 490 in black females [25]. In 2004, the stroke death rate per 100,000 was 48.1 for white males, 74.9 for black males, 47.2 for white females, and 65.5 for black females [4].

Table 1
Risk factors for ischemic stroke that are not modifiable

Risk factors	Highest-risk individuals
Age	Elderly, especially >80 years of age
Race	Blacks > Hispanics > whites
Sex	Men > women, except in the young (35–44 years)
Family history of stroke	Monozygotic twins; dominant genetic disorders (CADASIL)

Table 2
Well-established modifiable risk factors for ischemic stroke

Risk factors	Highest-risk individuals
Hypertension	Blood pressure >140/90
Diabetes	Multiple comorbidities, especially hypertension
Smoking	Smokers <55 years of age
Atrial fibrillation	Elderly, >80 years of age

Sex

In general, stroke is more prevalent in men than in women [26]. The incidence of stroke in the young (aged 35–44) is highest in women, however [27]. The increased risk associated with pregnancy is most significant post-partum [28]. Women accounted for 61% of stroke deaths in 2004, which is likely because of their greater longevity than men.

Family history

Parental history of stroke, TIA, or myocardial infarction is associated with 1.4 to 3.3 fold increased risk for stroke [29]. The increased prevalence of stroke between monozygotic and dizygotic twins is almost fivefold [30]. Cerebral autosomal dominant arteriopathy with subcortical infarcts and leukoencephalopathy (CADASIL), a rare genetic disorder, has been reported to cause recurrent strokes with typical onset between the ages of 30 to 50 years [31].

Table 3
Potentially modifiable risk factors for ischemic stroke

Risk factors	Highest-risk individuals
Asymptomatic carotid stenosis	Stenosis >80%
Dyslipidemia	Individuals who have established coronary artery disease
Cardiac disease	Recent MI with poor EF
Sickle cell disease	Young children who have homozygous SCD; adults who have multiple stroke risk factors
Dict	High-sodium, low-potassium diet in overweight or elderly individuals
Physical inactivity	Women; individuals who have multiple comorbidities
Obesity	Body mass index >30
Alcohol use	Heavy or binge drinkers
Hormone replacement therapy	Postmenopausal women on HRT
Hyperhomocysteinemia	Elderly; young males
Hypercoagulability	Young women who have antiphospholipid antibody
Elevated lipoprotein	Elevated Lp-PLA2 levels in men and women
Inflammation	Women who have CRP in highest quartile
Infection	Increased pathogen burden
Geography	Coastal plain states

Abbreviations: CRP, C-reactive protein; EF, ejection fraction; HRT, hormone replacement therapy; MI, myocardial infarction; SCD, sickle cell disease.

Hypertension

There is a well-established relationship between blood pressure and the risk for developing stroke. The relationship is continuous, consistent, and independent of other risk factors. Data from observational studies indicate that risk for death from both ischemic heart disease and stroke increases steadily beginning at systolic blood pressure as low as 115 mm Hg. The mortality of heart disease and stroke double with each increment of 20 mm Hg systolic blood pressure [32]. This risk is increased because hypertension accelerates the development of atherosclerosis, ultimately leading to an increased number of atherothrombotic events [33]. Longitudinal studies indicate that individuals who have high-normal blood pressure (130–139 mm Hg systolic, 85–89 mm Hg diastolic, or both) have a twofold increased risk for developing heart disease and stroke than those who have blood pressure less than 120/80 mm Hg [34].

Diabetes

Individuals who have known diabetes and elevated glucose are at increased risk for thromboembolic stroke independent of other cardiovascular risk factors [35]. Several epidemiologic studies have indicated an independent association between diabetes and ischemic stroke with a twofold to sixfold increased risk [27,35]. It is estimated that nearly 40% of all ischemic strokes can be attributed to the effects of diabetes either alone or in combination with hypertension [36]. This risk may be due to both the accelerated development of atherosclerosis over time and to the increased prevalence of other risk factors, including central obesity, elevated cholesterol, and hypertension associated with diabetes [27]. A longitudinal study of 13,999 people who had coronary heart disease suggests impaired glucose tolerance, defined as glucose levels between 140 and 199 mg/dL after a 2-hour glucose tolerance test, is associated with increased stroke risk in patients who have heart disease [37]. Also, more recent clinical studies have identified impaired glucose tolerance as an independent risk factor for recurrent stroke in patients who have TIA or minor ischemic stroke [38].

Smoking

Smoking has been identified as an independent risk factor for stroke in a plethora of studies over the years. The relative risk for stroke ascribed to cigarette smoking is 1.5. Relative risk varies among stroke subtypes with ischemic stroke having a relative risk of 1.9. Smokers younger than 55 years of age have a relative risk of 2.9, which is considerably higher than smokers older than 55 years; relative risk for smokers aged 55 to 74 years is 1.8, and relative risk is 1.1 for smokers older than 70 years. Ex-smokers continue to have an increased risk for stroke despite cessation [39]. Exposure to environmental tobacco smoke also increases the risk for stroke, with some studies reporting a nearly twofold increment of risk [40,41].

Atrial fibrillation

Atrial fibrillation is an independent risk factor for stroke with a threefold to fivefold increased risk [42]. Atrial fibrillation causes stagnation of blood flow within the left atrial appendage, which may lead to thrombus formation and embolism. Nonvalvular atrial fibrillation is the most common cause of cardioembolic stroke [43]. Nearly 30% of strokes in those aged 80 years or older are attributable to atrial fibrillation [42]. In addition to the morbidity associated with atrial fibrillation, there is 1.5 to1.9 fold increased risk for mortality [44]. Individuals who survive a stroke associated with atrial fibrillation may have increased frequency of recurrence and more severe functional deficits [43].

The CHADS2 criterion offers a risk stratification scheme for individual stroke risk factors in patients who have atrial fibrillation. The CHADS2 acronym stands for congestive heart failure, hypertension, age older than 75 years, diabetes mellitus, and prior stroke or TIA. Individuals receive 1 point for each risk factor except prior stroke or TIA, which receives 2 points [45]. The stroke rate increases by 1.5 with each 1-point increase on the CHADS2 score. Subsequent studies have validated this risk scheme and the study's ability to correctly identify those at high or low risk [46].

Asymptomatic carotid stenosis

Asymptomatic carotid stenosis greater than 50% is detected on average in 5% to 10% of adults 65 years of age or older, and stenosis greater than 80% is found in approximately 1% [27,47]. In the SMART study (Second Manifestations of ARTerial disease) of 2684 patients who had clinical manifestations of arterial disease or type 2 diabetes mellitus, but who did not have a history of cerebral ischemia, asymptomatic carotid stenosis was independently associated with vascular events [48]. In another longitudinal study of 715 patients who had asymptomatic cervical bruits, the annual rate of stroke for individuals who had carotid stenosis 80% or greater was 4.2%, and 1.4% in those who had stenosis less than 80%. The main predictor for vascular events was the severity of stenosis; specifically, progression to greater than 80% stenosis [49]. Studies assessing the long-term risk for stroke in asymptomatic carotid stenosis reveal that the risk is low and remains relatively stable in follow-up over 15 years. In patients who had 50% to 99% carotid stenosis, the 10- and 15-year risk for stroke was 9.3% and 16.3%, respectively [50].

Dyslipidemia

Elevated serum cholesterol and stroke is not a well-established risk factor for stroke. Previous studies were confounded by the inverse association of total cholesterol and cerebral hemorrhage, but more recent trials are specific to ischemic stroke. The Asia Pacific Cohort Studies Collaboration suggests a 25% increased risk for ischemic stroke with each 1-mmol/L (38.7-mg/dL) increase in total cholesterol [51]. The Women's Pooling Project of 24,343 women reported a 25% increase in fatal stroke with each 1-mmol/L increase in total cholesterol in women aged 30 to 54 years [52]. The 10-year follow-up of the Copenhagen Stoke Study revealed than an increase of 1 mmol/L in total serum cholesterol resulted in an increase in the Scandinavian Stroke Scale score. Specifically, high cholesterol levels were primarily associated with minor strokes and lower mortality [53]. Additional studies have also failed to show an association between serum cholesterol and risk for stroke [54,55]. Higher levels of HDL cholesterol have been associated with decreased risk for nonfatal stroke in men [56].

Cardiac disease

Multiple cardiac conditions, in addition to atrial fibrillation, are associated with increased stroke risk. There is a considerable risk for ischemic stroke in the first 5 years after a myocardial infarction, which is estimated to be 8.1% over 5 years. The increased risk is related to the extent of left ventricular dysfunction with an 18% increase of stroke risk with every 5% decrease of ejection fraction [57]. Also, there is a reported risk for cardioembolic stroke with valvular disease, left ventricular thrombi, and congenital defects, such as patent foramen ovale (PFO) and atrial septal aneurysm (ASA). PFO can develop when this small hole in the atrial septum fails to close properly at birth, and leads to a right-to-left shunt. ASA is characterized by excessive atrial septal motion.

The causal relationship between PFO/ASA and stroke is highly debated. The most commonly accepted pathophysiology is paradoxical embolism, but other possibilities may include an increased association with thrombus formation or atrial arrhythmias [58]. Despite these presumed mechanisms, some studies have failed to show an association between increased risk for initial stroke in individuals who have PFO or PFO in combination with ASA [59].

Sickle cell disease

Sickle cell disease (SCD) is an autosomal recessive disorder that causes an alteration in the hemoglobin β chain. The red blood cells have decreased oxygen carrying capacity and have a tendency to adhere to blood vessel walls [27]. By 20 years of age, 11% of children who have homozygous SCD suffer a stroke, with greatest risk in early childhood [60]. More than 22% of children who have homozygous SCD have evidence of stroke, either clinical or subclinical, on MRI [61]. Children who have high cerebral blood flow velocities determined by transcranial Doppler ultrasound have approximately a 10% risk for stroke per year, which is significantly reduced by up to 90% with frequent blood transfusions [62].

Diet

Studies have shown that there is a protective relationship between fruit and vegetable consumption and ischemic stroke risk [63,64]. This relationship is especially evident with consumption of cruciferous vegetables, green leafy vegetables, and citrus fruit. There is a 6% reduction in risk for ischemic stroke with each one-serving increase of fruits and vegetables daily [63].

In overweight individuals, higher sodium intake is associated with approximately 89% increased risk for stroke mortality [65,66]. Analyses also reveal that a 10 mmol increase in daily potassium is associated with 40% reduction in stroke mortality independent of other cardiovascular risk factors [67]. Potassium supplementation has shown a decrease in mean systolic and diastolic blood pressures [68]. The association between alterations in sodium and potassium intake and the reduction in stroke mortality is hypothesized to be achieved primarily by blood pressure lowering.

Physical inactivity

Moderate to high levels of physical activity have proved protective against stroke in middle-aged men [67,69]. The relative risk for stroke is 1.82 in women aged 65 to 74 years who have low physical activity [70]. In NOMASS, increased leisure time physical activity was protective against stroke across race, sex, and age. This decreased risk was related to level of intensity and duration [71].

Obesity

Obesity is a risk factor for ischemic stroke in women and men [72,73]. After adjustment for cardiovascular risk factors, women who had a body mass index (BMI) greater than 27 had significantly increased risk for ischemic stroke. Relative risk for BMI 27 to 28.9 was 1.75, for BMI 29 to 31.9 was 1.9, and for BMI greater than 32 was 2.37. Also, the risk for stroke was associated with the amount of weight gained after 18 years of age with relative risk of 1.69 for a gain of 11 to 19.9 kg and relative risk of 2.52 for a gain of 20 kg or greater (P trend $<.001$) [73]. Men who have BMI greater than 30 have a 1.95 relative risk for ischemic stroke, and with each unit increase in BMI there is a 6% increase in adjusted relative risk [72].

In addition to the relationship between BMI and stroke risk, studies have examined the relationship between abdominal adiposity and stroke risk. Abdominal adiposity may be defined as the highest quartile of waist circumference or hip/waist ratio, with obesity defined as greater than 102 cm in men and greater than 88 cm in women. Abdominal obesity is only found to be a risk factor for ischemic stroke in men [74].

Alcohol use

Studies have shown an increased risk for stroke with "irregular" drinking, including heavy and binge drinking [75]. Acute consumption of an intoxicating amount of alcohol is suggested to be an independent risk for stroke with a relative risk of 1.82. Consumption of 151 g to greater than 300 g of alcohol is significantly associated with increased risk for cardioembolic and cryptogenic stroke. Drinking more than 40 g of alcohol may trigger a cardiogenic embolism in those who have a high-risk source [76]. Moderate drinking (more than one drink in the past month to two drinks per day) is associated with decreased risk for ischemic stroke compared with individuals who had no drinks in the past year after adjusting for other risk factors [77].

Hormone replacement therapy

Hormone replacement therapy was previously hypothesized to reduce stroke risk, but recent clinical trials have failed to show benefit of postmenopausal hormone replacement therapy in reduction of stroke or severity [78,79]. In a clinical trial, women who received estrogen replacement therapy had a 2.9 relative risk for fatal strokes, and the nonfatal strokes that occurred were associated with increased functional deficits [79].

Hyperhomocysteinemia

Elevated serum total homocysteine level ($\geq$12.1 μmol/L) is independently associated with risk for nonfatal stroke [80]. The Homocysteine Studies Collaboration calculated that homocysteine levels reduced by 25% (about 3 μmol/L) are associated with a 19% reduction in stroke risk [81]. Higher homocysteine levels are found with increasing age [82]. Men, especially at younger ages, have higher homocysteine concentrations than women [83].

Hypercoagulability

Inherited thrombophilias, specifically factor V Leiden mutation, are associated with increased risk for venous thrombosis [84,85]. Inherited thrombophilias, including protein C deficiency, protein S deficiency, antithrombin III deficiency, factor V Leiden mutation, and prothrombin 20,210A mutation, have not been associated with increased risk for ischemic stroke on a consistent basis, however [84–86]. The presence of an antiphospholipid antibody, which includes anticardiolipin and lupus anticoagulant antibodies, is typically an acquired thrombophilia, but can also be inherited [87]. The Antiphospholipid Antibodies and Stroke Study (APASS) did not show an association between antiphospholipid antibodies and recurrent ischemic strokes [88]. Other trials suggest that the presence of antiphospholipid antibodies is an independent risk factor for stroke in young women [89].

Lipoprotein (a)

Lipoprotein (a) is strongly associated with atherosclerosis and is an independent risk factor for cardiovascular disease [90]. Lipoprotein (a) levels are significantly higher in ischemic stroke patients, but there has been no consistent association between lipoprotein level and initial ischemic stroke risk [90,91]. Individuals in the highest lipoprotein (a) quartile may have a greater extent of intracranial large-artery stenosis and increased number of stenotic lesions [89,92].

Lipoprotein-associated phospholipase A2

Lipoprotein-associated phospholipase A2 (Lp-PLA2) is a serine lipase that is produced by inflammatory cells and is associated with circulating low density lipoprotein [93]. Higher Lp-PLA2 levels are associated with increased cardiovascular events [94]. A significant association between Lp-PLA2 activity and ischemic stroke is reported in the Rotterdam study and many other epidemiologic studies [95,96]. Lp-PLA2 is specific for vascular inflammation.

Inflammation

Atherosclerosis is a chronic inflammatory process that is initiated by endothelial dysfunction [97]. C-reactive protein (CRP) is an acute phase reactant that serves as a marker of systemic inflammation [98]. Studies show that CRP is a strong predictor of cardiovascular events [99,100]. Several studies have indicated that there is a twofold increase of TIA/stroke for men in the highest quartile ($P = .027$) and almost a threefold risk for ischemic stroke/TIA for women in the highest quartile ($P = .0003$); however, after multivariant adjustment, the relative risk in men was statistically insignificant. The relative risk for women in the highest quartile was 2.1 after multivariate adjustment ($P = .008$) [101]. There is a synergism between CRP and Lp-PLA2 in stroke risk [95].

High-sensitivity C-reactive protein (Hs-CRP) levels have been shown to increase with severity of stroke [102]. More recent studies continue to show the association between stroke and hsCRP, but after adjustment for other risks, hsCRP was not an independent risk factor for stroke. Furthermore, evaluating hsCRP levels in combination with other risk factors did not improve the predictive value of stroke risk [103].

The CD40/CD40 ligand (CD40L) dyad is a powerful immune mediator and an inflammatory marker in the serum [104]. CD40L is implicated in multiple stages of atherogenesis [105]. Studies have shown that interruption of CD40 signaling is associated with plaque stabilization [106]. High plasma concentration of sCD40L may be associated with increased risk for cardiovascular events in apparently healthy women [104]. A study of patients who had atrial fibrillation revealed that elevated CD40L levels were not related to occurrence of stroke, vascular events, or mortality [107].

Infection

Infection has long been implicated as a cause of atherosclerosis. Recent studies have shown an association between acute bacterial or viral infections and increased risk for ischemic stroke, especially among infections occurring within the week before the stroke [108]. An additional study revealed an association between chronic infections, specifically bronchitis and periodontal disease, and increased ischemic stroke risk [108]. Infectious mechanisms for stroke pathogenesis remains unclear, but proposed mechanisms include increased cytokine expression and procoagulant effects [109].

Chlamydia pneumoniae has been isolated in atherosclerotic plaques of individuals who had cerebrovascular disease [110]. In a multiethnic population study, there was an association between elevated *C pneumoniae* IgA titers and ischemic stroke risk (odds ratio 4.51, 95% CI, 1.44 to 14.06) [111,112]. Despite the association between IgA serology titers and symptomatic disease, there was no association between presence of polymerase chain reaction (PCR)-positive *C pneumoniae* and severity of stenosis or symptomatic disease ($P = 1.0$) [110]. Many other infectious agents have been implicated in stroke pathogenesis, such as herpes viruses and cytomegalovirus [113].

Geography

Geographic differences in stroke mortality have been recognized in the United States since the 1940s. The term "stroke belt" has become obscure, but generally referred to the increased stroke mortality in the southeastern United States. More selective definitions referred to the coastal plain states where stroke mortality rates were reported to be extreme. The etiology of regional variations in stroke mortality is unknown, but proposed theories are multifactorial, and implicate distribution of risk factors, such as hypertension, smoking, and diet [114]. An ongoing large population-based epidemiologic study (REGARDS) is currently exploring reasons behind geographic variations in stroke mortality, but more importantly, if geographic differences still exist.

Risk factors for hemorrhagic strokes

ICH is the most common cause of hemorrhagic stroke in the United States. Age, ethnicity, and hypertension are strongly linked to ICH. Associations have been equivocal with other risk factors. Conditions of nature and environment that contribute to ICH are listed in Tables 4 and 5.

Age

A review of five cohort studies addressing age and ICH revealed escalating risk for older individuals. The risk approximately doubled with each decade of life [115]. Similar associations were found in cohort analysis of

Table 4
Nonmodifiable risk factors for intracranial hemorrhage

Risk factors	Highest-risk individuals
Age	Elderly
Sex	No significant difference between women and men, except during pregnancy and postpartum
Race/ethnicity	Asians > African Americans > Hispanics/ Native Americans > whites
Genetics	Icelandic CAA; Dutch CAA

Abbreviation: CAA, Cerebral amyloid angiopathy.

the ARIC study, the Cardiovascular Health Study (CHS), and the Kaiser Permanente database.

Race

The risk for ICH varies with race. The proportion of ICH of all stroke admissions in a multicenter population-based study in China varied from 17.1% to 39.4% [116]. Similarly, the percentage of ICH of all strokes in rural Japan was 26% in men and 29% women [117]. High rates of ICH in Asian populations have traditionally been explained by the high prevalence of hypertension or poorer control of hypertension in these people. In the NOMASS, Hispanics and blacks had a higher relative risk (2.3 and 3.5, respectively) of incident ICH compared with whites [118]. An epidemiologic follow-up study reported the incidence of intracerebral hemorrhage among blacks as 50 per 100,000, which is twice the incidence among whites

Table 5
Modifiable risk factors for intracerebral hemorrhage

Risk factors	Highest-risk individuals
Hypertension	Most common risk factor; especially age > 55 years, smokers, and noncompliance with medication.
Cerebral amyloid angiopathy	Elderly; concomitant hypertension and warfarin use
Cholesterol	Lower levels of total cholesterol (< sex-specific 10th percentile) and LDL-C
Anticoagulation	All patients have 7 to 10 fold increased ICH risk
Antiplatelets	Slight increase in ICH risk
Alcohol	Heavy consumption
Smoking	Asians with subarachnoid hemorrhage; link to primary ICH not well established.
Diabetes	Contributes to increased morbidity and mortality
Microbleeds	Prevalence ≥60% among ICH patients
Dialysis	Five times greater incidence of ICH than the general population
Drugs	Sympathomimetic agents and phenylpropanolamine use in those aged 18–49 years

Abbreviation: LDL-C, Low density lipoprotein cholesterol.

[119]. The percentage of stroke deaths from hemorrhage has been greater in Native Americans than in whites, 14.9% and 13.5%, respectively [120].

Sex

Overall, women are at a lower risk for ICH than men. There seems to be an age and sex interaction in the overall risk for ICH. A woman's risk for ICH is generally lower than a man's risk before age 65, but this disparity may not exist past the age of 64 [118]. Sturgeon and colleagues [121] did not find a significant difference in incident ICH events between sexes in a pooled cohort of the ARIC and the CHS. The Women's Health Initiative found no effect on hemorrhagic stroke risk for postmenopausal women taking an estrogen plus progestin combination pill [122]. During pregnancy the risk for ICH is significantly higher and is 28-fold more during the 6-week postpartum period [28].

Hypertension

Hypertension contributes to the majority of primary intracerebral hemorrhages. Numerous studies document this relationship, and it is consistent throughout America, Europe, and the Asia-Pacific region. The risk is common among individuals older than 55 years of age, smokers, and those not compliant with antihypertensive medications [123]. The Hemorrhagic Stroke Project, a matched case-control study of risk factors for ICH covering 44 hospitals in the United States, reported an adjusted odds ratio of 5.71 for hypertension among ICH cases than age-matched controls [124]. Recurrent hemorrhages are also reported to be more common in patients who had hypertension [125].

Diabetes

The data regarding diabetes as a risk factor for intracerebral hemorrhage vary. Pooled analysis of the ARIC and the CHS data show an age-adjusted relative rate of 1.11 for people who had diabetes and ICH [121]. A comparison of men in the Honolulu Heart Program and the Framingham Study revealed analogous rates of bleeds, but increased risk for ICH in patients who had diabetes was seen only in the Framingham group (relative risk, 3.1) [126].

Hyperglycemia on admission may increase the risk for early death. Admission plasma glucose level greater than 150 mg/dL and ICH volume greater than 20 mL are associated with death within 14 days of hospitalization [127]. In-hospital mortality rate is almost doubled in patients who have diabetes compared with those who do not [127,128].

Smoking

Smoking has been reported as a risk factor for cerebral hemorrhage in several studies. The link to subarachnoid hemorrhage, especially in the

Asian population, is well established [129]. The correlation between primary intracranial bleeds and smoking is not as strong, however. Current cigarette smokers had an odds ratio of 1.58 compared with those who never smoked [124]. Similar results were obtained in studies from Poland, Norway, and Australia [130,131]. A case-cohort study in Japan following 242 patients and a population-based case-control study from central Finland did not observe an association with smoking and primary intracranial hemorrhage, however [132,133]. These findings were consistent with the pooled cohort data of the ARIC and the CHS [121].

Dyslipidemia

An inverse relationship between total serum cholesterol and low density lipoprotein cholesterol (LDL-C) and hemorrhages is consistently being reported [134–137]. Total serum cholesterol level less than 4.62 mmol/L (178 mg/dL) was associated with a significantly increased risk for intracerebral hemorrhage in men aged 65 years or older (relative risk, 2.7; 95% CI, 1.4 to 5.0) in the Kaiser Permanente Study [135]. Increased in-hospital mortality within 48 hours of admission has been reported in patients who had lower total serum cholesterol levels [138].

Alcohol use

Consumption of excess amounts of alcohol has been established as a risk factor for hemorrhagic stroke. It is postulated that alcohol affects the coagulation pathway and cerebral vessel integrity [119,139].

Antithrombolytics

Oral anticoagulation increases the risk for spontaneous ICH. Several studies have shown a 7 to 10 fold higher risk for ICH in patients on oral anticoagulation compared with those who are not on treatment. It is estimated that 10% to 12% of all intracerebral hemorrhages may be related to anticoagulant medications. The mortality from oral anticoagulation–related ICH is approximately 50%, and typically occurs early in the hospital course. In contrast to spontaneous ICH, the duration of bleeding extends to 12 to 24 hours after the initial event [13,140].

The impact of antiplatelet medication on intracerebral hemorrhage is less than that of anticoagulants. Gorelick and Weisman calculated the risk for patients using aspirin for primary prevention of myocardial infarction to be 0.2 events per 1000 patient-years [141]. Multiple studies have shown increased adverse outcomes with antiplatelet use [142–144].

Cerebral amyloid angiopathy

Approximately 12% to 15% of all cerebral hemorrhages in elderly people are related to the presence of cerebral amyloid angiopathy (CAA). The most common form is amyloid β precursor protein–associated CAA, which is present in many nonhypertensive elderly patients who have sporadic lobar cerebral hemorrhage. Cerebral amyloid angiopathy was reported during autopsy in more than 50% of people aged 90 years or older [145]. Clinical series suggest that CAA-related intracerebral hemorrhage may preferentially affect the frontal lobe, although posteriorly located hemorrhages in the brain hemisphere are believed to be common [146]. Apolipoprotein epsilon 4/4 in patients who have lobar hemorrhages may contribute to increased risk [147]. Amyloid angiopathy is also associated with recurrent intracerebral hemorrhages and warfarin-associated bleeds [125,148]. Genetic forms of CAA, including Icelandic, Dutch, and Flemish CAA, predispose younger individuals to bleeds [149].

Microbleeds

Cerebral microbleeds found on MRI could be an emerging risk factor for hemorrhages [150,151]. A Swedish prospective study of 45 patients who had intraparenchymal hemorrhages found microbleeds in 64% of patients [152]. The presence of microbleeds may result in threefold larger volume of hemorrhage [153]. The quantity of microbleeds increases in older patients.

Illicit drugs

Sympathomimetic agents, such as cocaine or amphetamines, have long been known to be associated with intracerebral hemorrhages. The literature is replete with case reports of amphetamine use and ICH, which are seen mostly in the younger population [154–156]. In a 1-year series of all fatal intracranial hemorrhage cases investigated by the Connecticut Office of the Chief Medical Examiner, 59% were associated with cocaine abuse [157].

Dialysis

Since the 1970s there has been documentation of intracerebral hemorrhages in chronic renal failure patients on dialysis [158,159]. A Japanese retrospective study of hemodialysis patients followed for 13 years indicated a fivefold increased incidence of cerebral hemorrhage in these patients compared with the general population [160]. Another prospective study conducted in Okinawa reported a relative risk of 10.7 in chronic dialysis patients compared with normal individuals [161].

Tumors

There are few data about prevalence of brain hemorrhage associated with primary or metastatic intracranial tumors. The hemorrhage rate in a retrospective review of 905 intracerebral tumors, excluding pituitary and recurrent lesions, was 14.6%. Metastatic melanomas were the most likely of all tumors to bleed. Of the primary brain tumors, mixed oligodendrogliomas and astrocytomas had a hemorrhage rate of 29.2% [162]. Among 23 melanoma patients who had brain metastases in China, 17 had acute bleeding into the tumor [163].

Subarachnoid hemorrhage

Approximately 5% to 10% of all strokes are due to nontraumatic SAH. The most frequent cause is rupture of an aneurysm. Actual rates vary because the term subarachnoid hemorrhage is frequently classified in epidemiologic studies under "hemorrhagic stroke," along with intracerebral hemorrhage. Despite different methodologies, data from Greater Cincinnati and Bernalillo County (New Mexico), suggest higher rates among blacks and Mexican Americans [14,164–166].

Summary

The epidemiology of ischemic and hemorrhagic stroke is an ongoing exploration to identify risk factors that continue to expand with the advent of technological advancements and preventative medical practices. Identification of risk factors that can or cannot be modified is a crucial step in determining stroke risk. Once risk factors are elucidated, modifiable risk factors can be treated to reduce the risk for stroke. Many of the modifiable risk factors are well established, and specific interventions to reduce stroke risk have been established. Some risk factors are less established, and intervention to reduce risk is yet to be determined by evidence-based medicine. Data from ongoing randomized clinical trials continue to enhance our ability to prevent a first stroke.

References

[1] Who. Global burden of stroke. Available at: http://www.who.int/cardiovascular_diseases/en/cvd_atlas_15_burden_stroke.pdf. Accessed July 26, 2008.
[2] Donnan GA, Fisher M, Macleod M, et al. Stroke. Lancet 2008;371(9624):1612–23.
[3] Bogousslavsky J, Aarli J, Kimura J. Stroke: time for a global campaign? Cerebrovasc Dis 2003;16(2):111–3.
[4] Rosamond W, Flegal K, Furie K, et al. Heart disease and stroke statistics—2008 update: a report from the American Heart Association Statistics Committee and Stroke Statistics Subcommittee. Circulation 2008;117(4):e25–146.
[5] Albers GW, Caplan LR, Easton JD, et al. Transient ischemic attack—proposal for a new definition. N Engl J Med 2002;347(21):1713–6.
[6] Johnston SC, Gress DR, Browner WS, et al. Short-term prognosis after emergency department diagnosis of TIA. JAMA 2000;284(22):2901–6.
[7] Rothwell PM, Warlow CP. Timing of TIAs preceding stroke: time window for prevention is very short. Neurology 2005;64(5):817–20.
[8] Wolf PA, D'Agostino RB, O'Neal MA, et al. Secular trends in stroke incidence and mortality. The Framingham Study. Stroke 1992;23(11):1551–5.
[9] Adams HP Jr, Bendixen BH, Kappelle LJ, et al. Classification of subtype of acute ischemic stroke. Definitions for use in a multicenter clinical trial. TOAST. Trial of Org 10172 in Acute Stroke Treatment. Stroke 1993;24(1):35–41.

[10] Petty GW, Brown RD Jr, Whisnant JP, et al. Ischemic stroke subtypes: a population-based study of incidence and risk factors. Stroke 1999;30(12):2513–6.
[11] Flaherty ML, D Woo, Haverbusch M, et al. Racial variations in location and risk of intracerebral hemorrhage. Stroke 2005;36(5):934–7.
[12] Carandang R, Seshadri S, Beuser A, et al. Trends in incidence, lifetime risk, severity, and 30-day mortality of stroke over the past 50 years. JAMA 2006;296(24):2939–46.
[13] Steiner T, Rosand J, Diringer M. Intracerebral hemorrhage associated with oral anticoagulant therapy: current practices and unresolved questions. Stroke 2006;37(1):256–62.
[14] Labovitz DL, Halim AX, Brent B, et al. Subarachnoid hemorrhage incidence among whites, blacks and Caribbean Hispanics: the Northern Manhattan Study. Neuroepidemiology 2006;26(3):147–50.
[15] Petty GW, Brown RD Jr, Whisnant JP, et al. Survival and recurrence after first cerebral infarction: a population-based study in Rochester, Minnesota, 1975 through 1989. Neurology 1998;50(1):208–16.
[16] Petty GW, Brown RD Jr, Whisnant JP, et al. Ischemic stroke subtypes: a population-based study of functional outcome, survival, and recurrence. Stroke 2000;31(5):1062–8.
[17] Hanger HC, Wilkinson TJ, Fayez-Iskander N, et al. The risk of recurrent stroke after intracerebral haemorrhage. J Neurol Neurosurg Psychiatry 2007;78(8):836–40.
[18] Rosamond WD, Folsom AR, Chambless LE, et al. Stroke incidence and survival among middle-aged adults: 9-year follow-up of the atherosclerosis risk in communities (ARIC) cohort. Stroke 1999;30(4):736–43.
[19] Casper ML, Barnett E, Williams GI Jr, et al. Atlas of stroke mortality: racial, ethnic, and geographic disparity in the United States. Atlanta (GA): Department of Health and Human Services, Center for Disease Control and Prevention; 2003. p. 10.
[20] Feigin VL, Lawes CM, Bennett DA, et al. Stroke epidemiology: a review of population-based studies of incidence, prevalence, and case-fatality in the late 20th century. Lancet Neurol 2003;2(1):43–53.
[21] Dennis MS, Burn JP, Sandercock PA, et al. Long-term survival after first-ever stroke: the Oxfordshire Community Stroke Project. Stroke 1993;24(6):796–800.
[22] Kleindorfer D, Broderick J, Khoury J, et al. The unchanging incidence and case-fatality of stroke in the 1990s: a population-based study. Stroke 2006;37(10):2473–8.
[23] Woo D, Broderick JP. Spontaneous intracerebral hemorrhage: epidemiology and clinical presentation. Neurosurg Clin N Am 2002;13(3):265–79, v.
[24] White H, Boden-Albala B, Wang C, et al. Ischemic stroke subtype incidence among whites, blacks, and Hispanics: the Northern Manhattan Study. Circulation 2005;111(10):1327–31.
[25] Incidence and Prevalence: 2006 chartbook on cardiovascular and lung diseases. Bethesda (MD): National Heart, Lung, and Blood Institute; 2006.
[26] Brown RD, Whisnant JP, Sicks JD, et al. Stroke incidence, prevalence, and survival: secular trends in Rochester, Minnesota, through 1989. Stroke 1996;27(3):373–80.
[27] Goldstein LB, Adams R, Alberts MJ, et al. Primary prevention of ischemic stroke: a guideline from the American Heart Association/American Stroke Association Stroke Council: cosponsored by the Atherosclerotic Peripheral Vascular Disease Interdisciplinary Working Group; Cardiovascular Nursing Council; Clinical Cardiology Council; Nutrition, Physical Activity, and Metabolism Council; and the Quality of Care and Outcomes Research Interdisciplinary Working Group. Circulation 2006;113(24):e873–923.
[28] Kittner SJ, Stern BJ, Freeser BR, et al. Pregnancy and the risk of stroke. N Engl J Med 1996; 335(11):768–74.
[29] Kiely DK, Wolf PA, Cupples LA, et al. Familial aggregation of stroke. The Framingham study. Stroke 1993;24(9):1366–71.
[30] Brass LM, Isaacsohn JL, Merikangas KR, et al. A study of twins and stroke. Stroke 1992; 23(2):221–3.
[31] Kalimo H, Viitanen M, Amberla K, et al. CADASIL: hereditary disease of arteries causing brain infarcts and dementia. Neuropathol Appl Neurobiol 1999;25(4):257–65.

[32] Chobanian AV, Bakris GL, Black HR, et al. The seventh report of the Joint National Committee on prevention, detection, evaluation, and treatment of high blood pressure: the JNC 7 report. JAMA 2003;289(19):2560–72.
[33] Sacco RL, Adams R, Albers G, et al. Guidelines for prevention of stroke in patients with ischemic stroke or transient ischemic attack: a statement for healthcare professionals from the American Heart Association/American Stroke Association Council on stroke: co-sponsored by the Council on Cardiovascular Radiology and Intervention: the American Academy of Neurology affirms the value of this guideline. Stroke 2006;37(2): 577–617.
[34] Vasan RS, Larson MG, Leip EP, et al. Impact of high-normal blood pressure on the risk of cardiovascular disease. N Engl J Med 2001;345(18):1291–7.
[35] Burchfiel CM, Curb JD, Rodriguez BL, et al. Glucose intolerance and 22-year stroke incidence. The Honolulu heart program. Stroke 1994;25(5):951–7.
[36] Kissela BM, Khoury J, Kleindorfer D, et al. Epidemiology of ischemic stroke in patients with diabetes: the greater Cincinnati/Northern Kentucky stroke study. Diabetes Care 2005;28(2):355–9.
[37] Tanne D, Koren-Morag N, Goldbourt U. Fasting plasma glucose and risk of incident ischemic stroke or transient ischemic attacks: a prospective cohort study. Stroke 2004; 35(10):2351–5.
[38] Vermeer SE, Sandee W, Algra A, et al. Impaired glucose tolerance increases stroke risk in nondiabetic patients with transient ischemic attack or minor ischemic stroke. Stroke 2006; 37(6):1413–7.
[39] Shinton R, Beevers G. Meta-analysis of relation between cigarette smoking and stroke. BMJ 1989;298(6676):789–94.
[40] Bonita R, Duncan J, Truelsen T, et al. Passive smoking as well as active smoking increases the risk of acute stroke. Tob Control 1999;8(2):156–60.
[41] You RX, Thrift AG, McNeil JJ, et al. Ischemic stroke risk and passive exposure to spouses' cigarette smoking. Melbourne Stroke Risk Factor Study (MERFS) Group. Am J Public Health 1999;89(4):572–5.
[42] Wolf PA, Abbott RD, Kannel WB. Atrial fibrillation as an independent risk factor for stroke: the Framingham Study. Stroke 1991;22(8):983–8.
[43] Lin HJ, Wolf PA, Kelly-Hayes M, et al. Stroke severity in atrial fibrillation. The Framingham study. Stroke 1996;27(10):1760–4.
[44] Benjamin EJ, et al. Impact of atrial fibrillation on the risk of death: the Framingham Heart study. Circulation 1998;98(10):946–52.
[45] Fuster V, Ryden LE, Asinger RW, et al. ACC/AHA/esc guidelines for the management of patients with atrial fibrillation: executive summary a report of the American College of Cardiology/American Heart Association Task Force on Practice Guidelines and the European Society of Cardiology Committee for Practice Guidelines and Policy Conferences (Committee to Develop Guidelines for the Management of Patients With Atrial Fibrillation) developed in collaboration with the North American Society of Pacing and Electrophysiology. Circulation 2001;104(17):2118–50.
[46] Gage BF, Waterman AD, Shannon W, et al. Validation of clinical classification schemes for predicting stroke: results from the National Registry of Atrial Fibrillation. JAMA 2001; 285(22):2864–70.
[47] Fine-Edelstein JS, Wolf PA, O'Leary DH, et al. Precursors of extracranial carotid atherosclerosis in the Framingham Study. Neurology 1994;44(6):1046–50.
[48] Goessens BM, Visseren FL, Kappelle LJ, et al. Asymptomatic carotid artery stenosis and the risk of new vascular events in patients with manifest arterial disease: the SMART study. Stroke 2007;38(5):1470–5.
[49] Mackey AE, Abrahamowicz M, Langlois Y, et al. Outcome of asymptomatic patients with carotid disease. Asymptomatic Cervical Bruit Study Group. Neurology 1997;48(4): 896–903.

[50] Nadareishvili ZG, Rothwell PM, Beletsky V, et al. Long-term risk of stroke and other vascular events in patients with asymptomatic carotid artery stenosis. Arch Neurol 2002;59(7): 1162–6.
[51] Zhang X, Patel A, Horibe H, et al. Cholesterol, coronary heart disease, and stroke in the Asia Pacific region. Int J Epidemiol 2003;32(4):563–72.
[52] Horenstein RB, Smith DE, Mosca L. Cholesterol predicts stroke mortality in the women's pooling project. Stroke 2002;33(7):1863–8.
[53] Olsen TS, Christensen RH, Kammersgaard LP, et al. Higher total serum cholesterol levels are associated with less severe strokes and lower all-cause mortality: ten-year follow-up of ischemic strokes in the Copenhagen Stroke Study. Stroke 2007;38(10):2646–51.
[54] Bots ML, Elwood PC, Nikitin Y, et al. Total and HDL cholesterol and risk of stroke. EUROSTROKE: a collaborative study among research centres in Europe. J Epidemiol Community Health 2002;56(Suppl 1):i19–24.
[55] Shahar E, Chambless LE, Rosamond W, et al. Plasma lipid profile and incident ischemic stroke: the Atherosclerosis Risk in Communities (ARIC) study. Stroke 2003;34(3):623–31.
[56] Wannamethee SG, Shaper AG, Ebrahim S. HDL-Cholesterol, total cholesterol, and the risk of stroke in middle-aged British men. Stroke 2000;31(8):1882–8.
[57] Loh E, Sutton MSJ, Wun CC, et al. Ventricular dysfunction and the risk of stroke after myocardial infarction. N Engl J Med 1997;336(4):251–7.
[58] Messe SR, Silverman IE, Kizer JR, et al. Practice parameter: recurrent stroke with patent foramen ovale and atrial septal aneurysm: report of the Quality Standards Subcommittee of the American Academy of Neurology. Neurology 2004;62(7):1042–50.
[59] Di Tullio MR, Sacco RL, Sciacca RR, et al. Patent foramen ovale and the risk of ischemic stroke in a multiethnic population. J Am Coll Cardiol 2007;49(7):797–802.
[60] Ohene-Frempong K, Weiner SJ, Sleeper LA, et al. Cerebrovascular accidents in sickle cell disease: rates and risk factors. Blood 1998;91(1):288–94.
[61] Armstrong FD, Thompson RJ Jr, Wang W, et al. Cognitive functioning and brain magnetic resonance imaging in children with sickle cell disease. Neuropsychology Committee of the Cooperative Study of Sickle Cell Disease. Pediatrics 1996;97(6 Pt 1):864–70.
[62] Adams RJ, Brambilla DJ, Granger S, et al. Stroke and conversion to high risk in children screened with transcranial Doppler ultrasound during the STOP study. Blood 2004; 103(10):3689–94.
[63] Joshipura KJ, Ascherio A, Manson JE, et al. Fruit and vegetable intake in relation to risk of ischemic stroke. JAMA 1999;282(13):1233–9.
[64] Sauvaget C, Nagano J, Allen N, et al. Vegetable and fruit intake and stroke mortality in the Hiroshima/Nagasaki Life Span Study. Stroke 2003;34(10):2355–60.
[65] He J, Ogden LG, Vupputuri S, et al. Dietary sodium intake and subsequent risk of cardiovascular disease in overweight adults. JAMA 1999;282(21):2027–34.
[66] Nagata C, Takatsuka N, Shimuzu N, et al. Sodium intake and risk of death from stroke in Japanese men and women. Stroke 2004;35(7):1543–7.
[67] Khaw KT, Barrett-Connor E. Dietary potassium and stroke-associated mortality. A 12-year prospective population study. N Engl J Med 1987;316(5):235–40.
[68] Whelton PK, He J, Cutler JA, et al. Effects of oral potassium on blood pressure. Meta-analysis of randomized controlled clinical trials. JAMA 1997;277(20):1624–32.
[69] Abbott RD, Rodriguez BL, Burchfiel C, et al. Physical activity in older middle-aged men and reduced risk of stroke: the Honolulu Heart Program. Am J Epidemiol 1994;139(9): 881–93.
[70] Gillum RF, Mussolino ME, Ingram DD. Physical activity and stroke incidence in women and men. The NHANES I Epidemiologic Follow-up Study. Am J Epidemiol 1996;143(9):860–9.
[71] Sacco RL, Gan R, Boden-Albala B, et al. Leisure-time physical activity and ischemic stroke risk: the Northern Manhattan Stroke Study. Stroke 1998;29(2):380–7.
[72] Kurth T, Gaziano JM, Berger K, et al. Body mass index and the risk of stroke in men. Arch Intern Med 2002;162(22):2557–62.

[73] Rexrode KM, Hennekens CH, Willett WC, et al. A prospective study of body mass index, weight change, and risk of stroke in women. JAMA 1997;277(19):1539–45.
[74] Hu G, Tuomilehto J, Silventoinen K, et al. Body mass index, waist circumference, and waist-hip ratio on the risk of total and type-specific stroke. Arch Intern Med 2007; 167(13):1420–7.
[75] Mazzaglia G, Britton AR, Altman DR, et al. Exploring the relationship between alcohol consumption and non-fatal or fatal stroke: a systematic review. Addiction 2001;96(12):1743–56.
[76] Hillbom M, Numminen H, Juvela S. Recent heavy drinking of alcohol and embolic stroke. Stroke 1999;30(11):2307–12.
[77] Elkind MS, Sciacca R, Boden-Albala B, et al. Moderate alcohol consumption reduces risk of ischemic stroke: the Northern Manhattan study. Stroke 2006;37(1):13–9.
[78] Hulley S, Grady D, Bush T, et al. Randomized trial of estrogen plus progestin for secondary prevention of coronary heart disease in postmenopausal women. Heart and Estrogen/ progestin Replacement Study (HERS) Research Group. JAMA 1998;280(7):605–13.
[79] Viscoli CM, Brass LM, Kernan WN, et al. A clinical trial of estrogen-replacement therapy after ischemic stroke. N Engl J Med 2001;345(17):1243–9.
[80] Giles WH, Croft JB, Greenlund KJ, et al. Total homocyst(e)ine concentration and the likelihood of nonfatal stroke: results from the Third National Health and Nutrition examination survey, 1988–1994. Stroke 1998;29(12):2473–7.
[81] Homocysteine Studies Collaboration. Homocysteine and risk of ischemic heart disease and stroke: a meta-analysis. JAMA 2002;288(16):2015–22.
[82] Selhub J, Jacques PF, Wilson PW, et al. Vitamin status and intake as primary determinants of homocysteinemia in an elderly population. JAMA 1993;270(22):2693–8.
[83] Jacques PF, Rosenberg IH, Rogers G, et al. Serum total homocysteine concentrations in adolescent and adult Americans: results from the third National Health and Nutrition examination survey. Am J Clin Nutr 1999;69(3):482–9.
[84] Hankey GJ, Eikelboom JW, van Bockxmeer F, et al. Inherited thrombophilia in ischemic stroke and its pathogenic subtypes. Stroke 2001;32(8):1793–9.
[85] Ridker PM, Hennekens CH, Lindpaintner K, et al. Mutation in the gene coding for coagulation factor V and the risk of myocardial infarction, stroke, and venous thrombosis in apparently healthy men. N Engl J Med 1995;332(14):912–7.
[86] Juul K, Tybjarg-Hansen A, Steffensen R, et al. Factor V Leiden: the Copenhagen City heart study and 2 meta-analyses. Blood 2002;100(1):3–10.
[87] Weber M, Hayem G, DeBandt M, et al. The family history of patients with primary or secondary antiphospholipid syndrome (APS). Lupus 2000;9(4):258–63.
[88] Levine SR, Brey RL, Tilley BC, et al. Antiphospholipid antibodies and subsequent thrombo-occlusive events in patients with ischemic stroke. JAMA 2004;291(5):576–84.
[89] Brey RL, Stallworth CL, McGlasson DL, et al. Antiphospholipid antibodies and stroke in young women. Stroke 2002;33(10):2396–400.
[90] Morrisett JD. The role of lipoprotein[a] in atherosclerosis. Curr Atheroscler Rep 2000;2(3): 243–50.
[91] Milionis HJ, Winder AF, Mikhailidis DP. Lipoprotein (a) and stroke. J Clin Pathol 2000; 53(7):487–96.
[92] Arenillas JF, Molina CA, Chacon P, et al. High lipoprotein (a), diabetes, and the extent of symptomatic intracranial atherosclerosis. Neurology 2004;63(1):27–32.
[93] Zalewski, Macphee AC. Role of lipoprotein-associated phospholipase A2 in atherosclerosis: biology, epidemiology, and possible therapeutic target. Arterioscler Thromb Vasc Biol 2005;25(5):923–31.
[94] Brilakis ES, McConnell JP, Lennon RJ, et al. Association of lipoprotein-associated phospholipase A2 levels with coronary artery disease risk factors, angiographic coronary artery disease, and major adverse events at follow-up. Eur Heart J 2005;26(2):137–44.
[95] Gorelick PB. Lipoprotein-associated phospholipase A2 and risk of stroke. Am J Cardiol 2008;101(12A):34F–40F.

[96] Oei HH, van der Meer IM, Hofman A, et al. Lipoprotein-associated phospholipase A2 activity is associated with risk of coronary heart disease and ischemic stroke: the Rotterdam study. Circulation 2005;111(5):570–5.
[97] Ross R. Atherosclerosis is an inflammatory disease. Am Heart J 1999;138(5 Pt 2):S419–20.
[98] Folsom AR, Aleksic N, Catellier D, et al. C-reactive protein and incident coronary heart disease in the Atherosclerosis Risk In Communities (ARIC) study. Am Heart J 2002; 144(2):233–8.
[99] Hage FG, Szalai AJ. C-reactive protein gene polymorphisms, C-reactive protein blood levels, and cardiovascular disease risk. J Am Coll Cardiol 2007;50(12):1115–22.
[100] Ridker PM, Rifai N, Rose L, et al. Comparison of C-reactive protein and low-density lipoprotein cholesterol levels in the prediction of first cardiovascular events. N Engl J Med 2002; 347(20):1557–65.
[101] Rost NS, Wolf PA, Kase CS, et al. Plasma concentration of C-reactive protein and risk of ischemic stroke and transient ischemic attack: the Framingham study. Stroke 2001;32(11): 2575–9.
[102] Elkind MS, Tai W, Coates K, et al. High-sensitivity C-reactive protein, lipoprotein-associated phospholipase A2, and outcome after ischemic stroke. Arch Intern Med 2006;166(19): 2073–80.
[103] Bos MJ, Schipper CM, Koudstaal PJ, et al. High serum C-reactive protein level is not an independent predictor for stroke: the Rotterdam Study. Circulation 2006;114(15): 1591–8.
[104] Schonbeck U, Varo N, Libby P, et al. Soluble CD40L and cardiovascular risk in women. Circulation 2001;104(19):2266–8.
[105] Graf D, Muller S, Korthauer U, et al. A soluble form of TRAP (CD40 ligand) is rapidly released after T cell activation. Eur J Immunol 1995;25(6):1749–54.
[106] Schonbeck U, Libby P. CD40 signaling and plaque instability. Circ Res 2001;89(12): 1092–103.
[107] Lip GY, Patel JV, Hughes E, et al. High-sensitivity C-reactive protein and soluble CD40 ligand as indices of inflammation and platelet activation in 880 patients with nonvalvular atrial fibrillation: relationship to stroke risk factors, stroke risk stratification schema, and prognosis. Stroke 2007;38(4):1229–37.
[108] Grau AJ, Buggle F, Ziegler C, et al. Association between acute cerebrovascular ischemia and chronic and recurrent infection. Stroke 1997;28(9):1724–9.
[109] Lindsberg PJ, Grau AJ. Inflammation and infections as risk factors for ischemic stroke. Stroke 2003;34(10):2518–32.
[110] LaBiche R, Koziol D, Quinn TC, et al. Presence of Chlamydia pneumoniae in human symptomatic and asymptomatic carotid atherosclerotic plaque. Stroke 2001;32(4):855–60.
[111] Elkind MS, Quinn I, Grayston JT, et al. Chlamydia pneumoniae and the risk of first ischemic stroke : The Northern Manhattan Stroke Study. Stroke 2000;31(7):1521–5.
[112] Elkind MS, Tondella ML, Feikin DR, et al. Seropositivity to Chlamydia pneumoniae is associated with risk of first ischemic stroke. Stroke 2006;37(3):790–5.
[113] Gorelick PB. Stroke prevention therapy beyond antithrombotics: unifying mechanisms in ischemic stroke pathogenesis and implications for therapy: an invited review. Stroke 2002; 33(3):862–75.
[114] Lanska DJ, Kuller LH. The geography of stroke mortality in the United States and the concept of a stroke belt. Stroke 1995;26(7):1145–9.
[115] Ariesen MJ, Claus SP, Rinkel GJ, et al. Risk factors for intracerebral hemorrhage in the general population: a systematic review. Stroke 2003;34(8):2060–5.
[116] Zhang LF, Yang J, Hong Z, et al. Proportion of different subtypes of stroke in China. Stroke 2003;34(9):2091–6.
[117] Kitamura A, Nakagawa Y, Sato M, et al. Proportions of stroke subtypes among men and women ≥ 40 years of age in an urban Japanese city in 1992, 1997, and 2002. Stroke 2006; 37(6):1374–8.

[118] Labovitz DL, Halim A, Boden-Albala B, et al. The incidence of deep and lobar intracerebral hemorrhage in whites, blacks, and Hispanics. Neurology 2005;65(4):518–22.
[119] Qureshi AI, Tuhrim S, Broderick JP, et al. Spontaneous intracerebral hemorrhage. N Engl J Med 2001;344(19):1450–60.
[120] Gillum RF. The epidemiology of stroke in Native Americans. Stroke 1995;26(3):514–21.
[121] Sturgeon JD, Folsom AR, Longstreth WT, et al. Risk factors for intracerebral hemorrhage in a pooled prospective study. Stroke 2007;38(10):2718–25.
[122] Wassertheil-Smoller S, Hendrix SL, Limacher M, et al. Effect of estrogen plus progestin on stroke in postmenopausal women: the Women's Health Initiative: a randomized trial. JAMA 2003;289(20):2673–84.
[123] Thrift AG, McNeil JJ, Forbes A, et al. Three important subgroups of hypertensive persons at greater risk of intracerebral hemorrhage. Melbourne Risk Factor Study Group. Hypertension 1998;31(6):1223–9.
[124] Feldmann E, Broderick JP, Kernan WN, et al. Major risk factors for intracerebral hemorrhage in the young are modifiable. Stroke 2005;36(9):1881–5.
[125] Yen CC, Lo YK, Li JY, et al. Recurrent primary intracerebral hemorrhage: a hospital based study. Acta Neurol Taiwan 2007;16(2):74–80.
[126] Rodriguez BL, D'Agostino R, Abbott RD, et al. Risk of hospitalized stroke in men enrolled in the Honolulu Heart Program and the Framingham Study: A comparison of incidence and risk factor effects. Stroke 2002;33(1):230–6.
[127] Kimura K, Iguchi Y, Inoue T, et al. Hyperglycemia independently increases the risk of early death in acute spontaneous intracerebral hemorrhage. J Neurol Sci 2007;255(1–2):90–4.
[128] Arboix A, Massons J, Garcia-Eroles L, et al. Diabetes is an independent risk factor for in-hospital mortality from acute spontaneous intracerebral hemorrhage. Diabetes Care 2000; 23(10):1527–32.
[129] Feigin V, Parag V, Lawes CM, et al. Smoking and elevated blood pressure are the most important risk factors for subarachnoid hemorrhage in the Asia-Pacific region: an overview of 26 cohorts involving 306,620 participants. Stroke 2005;36(7):1360–5.
[130] Jamrozik K, Broadhurst RJ, Anderson CS, et al. The role of lifestyle factors in the etiology of stroke. A population-based case-control study in Perth, Western Australia. Stroke 1994; 25(1):51–9.
[131] Klimowicz-Mlodzik I, Pietrzykowska I, Chodakowska-Zebrowska M, et al. [Cigarette smoking and alcohol abuse effects on stroke development]. Neurol Neurochir Pol 1995; 29(2):151–8 [In Polish].
[132] Fogelholm R, Murros K. Cigarette smoking and risk of primary intracerebral haemorrhage. A population-based case-control study. Acta Neurol Scand 1993;87(5):367–70.
[133] Inagawa T. Risk factors for primary intracerebral hemorrhage in patients in Izumo City, Japan. Neurosurg Rev 2007;30(3):225–34 [discussion: 234].
[134] Cui R, Iso H, Toyoshima H, et al. Serum total cholesterol levels and risk of mortality from stroke and coronary heart disease in Japanese: the JACC study. Atherosclerosis 2007; 194(2):415–20.
[135] Iribarren C, Jacobs DR, Sadler M, et al. Low total serum cholesterol and intracerebral hemorrhagic stroke: is the association confined to elderly men? The Kaiser Permanente Medical Care Program. Stroke 1996;27(11):1993–8.
[136] Okumura K, Iseki K, Wakugami K, et al. Low serum cholesterol as a risk factor for hemorrhagic stroke in men: a community-based mass screening in Okinawa, Japan. Jpn Circ J 1999;63(1):53–8.
[137] Taira S, Kuniyoshi H, Makishi M, et al. [A case-control study of risk factors for cerebral hemorrhage in Hirara-City, Okinawa Prefecture]. Nippon Koshu Eisei Zasshi 1994; 41(12):1142–51 [In Japanese].
[138] Roquer J, Rodriguez Campello A, Gomis M, et al. Serum lipid levels and in-hospital mortality in patients with intracerebral hemorrhage. Neurology 2005;65(8):1198–202.
[139] Gorelick PB. Alcohol and stroke. Stroke 1987;18(1):268–71.

[140] Aguilar MI, Hart RG, Kase CS, et al. Treatment of warfarin-associated intracerebral hemorrhage: literature review and expert opinion. Mayo Clin Proc 2007;82(1):82–92.
[141] Gorelick PB, Weisman SM. Risk of hemorrhagic stroke with aspirin use: an update. Stroke 2005;36(8):1801–7.
[142] Foerch C, Sitzer M, Steinmetz H, et al. Pretreatment with antiplatelet agents is not independently associated with unfavorable outcome in intracerebral hemorrhage. Stroke 2006; 37(8):2165–7.
[143] Lacut K, Le Gal G, Seizeur R, et al. Antiplatelet drug use preceding the onset of intracerebral hemorrhage is associated with increased mortality. Fundam Clin Pharmacol 2007; 21(3):327–33.
[144] Toyoda K, Okada Y, Minematsu K, et al. Antiplatelet therapy contributes to acute deterioration of intracerebral hemorrhage. Neurology 2005;65(7):1000–4.
[145] Kalimo H. Pathology and genetics: cerebrovascular disease. Basel (Switzerland): ISN Neuropath press; 2005. p. 95.
[146] Sucker C, Hetzel GR, Grabensee B, et al. Amyloidosis and bleeding: pathophysiology, diagnosis, and therapy. Am J Kidney Dis 2006;47(6):947–55.
[147] Auer RN, Sutherland GR. Primary intracerebral hemorrhage: pathophysiology. Can J Neurol Sci 2005;32(Suppl 2):S3–12.
[148] Rosand J, Hylek EM, O'Donnell HC, et al. Warfarin-associated hemorrhage and cerebral amyloid angiopathy: a genetic and pathologic study. Neurology 2000;55(7):947–51.
[149] Ellison D, Love S. Neuropathology. St. Louis, MO: Mosby Press; 2000.
[150] Cordonnier C, Al-Shahi Salman R, Wardlaw J. Spontaneous brain microbleeds: systematic review, subgroup analyses and standards for study design and reporting. Brain 2007; 130(Pt 8):1988–2003.
[151] Koennecke HC. Cerebral microbleeds on MRI: prevalence, associations, and potential clinical implications. Neurology 2006;66(2):165–71.
[152] Alemany M, Stenborg A, Terent A, et al. Coexistence of microhemorrhages and acute spontaneous brain hemorrhage: correlation with signs of microangiopathy and clinical data. Radiology 2006;238(1):240–7.
[153] Lee SH, Kim BJ, Roh JK. Silent microbleeds are associated with volume of primary intracerebral hemorrhage. Neurology 2006;66(3):430–2.
[154] Cahill DW, Knipp H, Mosser J. Intracranial hemorrhage with amphetamine abuse-Neurology 1981;31(8):1058–9.
[155] Cantu C, Arauz A, Murillo-Bonilla LM, et al. Stroke associated with sympathomimetics contained in over-the-counter cough and cold drugs. Stroke 2003;34(7):1667–72.
[156] El-Omar MM, Ray K, Geary R. Intracerebral haemorrhage in a young adult: consider amphetamine abuse. Br J Clin Pract 1996;50(2):115–6.
[157] Nolte KB, Brass LM, Fletterick CF. Intracranial hemorrhage associated with cocaine abuse: a prospective autopsy study. Neurology 1996;46(5):1291–6.
[158] Ewald RW, Huber W, Wittenmeier KW, et al. [Problem of intracranial bleeding in chronically hemodialysed patients]. Verh Dtsch Ges Inn Med 1971;77:237–9 [In German].
[159] Siddiqui JY, Fitz AE, Lawton RL, et al. Causes of death in patients receiving long-term hemodialysis. JAMA 1970;212(8):1350–4.
[160] Onoyama K, Kumagai H, Miishima T, et al. Incidence of strokes and its prognosis in patients on maintenance hemodialysis. Jpn Heart J 1986;27(5):685–91.
[161] Iseki K, Kinjo K, Kimura Y, et al. Evidence for high risk of cerebral hemorrhage in chronic dialysis patients. Kidney Int 1993;44(5):1086–90.
[162] Kondziolka D, Bernstein M, Resch L, et al. Significance of hemorrhage into brain tumors: clinicopathological study. J Neurosurg 1987;67(6):852–7.
[163] Wang YC, Lee ST. Brain metastases of malignant melanoma in Chinese: report of 23 cases. Chin Med J (Engl) 2007;120(12):1058–62.

[164] Bruno A, Carter S, Qualls C, et al. Incidence of spontaneous subarachnoid hemorrhage among Hispanics and non-Hispanic whites in New Mexico. Ethn Dis 1997;7(1):27–33.
[165] Kissela B, Schneider A, Kleindorfer D, et al. Stroke in a biracial population: the excess burden of stroke among blacks. Stroke 2004;35(2):426–31.
[166] Morgenstern LB, Smith MA, Lisabeth LD, et al. Excess stroke in Mexican Americans compared with non-Hispanic Whites: the Brain Attack Surveillance in Corpus Christi Project. Am J Epidemiol 2004;160(4):376–83.

ELSEVIER
SAUNDERS

Neurol Clin 26 (2008) 897–921

NEUROLOGIC
CLINICS

MRI in the Management of Cerebrovascular Disease to Prevent Stroke

Keith R. Thulborn, MD, PhD

Center for Magnetic Resonance Research, University of Illinois Medical Center at Chicago, 1801 West Taylor Street, Suite 1307, Chicago, IL 60612, USA

The capability of MRI to make a diagnosis of acute stroke is not in dispute although its role in management of acute stroke is still limited. Ready access to CT in emergency departments with 24-hour-a-day, 7-day-a-week coverage by technologists has marginalized MRI. The primary management decision as to whether or not to use thrombolytic therapy for stroke is made based on randomized clinical trials that demonstrate improved outcome when used within 3 hours from time of symptom onset and the absence of hemorrhage on CT images. Thus, early clinical decisions do not require the use of MRI despite the limited use of thrombolysis, currently the only Food and Drug Administration–approved pharmacologic treatment. The historical precedent of CT in emergency departments hinders changes in practice and leaves MRI in a secondary role for stroke management in most medical facilities. Early adopters are moving toward customized patient treatment with decision making directed by diffusion and perfusion MRI.

In patients who have known cerebrovascular disease and are being evaluated for stroke etiology and prevention, MRI and magnetic resonance angiography (MRA) have a central role in medical decision making. This application of MRI, away from the access and time constraints of acute treatment, is discussed based on the author's experience. The use of quantitative perfusion and functional measurements is emphasized through the use of representative case examples.

Funding support: The author acknowledges financial support from PHS PO1 NS35949.

E-mail address: kthulbor@uic.edu

doi:10.1016/j.ncl.2008.08.001 **neurologic.theclinics.com**

Acute and early subacute stroke

The occlusion of an arterial vessel supplying oxygenated blood to a region of brain tissue that lacks sufficient collateral circulation to maintain hemodynamic reserve leads to a cascade of physiologic, metabolic, and functional changes (described elsewhere) [1–5]. From the perspective of MRI, the immediate change in an acute nonhemorrhagic stroke can be visualized within a few minutes on diffusion-weighted images [6–14]. Although the mechanism of signal change remains controversial, the restricted diffusion of water in the stroke results in increased signal intensity on diffusion-sensitized images [6,14]. One working hypothesis is that this signal increase is the result of rapid development of cytotoxic edema after compromise of aerobic metabolism resulting from cessation of blood flow with its supply of oxygen. This phenomenon can be characterized by the calculation of the apparent diffusion coefficient (ADC) map. Other MRIs, such as T2- and T1-weighted images and CT images, may remain normal until hours later when vasogenic edema develops. If hemorrhage is present, signal loss is readily apparent on magnetic susceptibility-sensitive gradient-echo images and less so on T1- and T2-weighted spin-echo images except through the mass effect from a hematoma and edema. Blood products from hemorrhage can persist in the brain parenchyma for decades and undergo an evolution of signal changes over days to months that reflect the changing biochemistry of iron metabolism [15–17]. CT readily detects most acute hemorrhages, although magnetic resonance (MR) is much more sensitive for small acute petechial hemorrhage and much more sensitive for detecting the iron storage products of hemosiderin and ferritin from old hemorrhages [18]. Once T2-weighted images show increased signal consistent with edema after a few hours, the diffusion-weighted imaging becomes ambiguous. The increased signal on diffusion-weighted images can be the result of the increased water content

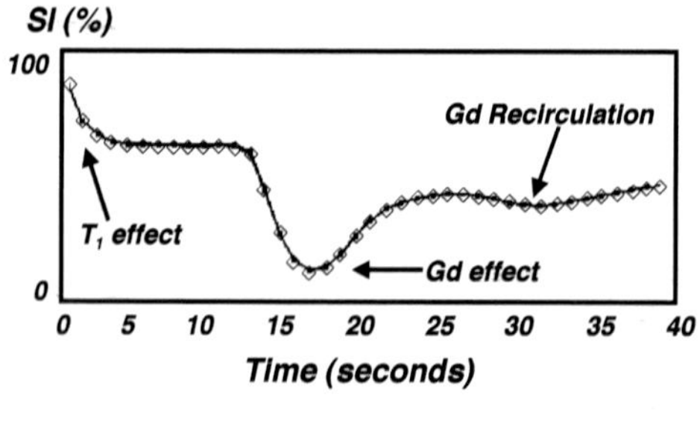

Fig. 1. Representative voxel-based time course of brain MR signal intensity for a bolus of gadolinium (Gd)-based MR contrast administered IV at the antecubital vein (5 mL/s, 20-gauge Angiocath, 0.1 mmol/kg). The initial decrease in the signal in the first 3 points is the result of progressive T1 relaxation spin saturation effects followed by the baseline (3–12 s) and then the arrival of the bolus at the capillary bed (TTA) when the signal intensity undergoes a rapid decrease and then recovers as the bolus washes out (TTT) of the capillary bed. Recirculation of contrast from the rest of the body prevents the signal intensity from returning completely to baseline and produces a second dip in the washout curve.

from vasogenic edema (so-called T2 shine through) rather than just restricted diffusion from cytotoxic edema. The ADC map derived from the diffusion-weighted imaging readily resolves this dilemma. Cytotoxic edema shows reduced ADC whereas vasogenic edema shows increased ADC values. This ADC map is calculated in a few seconds on clinical MR scanners after acquiring the diffusion-weighted imaging at two different levels of diffusion weighting and always is readily available. The ADC map in acute and early subacute stroke shows low ADCs, readily identified by comparing the abnormal side to the contralateral side. The differences can be 50% or more in most strokes but the region of stroke also can be heterogeneous. The ADC values remain low for a few days, begin to pseudonormalize by 5 to 10 days, and then become permanently supernormal as encephalomalacic changes take place [19]. During this early subacute time, the increasing edema initially produces mass effect that then resolves in the late subacute phase.

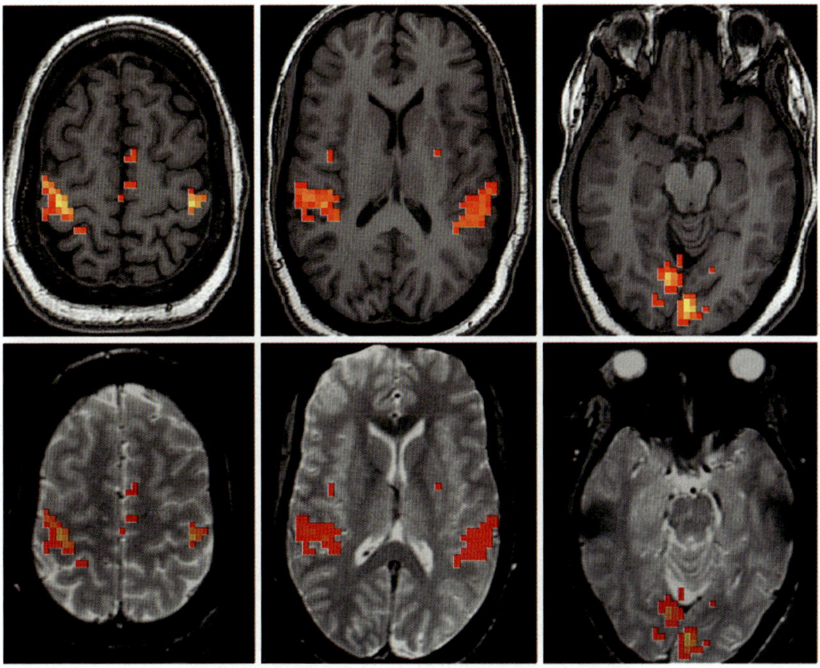

Fig. 2. Representative slices from an activation map superimposed over high-resolution, T1-weighted (*upper row*, dark cerebrospinal fluid [CSF]) and T2-weighted (*lower row*, bright CSF) anatomic images for a subject performing the audiovisual motor paradigm showing bilateral primary motor and somatosensory activation in superior MCA territory (lateral) (*left column*) and supplementary motor activation in anterior cerebral artery territory (medial) (*left column*), bilateral auditory activation in distal inferior MCA territory (*middle column*), and bilateral visual activation in PCA territory (posteriomedial) (*right column*). These activations interrogate each of the cerebral artery vascular territories.

Patients who have a nonhemorrhagic stroke by CT criteria and who are still within 3 hours of symptom onset may be eligible for thrombolysis therapy [20]. Such lesions typically show increased T2 signal changes, low ADC values, and no signal loss on gradient-echo images on MRI. The rationale for not using MRI routinely is to avoid delaying treatment when CT usually is more readily available.

Only approximately 5% of eligible patients receive thrombolytic treatment in the United States because of the potential that a devastating hemorrhage, a known risk for thrombolytic therapy, may occur within the lesion and further compromise the patient [20]. Attempts have been made to stratify risks by examining perfusion and diffusion MRI [21]. This concept is that large diffusion-perfusion mismatches identify patients who may benefit from treatment [22]. The mismatch has been conceptualized as being the ischemic penumbra—the region at risk for stroke progression. The mismatch paradigm has been used in ongoing research efforts to extend the treatment window for intravenous (IV) thrombolysis beyond 3 hours.

An alternative approach has been proposed in which sodium imaging is used to measure tissue sodium concentration (TSC) as a measure of tissue

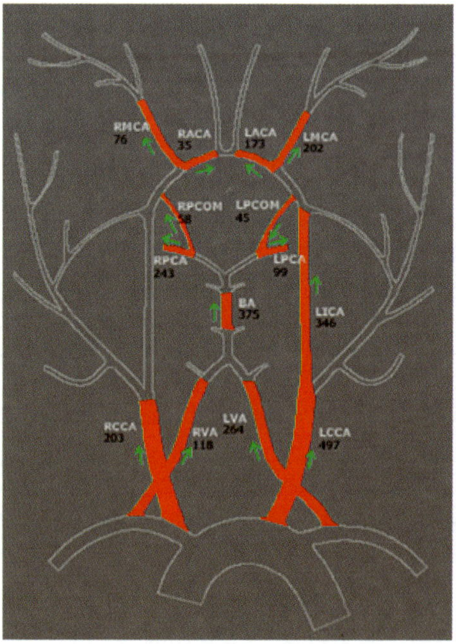

Fig. 3. Schematic summary (NOVA software, VasSol, Chicago) of the quantitative phase-contrast MRA measurements of blood flow for the large intracranial vessels for a patient who had right MCA stenosis. Flow through the right MCA is only 76 mL/min compared with that of the left MCA flow of 202 mL/min. Collateral pial-pial circulation from the right PCA explains its increased flow of 243 mL/min compared with that of 99 mL/min in the left PCA.

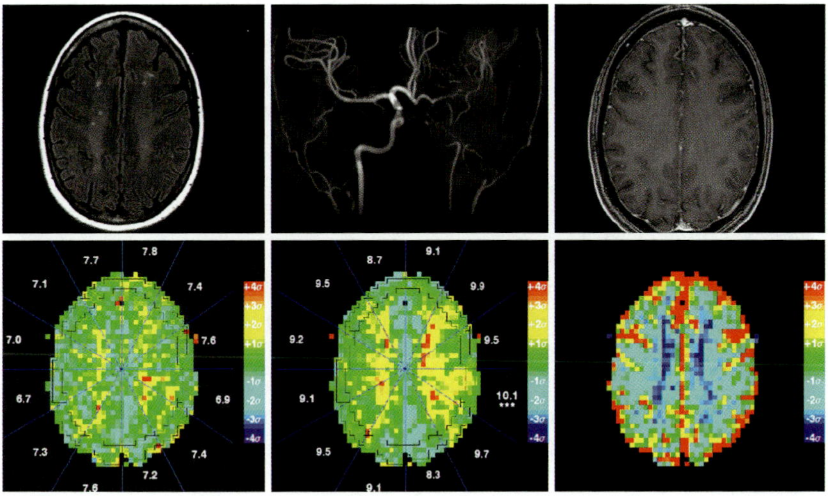

Fig. 4. Anatomic, angiographic, and perfusion MRI of patient in Case 1. T2-weighted fluid-attenuated inversion recovery (FLAIR) image showing multiple foci of high T2 signal abnormalities (*upper left*); MRA of the anterior circulation showing attenuation of flow enhancement in the left internal carotid artery and left MCA (*upper middle*); and IV contrast-enhanced T1-weighted image showing no enhancement (*upper right*). The perfusion maps are shown on the lower row with TTT (*lower left*), TTA (*lower middle*), and rCBV (*lower right*). No large asymmetries between left and right cerebral hemispheres and between anterior and posterior circulation are identified.

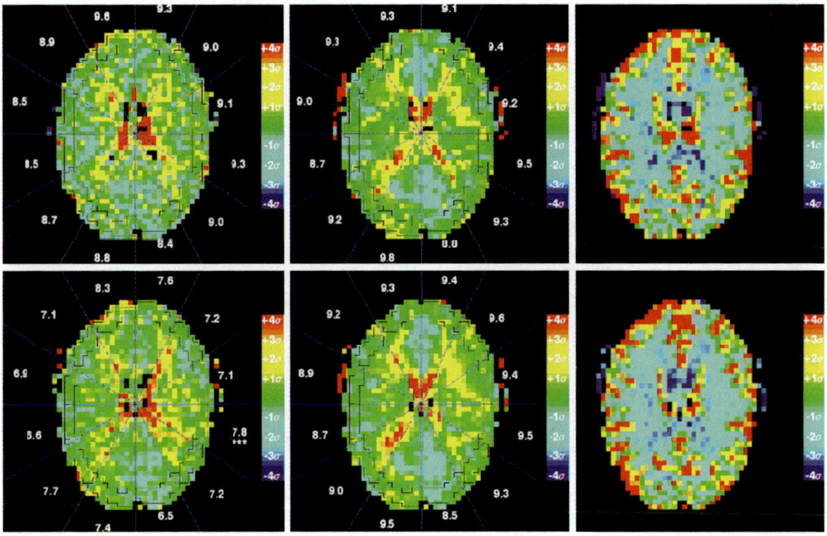

Fig. 5. The perfusion maps for patient in Case 1 before (*upper*) and after (*lower*) vasodilation with acctazolamide showing no significant asymmetries and normal perfusion parameters for TTT and TTA. Hemodynamic reserve remains intact in all vascular territories.

viability. Sodium ion homeostasis may directly reflect if tissue can be salvaged by appropriate treatment and indicate risk for hemorrhage. A quantitative TSC threshold of tissue viability would be an objective means of customizing treatment decisions in individual patients [19,23,24].

Management of stroke risk in patients who have known cerebrovascular disease

Every patient surviving a stroke or presenting with symptoms that may be explained by cerebral ischemia should undergo a thorough work-up to determine the extent of intracranial and extracranial etiologies that may underlie those signs and symptoms. This work-up, away from the urgency of the acute stroke setting, should include quantitative evaluation of the integrity of the large vessels of the neck and head and estimation of the

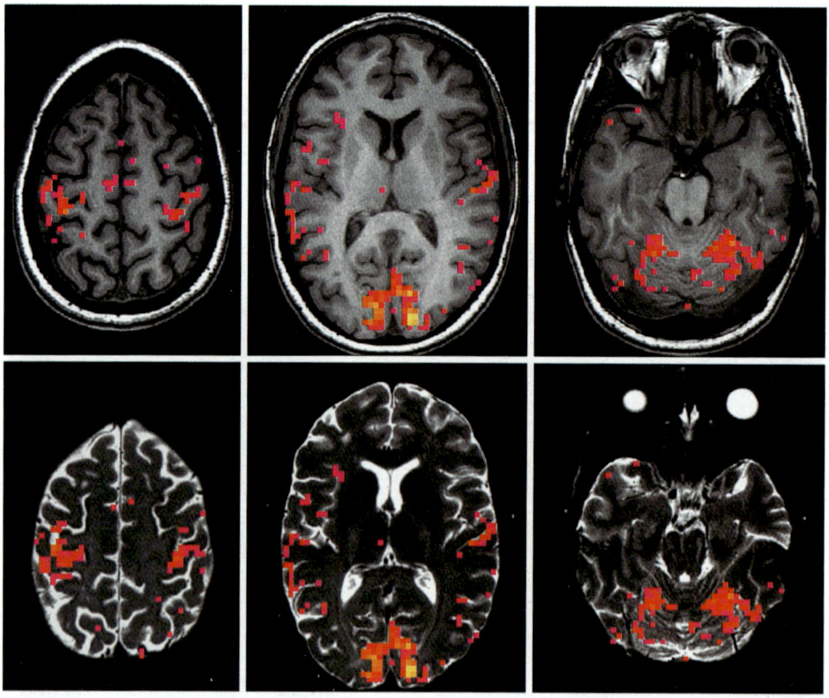

Fig. 6. The activation maps using the bilateral motor, auditory, and visual stimulus paradigm for patient in Case 1 superimposed over dark CSF T1-weighted images (*upper*) and over bright CSF T2-weighted images (*lower*). Somatosensory, primary motor, and supplementary motor cortex (*upper and lower left*); auditory and visual cortex (*upper and lower middle*); and cerebellar motor activation (*upper and lower right*) demonstrate sufficient hemodynamic reserve to maintain BOLD contrast responses in all vascular territories.

cerebral hemodynamic reserve. The lack of hemodynamic reserve puts patients at high risk for subsequent stroke [25,26].

Different centers may elect to obtain such information in a variety of ways. As these patients may require ongoing monitoring with subsequent follow-up imaging studies, quantitative parameters are valuable for temporal comparisons to measure disease progression. Methods using ionizing radiation should be minimized to avoid an accumulating radiation burden. For this reason, the roles of xenon CT, positron emission tomography, and single photon emission CT with vasodilatory challenges, such as with acetazolamide, are not discussed in this article. The more invasive strategies, such as conventional catheter angiography, should be used sparingly and also are not discussed further. MRI, MRA, MR perfusion, and diffusion measurements all are readily available on clinical MR scanners, quantitative, can be repeated over time without concern for increasing ionizing radiation burden, and noninvasive. These currently commercially available techniques are described. Newer research protocols are discussed only briefly, although these may soon enter clinical practice.

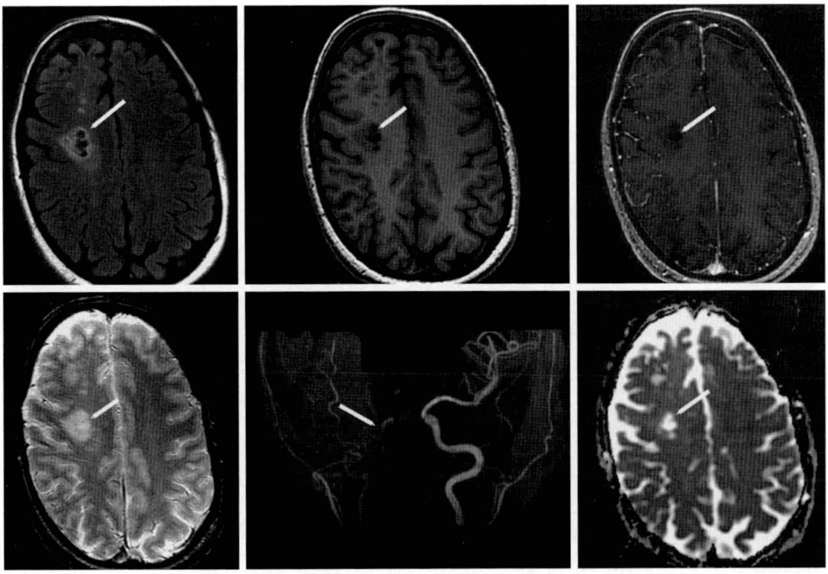

Fig. 7. MR anatomy and intracranial MRA obtained at 3.0 T of a patient who had history of stroke and known right internal carotid artery occlusion who currently is asymptomatic. T2-weighted FLAIR image showing ischemic lesions (*white arrow*) in the white matter of the right frontal lobe (*upper left*); unenhanced, T1-weighted, 3-D, gradient-echo image showing ischemic lesions (*white arrow*) (*upper middle*); IV contrast-enhanced, T1-weighted, 3-D, gradient-echo image showing no enhancement in lesions (*white arrow*) (*upper right*); T2-weighted, gradient-echo image showing no hemorrhage in lesions (*white arrow*) (*lower left*); and TOF MRA of the anterior circulation showing absence of flow enhancement in the right internal carotid artery (*white arrow*) and in the bilateral anterior and right MCAs and ADC map showing ischemic, CSF-filled, cavitary lesions (*white arrow*) (*lower middle*).

Magnetic resonance techniques for evaluation of cerebrovascular physiology in the setting of stroke prevention

Magnetic Resonance Perfusion

Dynamic susceptibility contrast (DSC) perfusion imaging exploits the magnetic susceptibility effects produced by the blood-brain barrier between the vascular space of the capillary bed and the surrounding brain parenchyma when a bolus of IV-administered paramagnetic gadolinium-based contrast agent passes through the capillary bed [27–29]. This method requires a rapid imaging technique that is sensitive to these magnetic susceptibility effects. Gradient-echo, echo-planar imaging at high temporal resolution (time to repeat = 1 to 1.5 s) usually is used. Using an IV bolus injection (5 mL/s, antecubital vein, 20-gauge Angiocath, standard full dose based on body weight [ie, 0.1 mmol/kg at 3.0 T]), the first passage of contrast through the brain is monitored as a washout curve in which the signal initially decreases and then increases as the contrast passes through the capillary bed (Fig. 1). This washout curve can be analyzed in several ways. As the arterial input function (AIF) is not readily available and, in the setting of vascular disease, varies across the different vascular territories of the brain, the simplest and fastest approach is the gamma variate fit to the experimental curve, introduced almost 3 decades ago [30], which allows the parameters

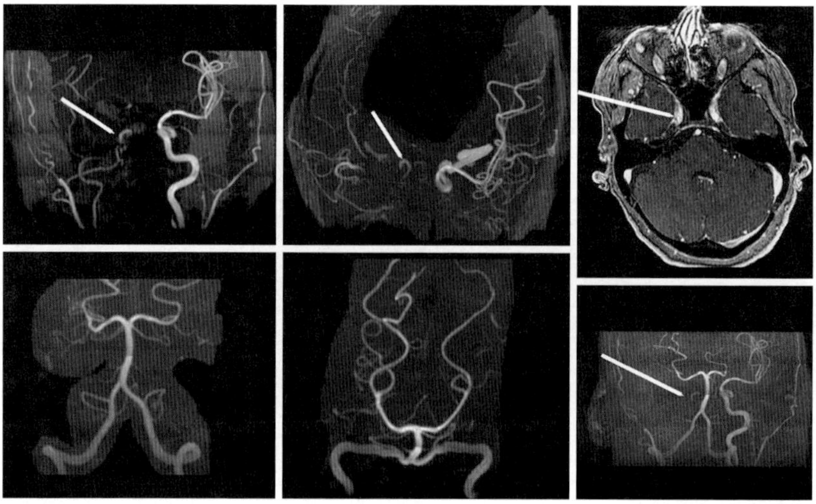

Fig. 8. MRA of patient in Case 2 from Fig. 7 showing (*upper left and middle*) maximum intensity projection reconstructed TOF angiogram of the (*upper left and middle*) anterior circulation in which the right internal carotid artery (*arrows*) is missing; (*upper right*) base images showing reduced flow (string sign) (*arrow*) in the precavernous portion of the right internal carotid artery; and (*lower left and middle*) normal posterior circulation and (*lower right*) combined anterior and posterior circulation showing the absence of flow enhancement in the right internal carotid artery (*arrow*), bilateral anterior cerebral arteries and the MCA.

of time to arrival (TTA), tissue transit time (TTT), and relative cerebral blood volume (rCBV) to be characterized. A relative cerebral blood flow (rCBF) can be estimated from the other parameters (rCBF = rCBV/TTT). These parameters are reproducible and can be used for studying disease progression over time. Details of this and similar methods are described elsewhere [27–30]. Although other methods of deconvolution of the AIF have theoretic value, these methods often fail to recognize that it is unique for each voxel and can vary widely across a brain with regional cerebrovascular pathology. No generally acceptable method for finding an AIF on a voxel-by-voxel basis currently exists and best estimates are computationally intensive without benefit over the gamma variate approach [30].

This perfusion method also can be enhanced using a vasodilatory challenge, such as acetazolamide (1 g IV injected slowly and a delay of 10 minutes to allow vasodilation) to measure hemodynamic reserve. Acetazolamide is a carbonic

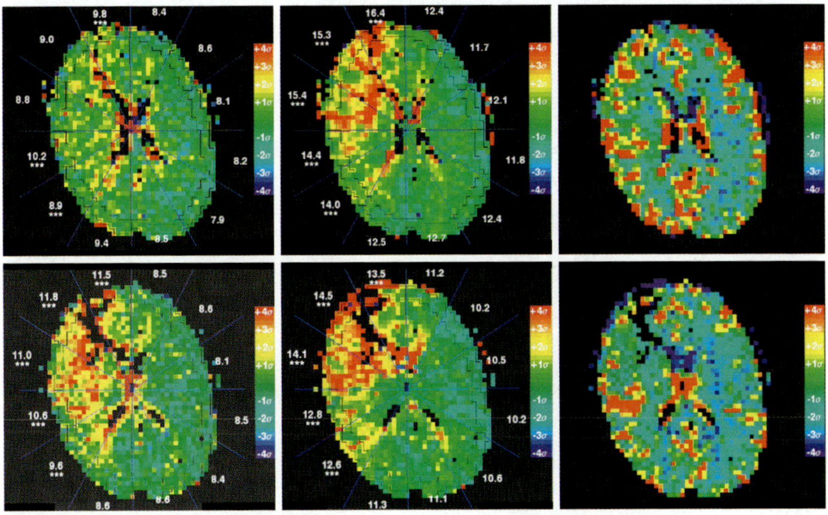

Fig. 9. MR perfusion maps before (*upper row*) and after vasodilation (*lower row*) with 1 g acetazolamide administered IV derived from DSC perfusion MRI of the same patient as in Fig. 7. TTT map with values for cortex showing slight asymmetry with longer values on right, especially in the posterior right MCA territory (*upper left*); TTA map showing prolonged arrival times in the right MCA territory (*upper middle*); rCBV map showing slightly increased right-sided values (*upper right*); TTT map after vasodilation shows markedly increased asymmetry with little change in the values in the left cerebral hemisphere (*lower left*); and TTA map shows increased asymmetry (*lower middle*) and rCBV map also shows asymmetry (*lower right*). The black voxels in the right frontal lobe are areas of such abnormal perfusion that the data cannot be fitted accurately. The worsening perfusion after vasodilation is indicative of lack of hemodynamic reserve in the right MCA territory and places the patient at high risk for a subsequent second stroke if aggressive management is not instituted. The color scales are based on standard deviations from the mean values of the whole brain for each parameter. Black voxels have insufficient contrast change during the first pass of the bolus to perform a gamma variate fit to obtain perfusion parameters.

anhydrase inhibitor that limits clearance of carbon dioxide (CO_2) from the brain by slowing its conversion to bicarbonate ions. This accumulated CO_2 causes cerebral vasodilation. This technique, requiring two perfusion studies, is demonstrated in the case examples (described later). Other approaches to measuring hemodynamic reserve using a CO_2 rebreathing technique soon may become available for clinical use [31].

Other perfusion methods also are available. Arterial spin labeling methods avoid the need for IV contrast but currently are more time consuming and not yet commercially available on all MR scanners [32].

Functional MRI

Functional MRI (fMRI) uses blood oxygenation level–dependent (BOLD) contrast to localize brain function [33]. When a region of the brain

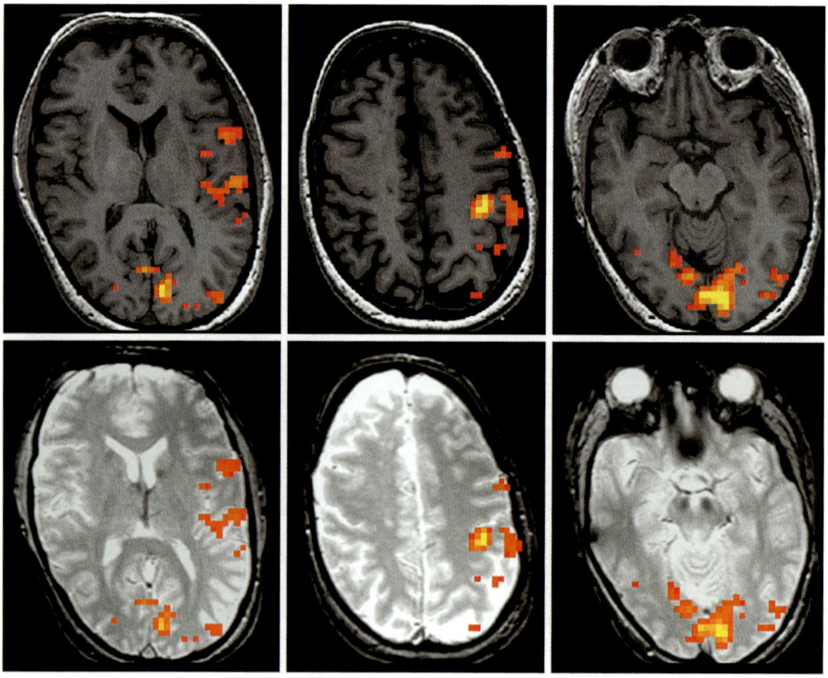

Fig. 10. Activation maps (color) superimposed over T1-weighted (dark CSF) images (*upper row*) and T2-weighted (bright CSF) images (*lower row*) for the bilateral audiovisual hand movement task. The maps show marked asymmetry with loss of activation in the right anterior and MCA territories, indicating loss of hemodynamic reserve, insufficient to maintain the BOLD hemodynamic response. Right auditory cortex (*upper and lower left*) fails to activate as does the right motor and somatosensory cortex (*upper and lower middle*), indicating compromised hemodynamic reserve in the anterior circulation on the right side compared with the left but no compromise in the posterior circulation as the visual cortex (*upper and lower right*) activates bilaterally.

increases its activity in response to a stimulus, there is a focal increase in blood flow and blood volume. The magnetic susceptibility of the blood in the capillary bed becomes more like the surrounding diamagnetic brain parenchyma as the increased blood flow displaces paramagnetic deoxyhemoglobin for diamagnetic oxyghemoglobin. This loss of the magnetic susceptibility difference between the capillaries and tissue eliminates one of the transverse relaxation mechanisms that cause loss of MR signal intensity. Thus, a small increase in MR signal intensity occurs that can be detected on magnetic susceptibility-weighted (T2*) images. This signal increase is small (1%–5% at 3 T) but can be detected statistically by comparing the average signal intensity of the control condition (without stimulus) with that of the active condition (with stimulus) after signal averaging of many images. Although this approach normally is used to map cortex for presurgical planning, the method also can be used to detect hemodynamic reserve. As the hemodynamic reserve decreases, the brain becomes more vasodilated. BOLD contrast is reduced and eventually undetectable when no further vasodilation can occur. The stimulus paradigm is designed to

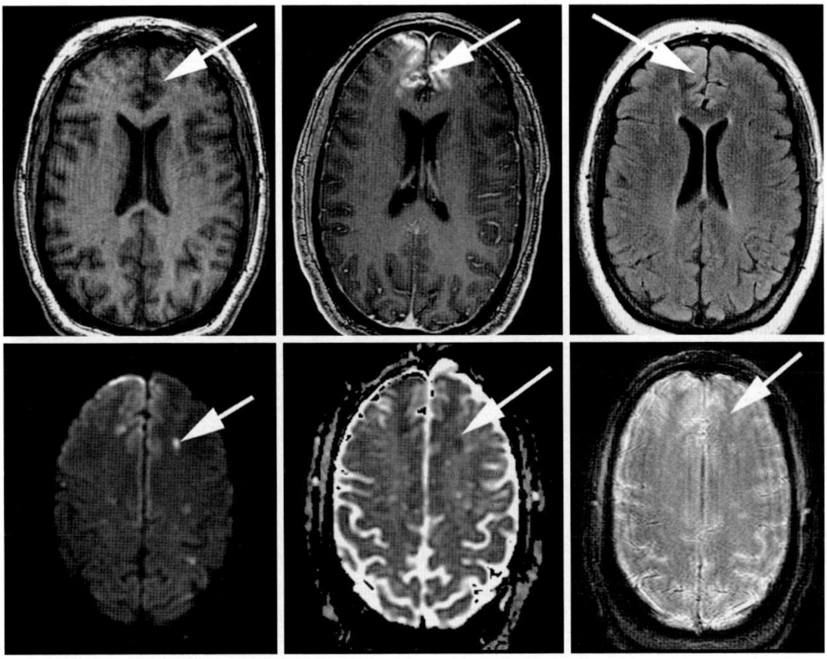

Fig. 11. Anatomic images of a young woman who had moyamoya disease who presented with bilateral subacute infarctions. Unenhanced T1-weighted image (*upper left*) with minimally visible bifrontal infarction (*arrow*); enhanced T1-weighted image (*upper middle*) showing enhancement (*arrow*) in the bilateral anterior cerebral artery territories; T2-weighted FLAIR image (*upper right*) showing edema/gliosis in the infarction; diffusion-weighted image (*lower left*) showing restricted diffusion (*arrow*) that is confirmed on ADC map (*arrow*) (*lower middle*); and T2-weighted, gradient-echo, weighted image showing no hemorrhage (*arrow*) (*lower right*).

efficiently interrogate all vascular territories. Motor, visual, and auditory stimuli are combined to allow assessment in the anterior (primary motor, somatosensory, and auditory) and posterior (visual and cerebellar motor) circulation in a single short paradigm.

The paradigm consists of a two-condition, block design with 4.5 cycles, each block with 30 seconds' duration. The control condition is a silent, static visual fixation on a central white cross (2° visual angle) on a black background, presented to the patient on a rear projection screen inside the magnet. The stimulus condition consists of audiovisual commands to open and close both hands at a fixed frequency (1 Hz). The words, OPEN and CLOSE, are presented visually and centrally with peripheral bilateral alternating black and white checkerboards on the same rear projection screen. The verbal commands also are simultaneously presented stereophonically through earphones. The activation map for this paradigm for healthy adults who do not have cerebrovascular disease is shown in Fig. 2.

Quantitative Magnetic Resonance Angiography

MRA can be performed with both time-of-flight (TOF) and phase-contrast (PC) techniques. Whereas the TOF method defines vascular

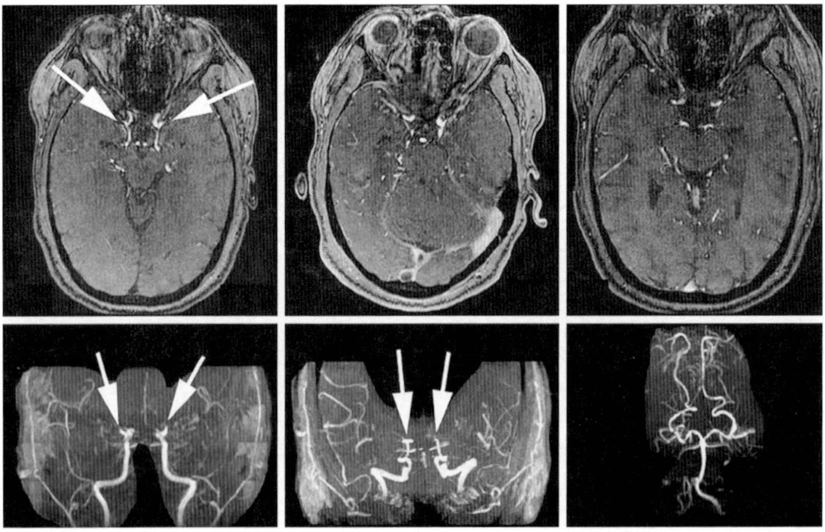

Fig. 12. MRA of the patient in Case 3 who had moyamoya disease showing the truncation of flow enhancement in the proximal middle and anterior cerebral arteries (*arrows*) but intact posterior communicating arteries (*upper row, arrows*) providing some collateral flow into the expanded PCAs (*lower right*), which provide pial-pial collateral circulation into the anterior circulation. The basilar artery is supplied by one dominant vertebral artery that is normal in caliber so that the expanded posterior circulation is the result of the posterior communicating arteries from the anterior circulation.

anatomy at high resolution in 3-D or 2-D modes in acceptable acquisition times, quantitative flow rates are not determined. The PC method is quantitative and able to determine blood flow (from flow velocity and vessel diameter) through specified large vessels but is time consuming. As these approaches were evolving in the preceding decades, the TOF technique became more popular for anatomic disease screening. The quantitative PC technique with improved analysis software, however, is again becoming recognized as potentially useful for following disease progression. The complete description of this method goes beyond the scope of this text and can be found elsewhere [34]. This technique provides large vessel conductance flow measurements for specified vessels (Fig. 3). Such flow measurements can be obtained before and after pharmacologic challenge with acetazolamide to assess hemodynamic reserve. Additionally, large vessel flow values can be used to determine

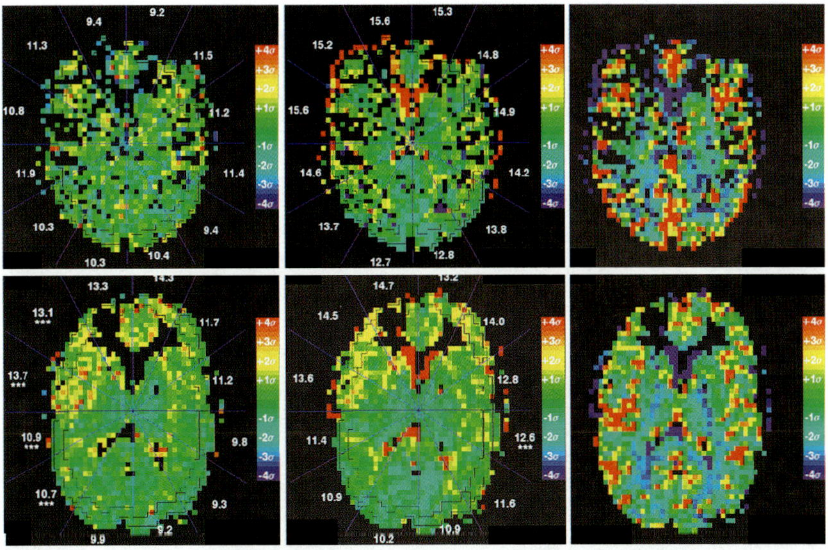

Fig. 13. Perfusion imaging of the patient in Case 3 who had moyamoya disease showing perfusion maps before vasodilation (*upper row*) and after vasodilation (*lower row*) with IV-administered acetazolamide. The TTT (*first column*) shows low values in the anterior cerebral artery territories (9.2–9.4 s) because of the infarction. Away from the infarctions, there are longer TTT values (right MCA: 10.8–11.9 s; left MCA: 11.2–11.4 s) in the MCA territories compared with values (10.3–10.4 s) in the PCA territories. These differences increase (right MCA: 10.9–13.7 s; left MCA: 9.8–11.2; PCA: 9.2–9.9 s) in right MCA after vasodilation, indicating compromised hemodynamic reserve. The TTA (*middle column*) values also show asymmetry between the anterior and posterior circulation that further widens after vasodilation. The rCBV (*right column*) is insensitive to the perfusion asymmetries. The color scales are based on standard deviations from the mean values of the whole brain for each parameter. Black voxels have insufficient contrast change during the first pass of the bolus to perform a gamma variate fit to obtain perfusion parameters.

the presence, quantity, and pattern of collateral flow and tissue level flows can be obtained directly by MR perfusion. The use of such measurements is illustrated in Cases 1 through 4.

Clinical cases

Case 1

A young, right-handed woman presented with variable complaints of right face numbness, left arm weakness, short-term memory loss, and migraine headaches. Her work-up included a conventional catheter angiogram that showed an occluded supraclinoid portion of her left internal carotid artery and significant stenosis of the distal right internal carotid artery. Many small collateral vessels at the circle of Willis were typical of moyamoya disease. Fig. 4 illustrates the anatomy, MRA, and perfusion

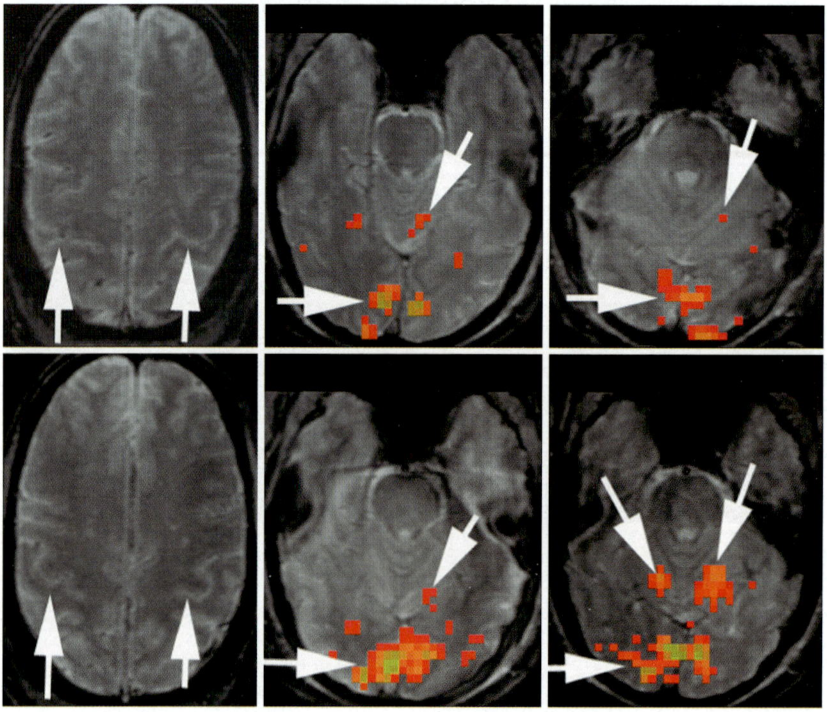

Fig. 14. Activation pattern for the audiovisual motor task showing no activation in the primary motor and somatosensory areas (*left column, vertical upward arrows*) but activation in the motor cerebellar regions (*right column, angled downward arrows*), indicating that the motor task was performed as also observed directly. The visual cortex activation (*horizontal arrows*) is readily apparent. The colored activation is superimposed over the T2-weighted, fast gradient-echo, echo-planar images.

studies for this patient. The anatomic images show diffuse cortical atrophy for age with multiple small foci of T2 hyperintense, nonenhancing, nonhemorrhagic, signal abnormalities in the white matter of both cerebral hemispheres, consistent with chronic small vessel distribution ischemia. The MRA shows diminished flow enhancement in the left internal carotid artery and left middle cerebral artery (MCA) compared with the right side. The perfusion studies show essentially normal TTT, TTA, and rCBV values without left-right or anterior-posterior asymmetries. The TTA values in the white matter seem slightly longer than normal, especially on the left side. The clinical question for the management of this symptomatic patient is whether or not the complaints and the anatomic changes resulted from emboli or reduced flow with concomitant loss of hemodynamic reserve. The perfusion study was performed before and after pharmacologic vasodilation with IV acetazolamide (Fig. 5). Vasodilation produces no left-right asymmetries with minimal change in TTA values and slightly reduced TTT values. Similarly, no gradient is present between the anterior and

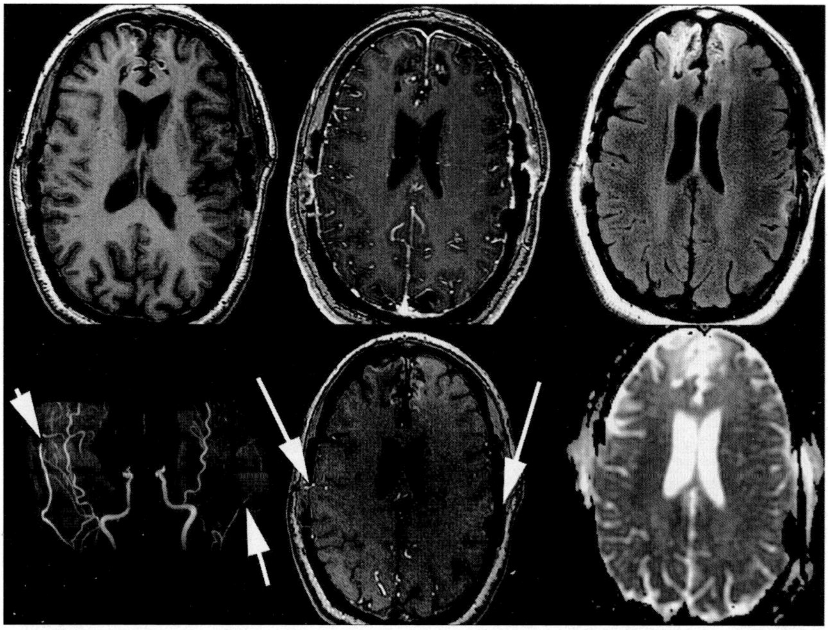

Fig. 15. Anatomic images and MRA after bilateral superficial temporal artery–MCA bypasses (*arrows*). T1-weighted image showing bilateral craniectomy postsurgical changes (*upper left*); contrast-enhanced T1-weighted image (*upper middle*); T2-weighted FLAIR images show progressive encephalomalacic changes in the frontal lobes from previous infarction (*upper right*); MRA (*lower left*) and a base image from that angiogram (*lower middle*) showing enhanced flow through the right superficial temporal artery compared with the left resulting from the susceptibility artifacts from the surgery; and ADC map showing no restricted diffusion to suggest acute or early subacute stroke (*lower right*).

posterior circulation. With bilateral disease, such as moyamoya, anterior-posterior circulation comparisons become important although no gradients are apparent in this case. As there is no redistribution and the perfusion values are in the normal range, collateral circulation through the multiple vessels at the circle of Willis and through the leptomeningeal collateral circulation is sufficient to maintain hemodynamic reserve. This is supported further by the fMRI activation map in Fig. 6. Activation is present in all vascular territories, indicating that there is sufficient hemodynamic reserve to support BOLD contrast. Close follow-up, however, is required as moyamoya disease often is progressive. This patient was treated with antithrombotic medication and instructed to maintain hydration.

Case 2

A middle-aged, right-handed, former smoker had a previous stroke with left-hand weakness and slurred speech that recovered to near baseline after 2 months. Initial work-up at an outside hospital suggested high-grade stenosis of the right internal carotid artery. Subsequent work-up was done several months later after referral to determine if there was adequate collateral circulation or reduced hemodynamic reserve. MRI identified chronic nonhemorrhagic small subcortical strokes in the right frontal lobe (Fig. 7) and right basal ganglia (not shown). The MRA showed the absence of flow

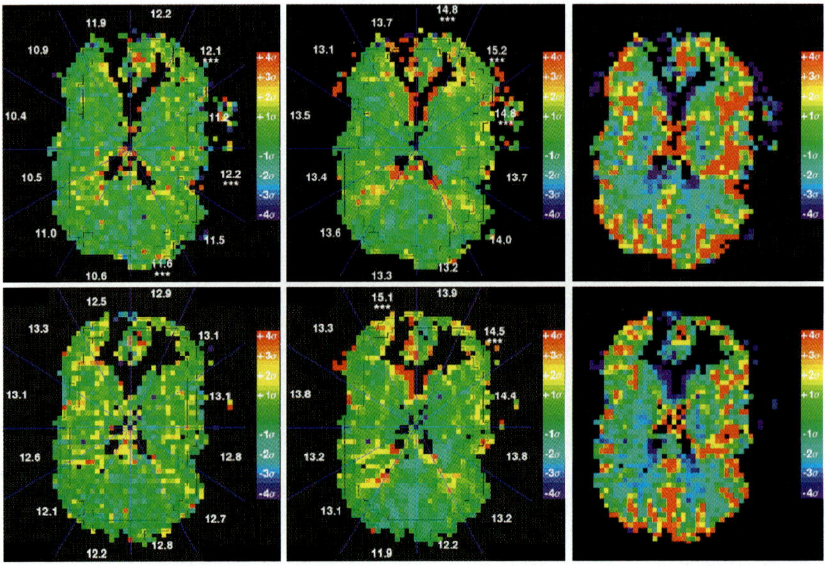

Fig. 16. The 6-week follow-up perfusion studies before (*upper row*) and after (*lower row*) vasodilation with acetazolamide show that the previous prebypass perfusion gradients in TTT (*left column*), TTA (*middle column*), and rCBV (*right column*) have been eliminated. Vasodilation results in no asymmetries, indicating that hemodynamic reserve has been restored.

enhancement in the right internal carotid artery and the bilateral anterior and MCAs (see Fig. 7; Fig. 8). The diffusion-weighted imaging showed no evidence of restricted diffusion to suggest acute or early subacute ischemia (see Fig. 7). This pattern of white matter involvement suggested limited hemodynamic reserve that affects white matter before gray matter. [35] The perfusion study was performed before and after vasodilation with IV acetazolamide and the perfusion maps are shown in Fig. 9. Before vasodilation, the rCBV is relatively symmetric and the TTT map is slightly asymmetric (1–2 s difference from right to left) and prolonged in the posterior aspect of the right MCA territory whereas the TTA is very asymmetric (2–3 s) being delayed on the right, more so in the white matter than the gray matter. These asymmetries all increase after vasodilation, as expected in the setting of limited hemodynamic reserve. The explanation for this effect is that once a territory is fully vasodilated, any further decrease in vascular resistance in other regions of the brain causes a selective redistribution of increased blood flow toward the regions of lower resistance. This finding is further supported by fMRI using BOLD contrast in which increased neuronal activity causes

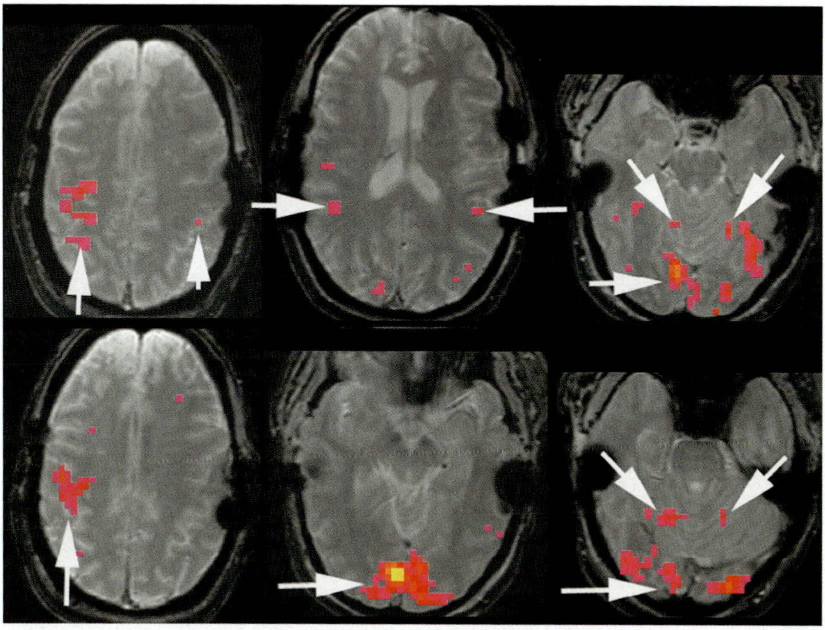

Fig. 17. The activation study at 6-week follow-up from the bilateral bypasses demonstrates restoration of activation in the motor and somatosensory cortex (*left column, vertical arrows*), in auditory cortex (*upper middle, arrows*), and maintained in the posterior circulation (*lower middle and right column*) (visual cortex [*horizontal arrows*] and cerebellar motor activation [*angled arrows*]). The asymmetry in activation with greater activation in the right cerebral hemisphere suggests that better flow augmentation was achieved on the right side. This is reflected in the better flow enhancement on the right side on the MRA in Fig. 15.

a localized increase in blood flow and blood volume [33]. The simple 4.5-minute audiovisual block-design paradigm (see Fig. 2) has been used to give the activation map (Fig. 10). Activation has been lost from the right anterior circulation.

Patients who have compromised hemodynamic reserve are at high risk for subsequent stroke. This patient requires aggressive medical management to limit emboli from the slow flow (string sign) in the right internal carotid artery. Vascular augmentation with angioplasty and stenting or a superficial temporal artery–MCA bypass could be considered if the patient's symptoms progress despite aggressive medical management.

Case 3

A young, right-handed woman presented with bifrontal nonhemorrhagic early subacute infarctions involving the anterior cerebral arteries (Fig. 11). The MRA (Fig. 12) confirmed the presence of moyamoya disease with the internal carotid arteries ending at the posterior communicating arteries that contribute to her expanded posterior circulation. Although present, the leptomeningeal collateral circulation from the posterior cerebral arteries (PCAs) had not been sufficient to reach the anterior cerebral artery territories leading to stroke. A perfusion study was performed before and after

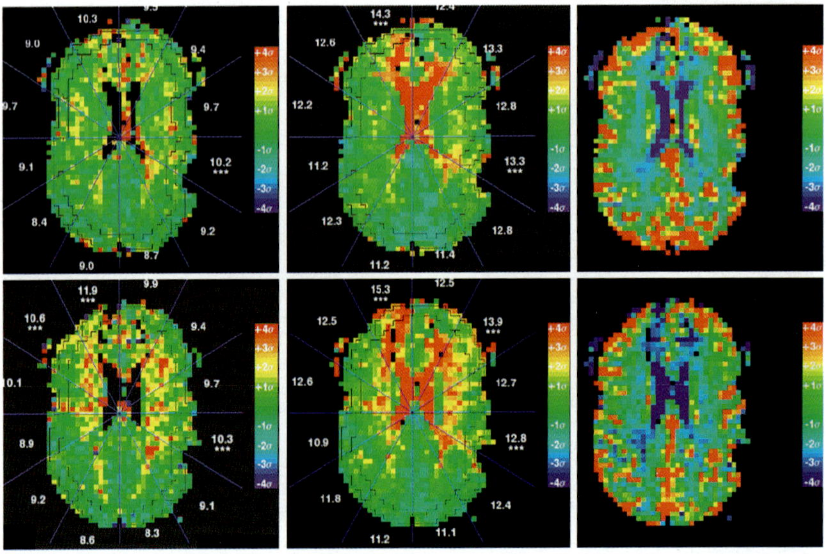

Fig. 18. The 6-month follow-up perfusion studies before (*upper row*) and after (*lower row*) vasodilation with acetazolamide show that some variability in distribution of perfusion has occurred since the 6-week follow-up study in TTT (*left column*); TTA values (*middle column*) are worsened by vasodilation especially in white matter and the rCBV maps (*right column*) remain insensitive to changes. This changes are more evident in the white matter but not in the gray matter after vasodilation.

vasodilation with IV administered acetozolamide (Fig. 13). Anteroposterior gradients in TTA and TTT are demonstrated. TTA becomes longer from the posterior to the anterior circulation indicative of the leptomeningeal collateral circulation. Vasodilation increases these gradients, indicating compromised hemodynamic reserve. This was confirmed with the functional activation map (Fig. 14) that fails to show detectable BOLD contrast in the anterior and MCA territories (motor, somatosensory, and auditory areas) but activation is present in the posterior circulation for the cerebrum (visual cortex) and cerebellum (motor). Quantitative flow measurements also confirm low flow and compromised hemodynamic reserve in the anterior circulation (eg, right and left MCA flow: preacetazolamide flows = 42 and 63 mL/min and postacetazolamide flows = 59 and 62 mL/min compared with basilar artery flows: preacetazolamide flows = 189 mL/min and postacetazolamide flows = 244 mL/min).

The recent stroke and the imaging demonstrating compromised hemodynamic reserve place this patient at high risk for further stroke.

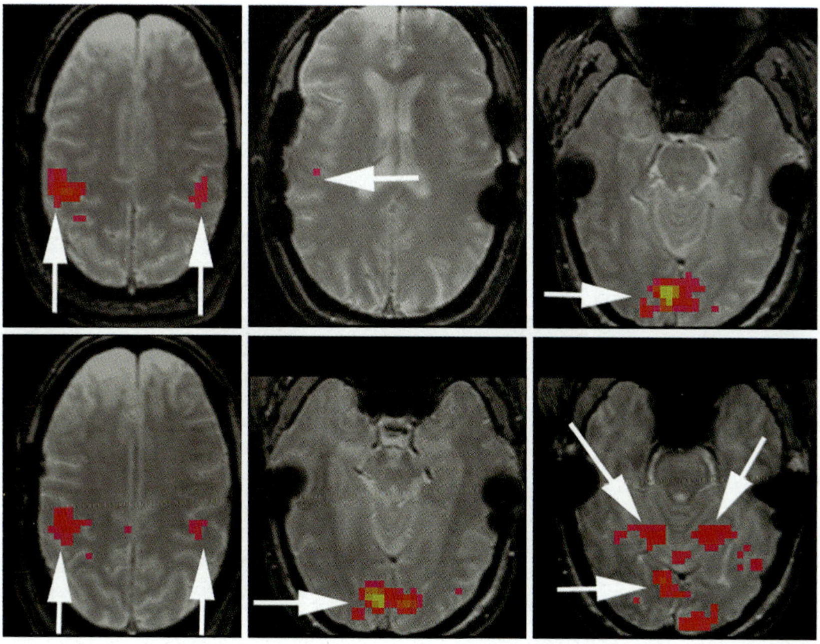

Fig. 19. The activation study at 6-month follow-up from the bilateral bypasses demonstrates further improvement with less asymmetry in the bilateral activation in the motor and somatosensory cortex (*left column, vertical arrows*) but with loss of activation in the auditory cortex (*upper middle, arrows*) since the 6-week follow-up study. Activation is maintained in the posterior circulation (*lower middle and right column*). The improved motor and somatosensory activation with loss of the auditory activation suggests that the distal MCA territories may be affected by the reduced hemodynamic reserve in the white matter evident on the perfusion study (see Fig. 18).

Cerebrovascular augmentation via bilateral superficial temporal artery–MCA bypasses and synangioses were performed. The follow-up studies were performed at 6 weeks and 6 months after the surgery.

The MRI and MRA at the 6-week follow-up (Fig. 15) demonstrate bilateral craniectomies and increased flow enhancement through the right superficial temporal artery. Flow through the left side does not seem augmented as much as the right side but this may be from the more severe surgical artifacts. All of the images show the magnetic susceptibility effects around the bilateral craniectomies that compromise delineation of the anastomoses of the bypasses. The perfusion studies (Fig. 16) also are affected immediately adjacent to the surgical bed but the previous perfusion gradients have normalized even after vasodilation. The activation studies (Fig. 17) show restored BOLD contrast in the previously compromised areas but with a left-right asymmetry that suggest that the left cerebral hemisphere has less reserve than the right side.

The MRI and MRA at the 6-month follow-up showed no significant changes (not shown). The perfusion study (Fig. 18) showed minor

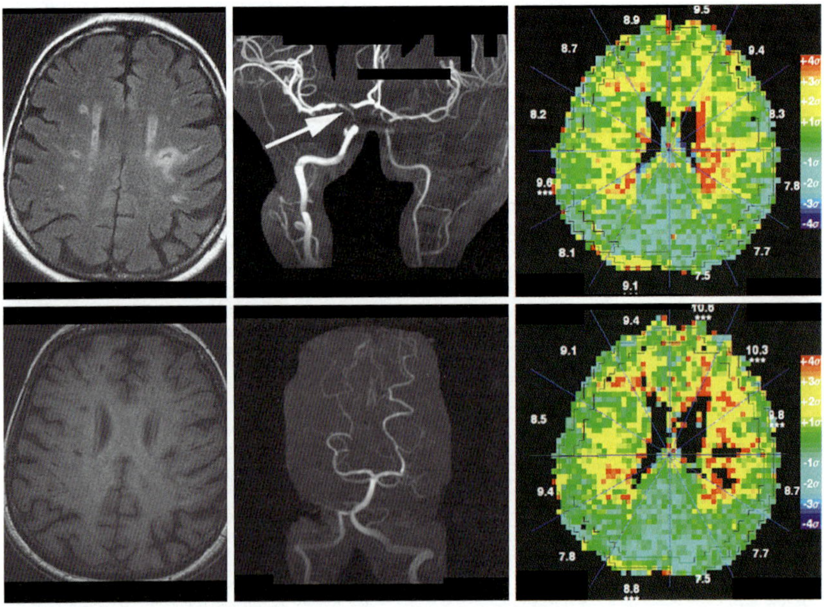

Fig. 20. Representative MRIs (*left column*), MRA (*middle column*), and MR perfusion TTT maps (*right column*) from Case 4. There are bilateral ischemic changes in the white matter of both cerebral hemispheres as shown on the T2-weighted FLAIR (*upper left*) and T1-weighted (*lower left*) images. There are very high-grade stenoses of the supraclinoid portions of the internal carotid arteries bilaterally but with greater flow remaining through the right internal carotid artery (*upper middle, arrow*). The posterior circulation (*lower middle*) shows expansion of the PCAs supplying pial-pial collateral flow, greater on the left side. The MR perfusion study shows longer TTT values in the white matter, especially on the left (*upper right*) and a worsening anterior-posterior gradient after vasodilation (*lower right*), also more severe in the white matter on the left.

variability in the perfusion parameters in the gray matter but the white matter showed perfusion asymmetries that worsened with vasodilation. This is consistent with the reduced hemodynamic reserve of the white matter compared with the gray matter and may be an early sign of recompromise. The activation study (Fig. 19) shows further improved BOLD contrast in the superior areas of the anterior circulation but reduction in activation in the distal more inferior MCA territories covering the auditory cortex. These patterns of change may reflect the ongoing readjustment of blood flow between white and gray matter and through the bypasses and the previously well-established leptomeningeal collateral circulation. These tissue level changes are not reflected in the qualitative flow patterns of the large vessels in the MRA.

Case 4

A young, right-handed woman was evaluated for bilateral stenoses of the supraclinoid portions of the internal carotid arteries consistent with moyamoya disease. The anatomic images (Fig. 20) show bilateral ischemic changes in the white matter, worse in the left cerebral hemisphere. The MRA (see Fig. 20) shows the bilateral internal carotid artery stenoses

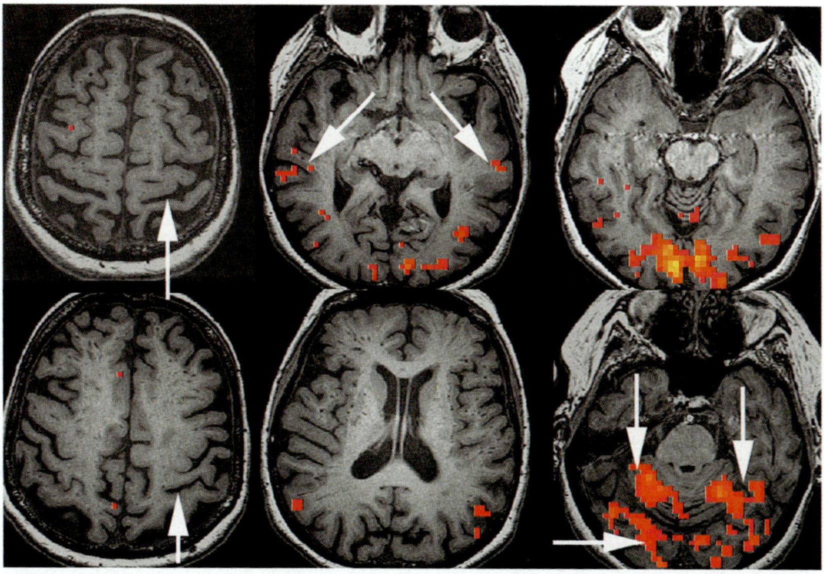

Fig. 21. Representative slices from the activation map of Case 4 showing no activation in the expected motor and somatosensory areas (*left column, upward arrows*), reduced activation in auditory cortex (*middle column, sloping arrows*), and normal activation in the visual (*right column, horizontal arrow*) and cerebellar motor (*right column, downward arrows*) areas. These observations indicate reduced hemodynamic reserve in the superior anterior circulation, insufficient to support BOLD contrast.

with expansion of the posterior circulation indicating leptomeningeal collateral flow. The MR perfusion study (see Fig. 20) demonstrates worsening gradients in TTT values between the anterior and posterior circulation, especially in the white matter, after vasodilation indicating compromise of the hemodynamic reserve in the anterior circulation, as expected from the anatomic changes. These findings are confirmed with the activation study (Fig. 21). No motor and somatosensory activation is detected in the superior portions of the cerebral hemispheres; markedly reduced auditory activation remains in the distal MCA territories of the superior temporal gyri; and normal visual activation and cerebellar motor activation persist in the occipital and cerebellar regions supplied by the posterior circulation.

This patient underwent angioplasty and stenting of the right-sided stenosis where the remaining flow was higher and which was more anatomically amenable to increase flow into the anterior circulation although the long-term outcome of this procedure remains to be determined. The poststent perfusion and activation results are shown in Figs. 22 and 23, respectively. The hemodynamic reserve was improved on the right side as indicated by the improved perfusion TTT and TTA parameters to match the posterior circulation (see Fig. 22) and restoration of the BOLD responses (see Fig. 23). The left side remains compromised in the distal MCA territory by asymmetric perfusion TTT and TTA values and loss of auditory

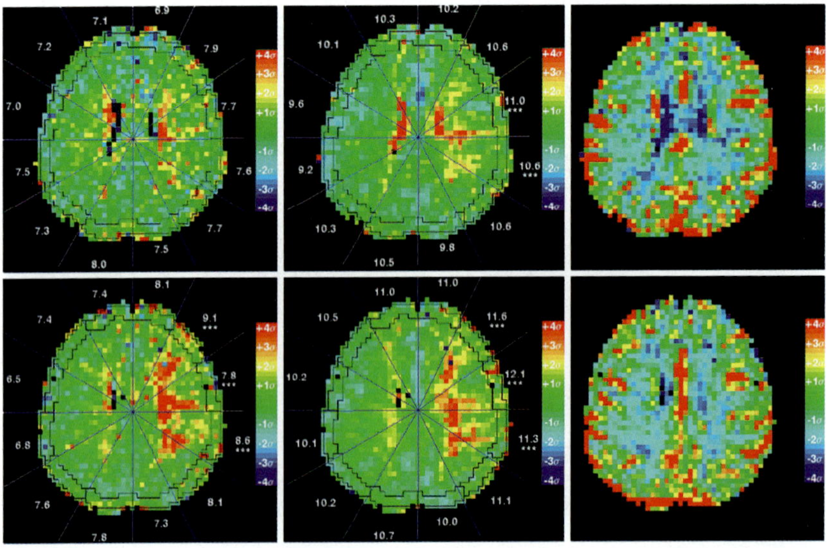

Fig. 22. Representative perfusion studies before (*upper row*) and after (*lower row*) vasodilation for Case 4 after angioplasty and stenting of the right internal carotid artery showing improved anterior-posterior symmetry in both TTT (*left column*) and TTA (*middle column*) values but residual asymmetries on the left, particularly in the white matter. The rCBV maps remain symmetric and insensitive to these changes.

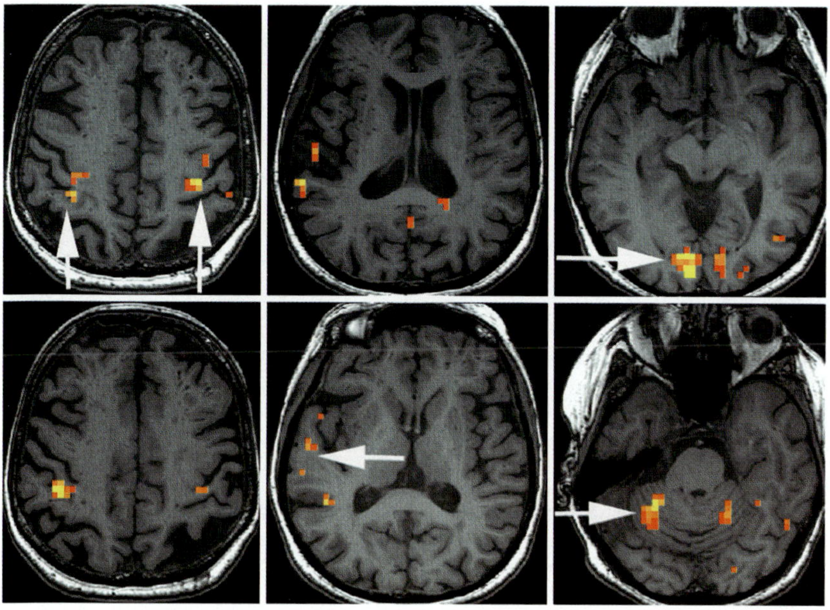

Fig. 23. Activation study after angioplasty and stenting of the right internal carotid artery showing restoration of activation in the motor and somatosensory areas (*left column, upward arrows*) but greater asymmetry in auditory activation (*middle column, horizontal arrow*) compared with prestenting (see Fig. 21). The activations in the visual (*upper right, arrow*) and cerebellar motor (*lower right, arrow*) cortex are unchanged.

activation compared with the right side. The quantitative flow measurements after stenting confirm that hemodynamic reserve was improved to the right cerebral hemisphere (eg, right MCA flow: preacetazolamide = 116 mL/min and postacetazolamide = 171 mL/min) but still compromised on the left side (eg, left MCA flow: preacetazolamide = 93 mL/min and postacetazolamide = 70 mL/min). Consideration was subsequently given to a left-sided flow augmentation procedure.

Summary

These four cases are representative of many hundreds of cases of cerebrovascular disease examined over the past 7 years in the Center for Magnetic Resonance Research in which management decisions have been guided by these MRI procedures. Symptoms in the presence of hemodynamic reserve suggest a need for aggressive medical treatment, such as risk factor control and antithrombotic medication. Symptomatic patients who have loss of hemodynamic reserve and who have recurrent symptoms despite medical management may be the optimal candidates for flow augmentation procedures, such as angioplasty with or without stenting and bypass surgery. The role of

MRI for initial evaluation and for following disease progression in these patients allows tailored care for patients based on the unique cerebrovascular pathophysiology of their disease. The long-term outcome of these medical and surgical interventions guided by MRI remains to be established. The cost of such imaging procedures for guiding clinical decisions toward appropriate management strategies is justified only if strokes are successfully prevented. These outcome measures are difficult to obtain without controlled clinical trials but warrant further investigation.

References

[1] Hossmann KA. Viability thresholds and the penumbra of focal ischemia. Ann Neurol 1994; 36:557–65.
[2] Ginsberg MD, Pulsinelli WA. The ischemic penumbra, injury thresholds and the therapeutic window for acute stroke. Ann Neurol 1994;36:553–4.
[3] Obrenovitch TP. The ischemic penumbra: twenty years on. Cerebrovasc Brain Metab Rev 1995;7:297–323.
[4] Astrup J, Siesjo BK, Symon L. Thresholds in cerebal ischemia—the ischemic penumbra. Stroke 1981;12:723–5.
[5] Kalafut MA, Saver JL. The acute stroke patient: the first 6 hours. In: Cohen SN, editor. Management of ischemic stroke. New York: McGraw-Hill; 2000. p. 17–52.
[6] Moseley M, Kucharczykk J, Mintorovitch J, et al. Diffusion-weighted MR imaging of acute stroke: correlation with T2-weighted and magnetic susceptibility-enhanced MR imaging in cats. AJNR Am J Neuroradiol 1990;11:423–9.
[7] Moseley M, Cohen Y, Mintorovitch J, et al. Early detection of stroke by diffusion MRI. Magn Reson Med 1990;14:330–43.
[8] Back T, Hoehn-Berlage M, Kohno K, et al. Diffusion nuclear magnetic resonance imaging in experimental stroke. Correlation with cerebral metabolites. Stroke 1994;25:494–500.
[9] Knight RA, Ordidge RJ, Helpern JA, et al. Temporal evolution of ischemic damage in rat brain measured by proton nuclear magnetic resonance imaging. Stroke 1991;2:802–8.
[10] Minematsu K, Li L, Fisher M, et al. Diffusion-weighted magnetic resonance imaging: rapid and quantitative detection of focal brain ischemia. Neurology 1992;42:235–40.
[11] deCrespigny A, Tsuura M, Moseley M, et al. Perfusion and diffusion MR imaging of thromboembolic stroke. J Magn Reson Imaging 1993;3:746–54.
[12] Desmond PM, Lovell AC, Rawlinson AA, et al. The value of apparent diffusion coefficient maps in early cerebral ischemia. AJNR Am J Neuroradiol 2001;22:1260–7.
[13] Wu O, Koroshetz WJ, Ostergaard L, et al. Predicting tissue outcome in acute human cerebral ischemia using combined diffusion and perfusion-weighted MR imaging. Stroke 2001;32:933–42.
[14] Roberts TP, Rowley HA. Diffusion weighted magnetic resonance imaging in stroke. Eur J Radiol 2003;45(3):185–94.
[15] Thulborn KR, Atlas SW. Intracranial hemorrhage. In: Atlas SW, editor. Magnetic resonance imaging of the brain and spine. New York: Raven Press; 1990. p. 175–222.
[16] Atlas SW, Thulborn KR. MR detection of hyperacute parenchymal hemorrhage of the brain. AJNR Am J Neuroradiol 1998;19(8):1471–7.
[17] Gomori JM, Grossman RI. Mechanisms responsible for the MR appearance and evolution of intracranial hemorrhage. Radiographics 1988;8(3):427–40.
[18] Thulborn KR, Sorensen AG, Kowell NW, et al. Biochemical correlation of the magnetic resonance appearance of experimentally induced cerebral hemorrhage in the rat. AJNR Am J Neuroradiol 1990;11:291–7.
[19] Thulborn KR, Gindin TS, Davis D, et al. Comprehensive MRI protocol for stroke management: tissue sodium concentration as a measure of tissue viability in a non-human primate model and clinical studies. Radiology 1999;139:26–34.

[20] The National Institutes of Neurological Disorders and Stroke rt-PA Stroke Study Group. Tissue plasminogen activator for acute ischemic stroke. N Engl J Med 1995;333:1581–7.
[21] Rowley HA. Extending the time window for thrombolysis: evidence from acute stroke trials. Neuroimaging Clin N Am 2005;15(3):575–87.
[22] Kidwell CS, Alger JR, Saver JL. Evolving paradigms in neuroimaging of the ischemic penumbra. Stroke 2004;35(11 Suppl 1):2662–5.
[23] Thulborn KR. Clinical sodium MR imaging of the brain. In: Latchaw RE, Kucharczyk J, Moseley ME, editors. Diagnostic and therapeutic imaging of the nervous system. Elsevier; 2004. p. 249–58.
[24] Thulborn KR, Davis D, Snyder J, et al. Sodium MR imaging of acute and subacute stroke for assessment of tissue viability. Neuroimaging Clin N Am 2005;15:639–53.
[25] Imaizumi M, Kitagawa K, Oku N, et al. Clinical significance of cerebrovascular reserve in acetazolamide challenge -comparison with acetazolamide challenge H2O-PET and Gas-PET. Ann Nucl Med 2004;18(5):369–74.
[26] Nemoto EM, Yonas H, Kuwabara H, et al. Differentiating hemodynamic compromise by the OEF response to acetazolamide in occlusive vascular disease. Adv Exp Med Biol 2005; 566:135–41.
[27] Ostergaard L, Sorensen AG, Kwong KK, et al. High resolution measurement of cerebral blood flow using intravascular tracer bolus passages. Part II: experimental comparison and preliminary results. Magn Reson Med 1996;36(5):726–36.
[28] Ostergaard L, Weisskoff RM, Chesler DA, et al. High resolution measurement of cerebral blood flow using intravascular tracer bolus passages. Part I: mathematical approach and statistical analysis. Magn Reson Med 1996;36(5):715–25.
[29] Thulborn KR, Uttecht S, Betancourt C, et al. A functional, physiological and metabolic toolbox for clinical magnetic resonance imaging: integration of acquisition and analysis strategies. Int J Imag Syst Tech 1997;8:572–81.
[30] Axel L. Cerebral blood flow determination by rapid-sequence computed tomography. Radiology 1980;137:679–86.
[31] Mandell DM, Han JS, Poublanc J, et al. Mapping cerebrovascular reactivity using blood oxygen level-dependent MRI in patients with arterial steno-occlusive disease: comparison with arterial spin labeling MRI. Stroke 2008;39(7):2021–8.
[32] Deibler AR, Pollock JM, Kraft RA, et al. Arterial spin-labeling in routine clinical practice, part 1: technique and artifacts. AJNR Am J Neuroradiol 2008;7:1228–34.
[33] Huettel SA, Song AW, McCarthy G, editors. Functional magnetic resonance imaging. Sunderland (MA): Sinauer Associates; 2003.
[34] Zhao M, Amin-Hanjani S, Ruland S, et al. Regional cerebral blood flow using quantitative MR angiography. AJNR Am J Neuroradiol 2007;28(8):1470–3.
[35] Fortanarosa J, Damen F, Flannery M, et al. Early hemodynamic compromise occurs in white matter, before gray matter, in patients with cerebral vaso-occlusive disease. In: Program of 45th Annual Meeting American Society of Neuroradiology. Chicago, June 9–14, 2007. (#273 presentation).

Section II

Diagnosis and Management of Acute Ischemic and Hemorrhagic Stroke

ELSEVIER
SAUNDERS

Neurol Clin 26 (2008) 923–942

NEUROLOGIC
CLINICS

Emergency Department Evaluation and Management of Stroke: Acute Assessment, Stroke Teams and Care Pathways

Alissa R. Gorelick, DO[a,*],
Philip B. Gorelick, MD, MPH, FACP[b],
Edward P. Sloan, MD, MPH, FACEP[c]

[a]*Emergency Medicine Residency Program, Department of Emergency Medicine, University of Illinois College of Medicine at Chicago, University of Illinois Medical Center, 1740 West Taylor Street, Chicago, IL 60612, USA*
[b]*Center for Stroke Research, Department of Neurology and Rehabilitation, University of Illinois College of Medicine at Chicago, University of Illinois Medical Center, 912 South Wood Street, Room 855N NPI, M/C 796, Chicago, IL 60612-7330, USA*
[c]*Department of Emergency Medicine, University of Illinois College of Medicine at Chicago, Mail Code 724, 808 South Wood Street, Chicago, IL 60612, USA*

Acute stroke recognition and intervention in the emergency department (ED) is crucial to improving outcomes for patients with this serious, yet treatable, cerebrovascular disorder. Nationwide, stroke is the third leading cause of death after heart disease and cancer; stroke fatalities occur every 3 to 4 minutes [1]. There are an estimated 780,000 new or recurrent strokes every year, with a stroke occurring approximately every 45 seconds. The majority of patients who experience stroke symptoms will present to the ED as their entry point into the health care system. The ED physician has the responsibility to assess, diagnose, and mobilize resources that will aid in the rapid treatment of stroke patients.

Currently, an estimated 1.8%–2.1% of acute ischemic stroke patients receive intravenous (IV) rt-PA [2]. Some of the reasons for the low frequency

---

Emergency Neurologic Education Resource: Foundation for Education and Research in Neurologic Emergencies (FERNE). FERNE is a Web-based system with targeted programs and resources for education of emergency department faculty and staff in neurologic emergencies. FERNE may be accessed at www.ferne.org.

* Corresponding author.
E-mail address: alissagorelick@hotmail.com (A.R. Gorelick).

doi:10.1016/j.ncl.2008.05.008

of IV rt-PA administration include lack of a well-developed local care system to implement treatment, delayed ED arrival times after stroke onset, lack of emergency medical services (EMS) delivery system use, poor physician motivation, and poor patient awareness [3–5].

Additionally, 3%–4% of Americans over the age of 65 may experience a transient ischemic attack (TIA) that carries a high subsequent stroke risk, especially in the period immediately following TIA. Ninety-day stroke rates after TIA have been estimated to be about 10% or higher with approximately half of the strokes occurring within several days of the sentinel event [1]. Stroke exacts a high financial burden with an estimated total cost of $62.7 billion in the United States [1].

Acute stroke management and prevention may begin in the ED. Fortunately, stroke systems are being developed that make it possible for the ED physician to facilitate patient care on multiple levels. This includes advanced notification of an incoming acute stroke patient, incorporating onset time by emergency medical services (EMS); rapid diagnosis with input from stroke team neurologists and radiologists; and telestroke for patients in areas of remote access. Further, the low usage rates of approved therapies may be improved upon in well-organized and coordinated acute stroke care systems. The Mississippi Stroke Education Consortium served as one of the first comprehensive templates for widespread, coordinated stroke care [6].

In this article, the authors review acute stroke management and organized approaches to stroke care from the perspective of the emergency medicine (EM) physician.

Prehospital care

Similar to acute myocardial infarction and trauma ("golden hour" concept), stroke must be treated in a timely manner. In acute stroke management the adage is "time is brain" as delays in diagnosis and treatment may render the patient neurologically impaired and disabled. Promptly implementing the "Stroke Chain of Survival" (seven Ds) (Box 1) [7–9] heightens the likelihood of early presentation and acute treatment of the ischemic or hemorrhagic stroke patient. An American Heart Association/American Stroke Association (AHA/ASA) policy statement emphasizes the implementation of EMS within stroke systems of care [10]. Several states and large communities have enacted legislation for EMS to preferentially triage acute stroke patients to appropriate "stroke centers" that are capable of rapid assessment and treatment.

Field identification: stroke scales

Several scales have been developed to identify stroke patients in the field (eg, Los Angeles Prehospital Stroke Scale [LAPSS] and Cincinnati Prehospital Stroke Scale). The LAPSS was designed to not only aid in the diagnosis

Box 1. Stroke chain of survival: the seven Ds

1. Detection of onset of stroke signs and symptoms
2. Dispatch through activation of the EMS and prompt response
3. Delivery of the patient to a pre-notified hospital, with appropriate pre-hospital care
4. Door (ED triage)
5. Data compilation including such ED evaluation as head CT scan
6. Decision regarding potential therapies
7. Drug therapy

Data from Refs. [7–9].

of stroke but also as a means to exclude diseases that may mimic the symptoms of stroke [11]. As part of the examination, EMS personnel are trained to identify the most common signs of stroke [12]. The Cincinnati Prehospital Stroke Scale is popular because it is simpler to administer than the LAPSS. There are three components: (1) facial asymmetry; (2) speech disturbance; and (3) upper extremity weakness [13,14]. This scale may be simply taught as the three Ds of "*d*rift (arm), *d*roop (facial weakness), and *d*ysarthria (slurred speech)" under the acronym "FAST" for *f*acial droop, *a*rm drift, and *s*peech (dysarthria and aphasia) with *T* for onset time [15].

Expediting stroke transport and care

Other systems that may be useful to bridge gaps in acute stroke care access in remote areas (eg, rural critical access hospitals) where stroke expertise is not available include air (eg, helicopter) transport systems [16] and telestroke [17]. These systems may serve as a remote arm or extension of an expert stroke treatment center. EMS participation in clinical trials of neuroprotective agents administered in the field has also been shown to be feasible [18].

Emergency department triage of the acute stroke patient and treatment goals

Advanced notification of an incoming acute stroke patient including onset time by EMS and rapid transport to the closest appropriate facility is essential to expeditious stroke care. An acute stroke victim should be transferred to the nearest center with access to stroke expertise, capable of performing a rapid brain imaging study, and able to render IV rt-PA if indicated. Published recommendations for primary stroke centers are listed in Box 2 [19]. Primary stroke center certification may be available through several hospital accrediting agencies and some state health departments.

The National Institute of Neurological Disorders and Stroke (NINDS) consensus conference issued the following recommendations for hospitals receiving acute stroke patients: (1) ED physician evaluation within 10 minutes of arrival; (2) stroke team notification within 15 minutes of arrival; (3) brain computed tomography (CT) within 25 minutes and interpretation within 45 minutes of arrival; and (4) if indicated, door-to-drug treatment time of less than 60 minutes from arrival in at least 80% of patients [20].

Emergency department management of the acute stroke patient

Once a patient arrives at the ED, expeditious triage, nursing, and physician assessments are paramount. This process may be facilitated by an ED stroke care map or plan. Prompt evaluation for reperfusion therapy in the case of ischemic stroke patients is vital as brain tissue becomes increasingly less salvageable as time progresses [21]. Additionally, identifying hemorrhagic stroke patients for whom early neurosurgical intervention may be beneficial is important. Ideally, every hospital should have an acute stroke care plan that uses all of the essential resources including EMS, EM physicians and consulting physicians nursing, radiology, and pharmacy to expedite the evaluation and initiate treatment of acute stroke patients.

Evaluation of the acute stroke patient

As with any critical ill patient, assessing the ABCs (airway, breathing, and circulation) and providing unstable patients with life support when

Box 2. Primary stroke center: essential components and stroke team members

1. Written stroke care protocols
2. Laboratory services
3. Stroke unit for centers that provide ongoing in-hospital care for stroke patients
4. Emergency medical services
5. ED physician and staff
6. Acute stroke team
7. Neurosurgical availability
8. 24-hour CT availability and interpretation by a neuroradiologist and staff

From Alberts MA, Hademenos G, Latchaw RL, et al. Recommendations for the establishment of primary stroke centers. JAMA 2000;283:3103; with permission.

indicated is essential. Concurrently, a "code stroke" should be activated to alert those involved with the acute stroke plan and to prepare for rapid brain imaging and subsequent treatment if indicated. In a busy ED, many of these steps occur in parallel.

Stroke history and determination of stroke subtype

First, a focused history of symptoms with emphasis on time of onset is established. Since onset time is critical to determining eligibility for acute reperfusion therapy, it is necessary to determine when the patient was last known to be asymptomatic [12]. For example, in a patient who awakens from sleep with stroke symptoms, the time window to thrombolytic treatment begins when they were last noted to be normal neurologically, not simply the time of awakening. Next, medical history is obtained to elucidate any contraindications for rt-PA use. One focuses on previous cerebrovascular events, stroke risk factors, recent invasive procedures, bleeding risks and medication use. The history may yield important factors that can influence etiologic diagnosis (eg, history of atrial fibrillation, coronary artery disease, carotid occlusive disease, intracranial aneurysm), acute reperfusion therapy eligibility (eg, warfarin use, history of intracranial hemorrhage, recent surgery or active bleeding) and recurrent stroke prevention strategy (eg, hypertension, dyslipidemia, cigarette smoking) [22].

Physical examination

Because the time to thrombolytic treatment is critical, the initial physical examination may be "strategic, rather than exhaustive" [12]. A focused neurologic examination to assess level of consciousness, mental status, localizing focal signs, and evaluation of stroke severity may be performed. The National Institute of Neurological Disorders and Stroke's "NIHSS" (ie, National Institute of Health stroke scale) is a preferred neurologic examination instrument to capture the neurologic function, which is discussed below. Before a NIHSS assessment, the ED physician should quickly assess the patient's mental status and ability to protect the airway.

Additionally, clues to stroke etiology may be found by auscultating the heart for murmurs and arrhythmias and the carotid arteries for bruits. Peripheral pulses should be palpated for strength and regularity. Fundoscopic examination should be performed to assess for retinal hemorrhage, papilledema, retinal infarction, or embolism (eg, Hollenhorst plaques or cholesterol emboli). Unexplained fever may suggest endocarditis and nuchal rigidity should raise suspicion for meningitis or subarachnoid hemorrhage.

National Institutes of Health stroke scale

The generally accepted neurologic examination for stroke patients is the NIHSS, which assesses neurologic domains such as level of consciousness, motor, sensory, speech, and language. This standardized tool aids in localizing the stroke lesion, quantifying the deficit, and it may guide thrombolytic therapy decision-making (Box 3) [12]. This tool is important for ED physicians because it allows them to accurately communicate with neurologic consultants who may not be present in real time during the examination as well as to make optimal decisions regarding treatment.

General diagnostic testing

Laboratory tests including complete blood count, electrolytes, renal function, glucose, cardiac enzymes, prothrombin, and partial thromboplastin times, should be drawn immediately to ensure rapid turnaround [12]. Disturbances in electrolytes, renal function, and serum glucose may worsen symptoms from previous stroke, mimic stroke symptoms, result from new stroke, or affect diagnostic and treatment decisions (eg, iodinated contrast administration with renal insufficiency) [12]. Elevation of cardiac enzymes may suggest concurrent myocardial infarction or be due to neurogenic cardiac dysfunction as may occur after hemorrhagic stroke, particularly subarachnoid hemorrhage. Abnormalities in the complete blood count or coagulation studies cannot only give clues as to the etiology of the stroke, but they also may influence treatment decisions.

General diagnostic testing should include a chest radiograph because aspiration is a concern in stroke patients with dysphagia and a 12-lead ECG to evaluate for pre-existing cardiac disease and concurrent myocardial injury. Patients should be placed on a continuous cardiac monitor for at least the first 24 hours and have frequent pulse oximetry [12]. In selected cases, pregnancy testing, blood alcohol level, urine or blood toxicology screen, liver function, and lumbar puncture may be considered [22].

Neuroimaging

CT

After a history and the initial physical examination have been completed and appropriate laboratory tests drawn, stroke patients should be sent immediately for a neuroimaging study. The most practical and widely available study to diagnosis acute stroke is noncontrast brain CT. CT can be obtained within minutes making it feasible for even critically ill patients [12]. When obtained within 3 hours of stroke symptom onset, CT can detect subtle parenchymal changes of early ischemic brain injury or disorders that may mimic stroke such as tumor or infection. Importantly, CT identifies parenchymal brain hemorrhage and subdural hematoma about 100% of the time as well as subarachnoid hemorrhage (85%–97% accuracy) [23,24].

Subtle signs of acute brain ischemia on noncontrast brain CT include: loss of gray-white matter differentiation (insular ribbon sign), blurring of the internal capsule, mild sulcal effacement and decreased clarity of the

Box 3. National Institutes of Health stroke scale

1a. Level of consciousness

0 = Alert; keenly responsive
1 = Not alert, but arousable by minor stimulation to obey, answer, or respond
2 = Not alert, requires repeated stimulation to attend, or is obtunded and requires strong or painful stimulation to make movements (not stereotyped)
3 = Responds only with reflex motor or autonomic effects or totally unresponsive, flaccid, areflexic

1b. Level of consciousness

Patient is asked the month and age

0 = Answers both questions correctly
1 = Answers one question correctly
2 = Answers neither question correctly

1c. Level of consciousness

Patient is asked to open and close eyes and to grip and release nonparetic hand

0 = Performs both tasks correctly
1 = Performs one task correctly
2 = Performs neither task correctly

2. Best gaze

0 = Normal
1 = Partial gaze palsy, when gaze is abnormal in one or both eyes, but where forced deviation or total gaze paresis is not present
2 = Forced deviation, or total gaze paresis not overcome by oculocephalic maneuver

3. Visual

0 = No visual loss
1 = Partial hemianopia
2 = Complete hemianopia
3 = Bilateral hemianopia

4. Facial palsy

0 = Normal symmetric movement
1 = Minor paralysis
2 = Partial paralysis
3 = Complete paralysis of one or both sides

5. Motor arm

Scored for right and left arm

0 = No drift, arm holds 90 degrees if sitting (or 45 degrees if supine) for full 10 s

1 = Drift, arm holds 90 degrees if sitting, (or 45 degrees if supine) but drifts down before full 10 s; does not hit bed or other support

2 = Some effort against gravity, arm cannot get to or maintain 90 degrees if sitting (or 45 degrees if supine), drifts down to bed, but has some effort against gravity

3 = No effort against gravity, arm falls

4 = No movement

X = Amputation, joint fusion

6. Motor leg

Scored for right and left leg

0 = No drift; leg holds 30 degrees position for full 5 s

1 = Drift; leg falls by the end of the 5-s period but does not hit bed

2 = Some effort against gravity; leg falls to bed by 5 s but has some effort against gravity

3 = No effort against gravity; leg falls to bed immediately

4 = No movement

X = Amputation, joint fusion

7. Limb Ataxia

0 = Absent

1 = Present in one limb

2 = Present in two limbs

8. Sensory

0 = Normal; no sensory loss

1 = Mild to moderate sensory loss; patient feels pinprick is less sharp or is dull on the affected side, or there is loss of superficial pain with pinprick but patient is aware of being touched

2 = Severe to total sensory loss; patient is not aware of being touched in the face, arm, and leg

9. Best language

0 = No aphasia; normal

1 = Mild to moderate aphasia; some obvious loss of fluency or facility of comprehension, without significant limitation of ideas expressed or form of expression; reduction of speech and/or comprehension makes conservation about provided material difficult or impossible

2 = Severe aphasia; all communication is through fragmentary expression; great need for inference, questioning and guessing by the listener; range of information that can be exchanged is limited; listener carries burden of communication

3 = Mute, global aphasia; no usable speech or auditory comprehension

10. Dysarthria

0 = Normal

1 = Mild to moderate; patient slurs at least some words and at worst can be understood with some difficulty

2 = Severe; patient's speech is so slurred as to be unintelligible in the absence of or out of proportion to any dysphasia, or is mute/anarthric

X = Intubation or other physical barrier

11. Extinction and inattention

0 = No abnormality

1 = Visual, tactile, auditory, spatial, or personal inattention or extinction to bilateral simultaneous stimulation in one of the sensory modalities

2 = Profound hemi-inattention or hemi-inattention to more than one modality. Does not recognize own hand or orients to only one side of space

Courtesy of NIH Neurological Institute, Bethesda, MD.

lentiform nucleus [21]. Although there may subtle signs of ischemia on brain CT, CT findings that contraindicate the use of rt-PA are equally as important. CT contraindications to IV rt-PA include: (1) presence of hemorrhage; (2) another lesion that might preclude rt-PA use; and (3) the presence of a large hypodense lesion in a distribution consistent with the neurologic examination (ie, middle cerebral artery infarct) and one that suggests that the acute stroke is more than 3 hours old [25].

As cerebral infarction matures, the area becomes increasingly hypodense on CT. Although the above early CT signs of cerebral ischemia may be subtle, non-neuroradiologists have been shown to have comparable success to neuroradiologists in detecting these changes [26]. Rapid time to and prompt, accurate evaluation of brain CT scan is an essential element of acute stroke care.

More recently, CT angiography and perfusion studies have been used [27]. The technology for such studies may be adapted to more standard CT techniques. It provides information about occlusive brain artery site and etiology, as well as brain perfusion, which may prove to identify the extent of salvageable ischemic brain tissue. Further studies are needed to validate its usefulness in practice. Noncontrast CT however remains the most efficacious and widely used imaging modality because it can rapidly assess and determine the presence of hemorrhage or nonvascular lesion that might explain the cause of the neurologic deficit or preclude the use of rt-PA.

MRI

Brain MRI has been used increasingly for acute stroke diagnosis. Prior brain MRI studies using T2-weighted images did not show significant advantages of MRI over CT for stroke detection [28]. Furthermore, older MRI sequences could not readily detect acute hemorrhage. However, as brain MRI has evolved, it has been shown to be better than CT for detection of acute ischemia; it can now easily detect acute and chronic hemorrhage [29]. The advent of diffusion-weighted imaging (DWI) has provided a sensitive MRI technology for detection of acute ischemic stroke. Furthermore, gradient echo (GRE) or susceptibility-weighted imaging (SWI) provides a means for the detection of recent hemorrhage. Although debate continues about the brain imaging modality of choice in acute stroke, CT offers certain advantages in terms of availability and ease of use, but MRI is likely the preferred test for accurate diagnosis in acute suspected stroke. Patients with pacemakers, metal implants or claustrophobia, however, cannot undergo MRI. Furthermore, MRI may not be readily available at all centers and its use may take longer to complete. Therefore, CT is an accepted initial imaging modality in acute stroke.

Magnetic resonance angiography (MRA) may be coupled with brain MRI to determine site and type of occlusive cerebrovascular disease. Furthermore, MR technology may be adapted to provide information about brain perfusion and possibly to determine the extent of salvageable brain tissue after acute ischemic infarction.

Therapy

Stabilization

Supplemental oxygen should be administered to those who have hypoxia [30]. Patients at risk for ventilatory compromise secondary to hypoventilation, aspiration, or inability to protect their airway should be immediately considered for endotracheal (ET) intubation with rapid sequence intubation. In the case that ET intubation becomes necessary, sedatives that do not elevate intracranial pressure such as propofol, thiopental, midazolam, or etomidate should be used [12]. Stroke patients who require intubation generally have poor outcomes [30]. As of yet, data do not support the use of hyperbaric oxygen.

Blood pressure management

After a secure airway has been established, blood pressure management should be undertaken. After a stroke, the regional autoregulatory mechanism that ensures consistent cerebral blood flow becomes impaired [12]. Consequently, systemic blood pressure largely dictates cerebral blood flow in and around the infarct. Thus, lowering systemic blood pressure too quickly or too soon in the stroke patient may intensify ischemia. For this reason, it is generally recommended that antihypertensive therapy should not be given unless two consecutive blood pressure measurements taken 5 min apart yield SBP > 220 or MAP > 130 (National Stroke Assoc Consensus Panel) unless there is a compelling indication for treatment (eg, acute myocardial infarction, aortic dissection, hypertensive encephalopathy) [30]. However, for a patient to be considered for treatment with rt-PA, they must have a blood pressure of ≤ 185/110 mm Hg [25]. Also, chronic hypertension is a known risk factor for ischemic stroke and patients with a past medical history of hypertension have baseline cerebral autoregulation set at a higher level than normotensive individuals [31]. Hypertensive patients may experience a drop in cerebral blood flow at a relatively higher MAP [12].

For acute ischemic stroke patients who have received rt-PA, blood pressure should be kept at less than 180/105 mm Hg to decrease the risk of brain hemorrhage. The NINDS rt-PA trialists recommended use of parenteral labetolol as a first-line antihypertensive and a nitroprusside infusion as second-line therapy [25]. The American Stroke Association recommends labetolol or a nicardipine infusion for blood pressure management after rt-PA has been given [30]. Nitroglycerin paste can be used to lower blood pressure before a patient has received rt-PA, however, it is not recommended for blood pressure management after rt-PA has been initiated. The benefit of a beta blocker such as labetolol is that it does not cause venodilation, which can increase cerebral blood volume [12]. Nitroprusside is a cerebral venodilator, however its effects are rapid and can be closely monitored.

The reader is referred to the recent American Heart Association/American Stroke Association guidelines for all aspects of early management of ischemic stroke [30]. Specifics regarding blood pressure management are reviewed in Box 4. A similar statement from the American Heart Association/American Stroke Association may be useful for the reader to review in relation to guidelines for the management of blood pressure in intracerebral hemorrhage (Box 5) [32].

Hypotension, hyperglycemia, and hyperthermia

Although uncommon in ischemic stroke, hypotension is possible when stroke is accompanied by heart failure, hypovolemia, MI, or arrhythmia [12]. The etiology of the hypotension must be identified for appropriate treatment [30]. Volume status should be assessed and dehydration corrected. To support cerebral perfusion while preventing cerebral edema, hypotonic IV fluid should be avoided and normal saline should be given as long as the patient can tolerate such fluids.

Other concerns include hyperglycemia, which is a common metabolic disturbance in acute ischemic stroke [30]. Acute hyperglycemia has been associated with poor stroke outcome [30]. Hence, insulin is recommended for glucose control when the glucose concentration is >140 to 185 mg/dL [30]. Clinical trial data has been mixed in relation to the risks and benefits

Box 4. Guidelines for blood pressure management in acute ischemic stroke

1. The management of arterial hypertension remains controversial and a cautious approach is recommended.
2. For recombinant tissue plasminogen activator (rt-PA) use, systolic blood pressure should be ≤185 mm Hg and diastolic blood pressure should be ≤110 mm Hg and maintained below 180/105 mm Hg for at least 24 hours after intravenous rt-PA treatment
3. For patients eligible for rt-PA with initial BP >185/110, the following therapeutic recommendations exist:
   a. Labetolol 10–20 mg IV over 1 minute which may be repeated once, or
   b. Nitropaste 1-2 in, or
   c. Nicardipine 5 mg/h, titrate up by 2.5 mg/h at 5- to 15-minute intervals with a maximum dose of 15 mg/h. After the desired BP is reached, decrease by 3 mg/h.
4. For those with markedly elevated blood pressures, a reasonable goal is to lower blood pressure by about 15% during the first 24 hours. Unless there is a compelling reason to lower blood pressure, medications may be withheld unless the systolic blood pressure is >220 mm Hg or the mean blood pressure is >120 mm Hg.

Data from Adams HP, del Zoppo G, Alberts M, et al. Guidelines for the early management of adults with ischemic stroke. Stroke 2007;38:1673–4.

of tighter glucose control in acute ischemic stroke, and more clinical trial data is needed to resolve the controversy [33].

Hyperthermia can be detrimental to acute ischemic stroke patients. Proposed mechanisms for injury include increases in neurotransmitters, damaging ischemic depolarization, and impaired energy metabolism [34]. Patients with fever or hyperthermia should be promptly treated with antipyretics and cooling blankets (if needed) to preserve brain function. Hypothermia may prove to be of therapeutic value in the future because it has been shown to be after cardiac arrest with ischemic hypoxia of the brain [30].

Intravenous thrombolytic therapy

The NINDS rt-PA stroke study milestone report in 1995 led to the FDA approval of rt-PA for treatment of acute ischemic stroke during the first 3 hours after onset [25]. The NINDS trial showed improvement in clinical

Box 5. Guidelines for blood pressure management in ICH

1. Hemorrhagic expansion or neurologic decline is not clearly related to isolated systolic blood pressure (SBP) ≤210 mm Hg
2. Reduction in cerebral flow does not occur with a decrease in mean arterial pressure by 15% or less
3. Patients with elevated SBP experience more hemorrhagic enlargement, however, this may be attributed to the increased growth of ICH with an associated increase in ICP as a contributing factor to the further development of ICH
4. A rapid decline in blood pressure during acute hospitalization may be associated with increased mortality
5. Preservation of cerebral perfusion pressure >60 mm Hg is recommended for patients with spontaneous ICH as well as traumatic brain hemorrhage

Abbreviations: ICH, intracranial hemorrhage; ICP, intracranial pressure.

Data from Broderick J, Connolly S, Feldmann E, et al. Guidelines for the management of spontaneous intracerebral hemorrhage in adults. 2007 update. Stroke 2007;38:2006–7.

outcome at 3 months with IV rt-PA administered within 3 hours of symptom onset when compared with placebo after acute ischemic stroke [25]. For every 18 stroke patients treated with IV rt-PA, two more will achieve as good an outcome as they would have without IV rt-PA and one will have significant intracerebral hemorrhage related to treatment. However, the NINDS trial demonstrated that the overall 90-day mortality was no different whether receiving IV rt-PA or placebo treatment. This underscores the risk of mortality in stroke [3,35].

Although there was a 6.4% risk of detrimental hemorrhagic infarction with about half of these patients dying in the NINDS trial, the absolute benefit of rt-PA (11%–13%) in improving clinical outcomes on the modified Rankin Scale, NIHSS and a global statistic, for example, conferred an overall advantage of administering rt-PA [21,25,36]. At 3 months, 31%–50% of patients in the trial had complete or near-complete recovery of stroke symptoms in contrast to the 20%–38% of patients receiving placebo [37]. Eligibility criteria for rt-PA administration in acute ischemic stroke are listed in Box 6 [27].

Many patients being screened for rt-PA administration, however, do not qualify for thrombolytic therapy based on their presentation time, which is outside the 3-hour treatment window and other exclusion criteria (see Box 6). It is within the skill set of the ED physician to make prompt, informed decisions concerning the use of rt-PA to stay within the critical 3-hour

Box 6. Eligibility criteria for rt-PA administration

Inclusion criteria

- Ischemic stroke with clearly defined onset time (<3 hours for symptom onset to bolus time)
- Measurable neurologic deficit (eg, on the NIHSS)
- No evidence of hemorrhage on brain CT or MRI

Exclusion criteria

- Stroke or serious head injury within 3 months
- Major surgery within 14 days
- History of intracranial hemorrhage
- Systolic blood pressure >185 mm Hg or diastolic blood pressure >110 mm Hg, or aggressive lowering of blood pressure to meet these limits
- Rapidly improving or minor symptoms
- Gastrointestinal or genitourinary hemorrhage within 21 days
- Arterial puncture within 7 days at a noncompressible site
- Seizure at onset of stroke
- Elevated partial thromboplastin time (PTT) for patients on heparin
- Prothrombin time (PT) >15 seconds
- International normalized ratio >1.4[a]
- Platelet count <100,000
- Glucose <50 mg/dL or >400 mg/dL

[a] The INR level recommended for use by the American Heart Association/American Stroke Association is <1.7 [30].

Data from Gorelick PB, Weber MA. Handbook of stroke prevention and treatment. London: Current Medicine Group; 2007.

window. It is therefore important for ED physicians to communicate effectively with consulting neurologists and radiologists to maximize ischemic stroke diagnosis and rt-PA delivery. National guidelines endorse intravenous rt-PA for acute ischemic stroke based on replication of the NINDS rt-PA findings in post-marketing studies when the treatment is administered according to protocol guidelines [36].

Perspectives on rt-PA administration

Delay in seeking treatment is a common reason for ineligibility for rt-PA therapy [38]. In a study from Calgary hospitals over a 3-year period, 73% of patients were ineligible due to presentation time beyond the 3 hours. Reasons for ineligibility included: patients not directly seeking medical attention and waiting to see if symptoms would improve; delays in transfer to a hospital capable of treating the patient; and indeterminate time of onset. Of 23% of patients who were admitted with a diagnosis of ischemic stroke within the allotted time frame, 27% received IV rt-PA. Acute ischemic stroke patients with rapid early improvement or mild symptoms may benefit from rt-PA administration as study has shown that these patients may still be at risk of dependency or death [38–41]. Routine use of rt-PA beyond the 3-hour time window is not recommended. It is, however, being studied to determine means for salvaging brain tissue at risk with advanced neuroimaging techniques and new approaches to administering thrombolytics, as well as using them in conjunction with clot retrieval devices.

Intra-arterial thrombolysis and clot retrieval devices

Intra-arterial thrombolysis (IAT) may as well prove to be an effective tool in acute ischemic stroke treatment. Studies such as Prolyse in Acute Cerebral Thromboembolism (PROACT) have shown the value of drugs such as intra-arterial recombinant prourokinase (r-proUK) for improving clinical outcomes in middle cerebral artery (M1 and M2) ischemic stroke within 6 hours of stroke onset [42]. The PROACT trial did show, however, a 10% risk of intracranial hemorrhage within 24 hours as compared with a 2% risk in the control group although this was not statistically significant [42]. IAT has not been approved in the United States for routine clinical use; it requires specialized catheter labs and skilled clinicians for administration. Combined intravenous and intra-arterial thrombolytic approaches are being studied as are the development of new agents that may be safer and concomitantly used with clot retrieval devices. A systematic review of published IAT series with 3-month follow-up shows considerable variability and lack of evidence for a net improvement in outcome after IAT compared with what might be predicted based on natural history [43]. These findings help to confirm the need for prospective studies comparing IAT with best medical therapy or other reasonable intervention.

Clot retrieval devices such as the MERCI endovascular embolectomy device, which was approved by the FDA in 2005, are an alternative to intravenous thrombolysis [44] or may be used as adjuvant therapy for reperfusion. The MERCI device is approved for clot retrieval within the first 8 hours of acute ischemic stroke, however, debate has ensued over its' efficacy [44]. The Penumbral System, a mechanical device to remove clot in acute ischemic stroke due to large vessel occlusion, was approved by the US FDA in 2007 for use in clinical practice [45].

In light of advancements in the treatment of ischemic stroke, it is important for the ED physician to remain informed about all of the available treatment options. This becomes increasingly important for patients who may not be good candidates for IV rt-PA (eg, who present beyond the 3 hour window) or in patients who receive IV-rt-PA but who do not appear to improve.

Anticoagulation and antiplatelet therapy

Anticoagulation with either unfractionated or low molecular weight heparin is not recommended in acute ischemic stroke unless it is being used for venous thromboembolism prophylaxis or there is a compelling cardiac or other indication [30]. Lack of substantial evidence of efficacy and risk of bleeding complications for the above treatments have led to these recommendations [46]. However, warfarin is indicated for patients who have atrial fibrillation due to high risk for subsequent ischemic infarction, although it is not typically initiated acutely in the ED. The use of IV heparin in acute ischemic stroke is discussed in detail elsewhere [30].

Aspirin 325 mg/d is indicated within 48 hours after acute ischemic stroke onset [30]. For patients who have received acute thrombolytic therapy, aspirin should not be administered until after 24 hours if there are no contraindications. There is no absolute contraindication to administering rt-PA in a patient who is taking daily aspirin. Aspirin administration has been shown to reduce the risk of recurrent stroke.

Management of transient ischemic attack in the emergency department

TIA constitutes about 0.3% of ED visits [47]. Transient neurologic attacks are important to recognize in the ED because they have a high risk of subsequent major vascular events [48]. Furthermore, it is estimated that up to 12.8% of TIA patients may present with stroke within 7 days [49]. The importance of timely diagnosis and treatment of TIA or minor stroke has been emphasized in the United Kingdom where rapid referral to TIA clinics has resulted in a substantial reduction of subsequent stroke [49]. In the United States, some have recommended an accelerated diagnostic protocol for patients who present to the ED with TIA. ED observation units can successfully evaluate TIA patients so as to shorten the length of stay, minimize costs, and also detect those who are at greatest risk of imminent stroke, requiring hospital admission [50]. ED physicians and staff, therefore, must assure that such patients receive rapid diagnosis and treatment. The reader is referred to an overall guide for management of TIA that has been established by the National Stroke Association [51].

Although no formal scale exists for risk stratification of TIA patients who present to the ED, it is the responsibility of the ED physician to consider the patient's overall clinical picture. Decisions to admit to the hospital, ED observation unit if available, or to discharge a patient with close follow-up should be based on past medical history (eg, history of recurrent TIAs or atrial fibrillation), physical examination findings (eg, carotid bruits), and diagnostic tests such as ECG and brain CT. In the case that a patient with TIA is discharged from the ED, it is critical to ensure that rapid follow-up for further diagnostics such as carotid ultrasound is available for the patient in a timely manner.

Prevention of recurrent cerebral ischemia in the emergency department

History of a first stroke or TIA is a major predictor of future stroke risk and must be managed appropriately [52]. Review of indications for antithrombotics, cardiovascular risk factor control, and other interventions that will be performed in the ambulatory care area is beyond the scope of this article and is described elsewhere in this text [53]. The reader is referred to a comprehensive guideline statement from the American Heart Association/American Stroke Association on the prevention of stroke in persons with stroke or TIA [54,55] or another published handbook for more information [22].

Summary

The ED and EMS serve as a front line for care of acute stroke patients. The ED physician plays an important role in evaluating stroke patients, communicating with neurology and radiology consultants, as well as mobilizing resources. Organized and comprehensive approaches to acute stroke care including standardized protocols to effectively transport, diagnose, and treat such patients need to be in place to assure successful treatment and prevention of stroke. The 3-hour window for administration of rt-PA is narrow and does not allow for system delays or patients may be excluded from treatment opportunities. The establishment of joint commission or state-certified primary stroke centers and the possible future development of comprehensive stroke centers have the potential to positively impact stroke outcomes on a large-scale level.

References

[1] American Heart Association. Heart Disease and Stroke Statistics: 2008 update. Available at: www.americanheart.org/statistics. Accessed July 7, 2008.

[2] Kleindorfer D, Lindsell CJ, Brass L, et al. National US estimates of recombinant tissue plasminogen activator use. ICD-9 codes substantially underestimate. Stroke 2008;39: 924–8.

[3] Marler JR, Goldstein LB. Stroke—tPA and the clinic. Science 2003;301:1677–9.

[4] Morris DL, Rosamond W, Madden K, et al. Prehospital and emergency department delays after acute stroke. The Genentech stroke prevention survey. Stroke 2000;31:2528–90.

[5] Schroeder EB, Rosamond WD, Morris DL, et al. Determinants of use of emergency medical services in a population with stroke symptoms. The second delay in accessing stroke healthcare [DASH II study]. Stroke 2000;31:2591–6.

[6] Gordon DL. The Mississippi Stroke Education Consortium: a state-based template to promote stroke awareness, prevention, and emergency treatment. Neuroepidemiology 2000;19: 1–12.

[7] Hazinski MF. Demystifying recognition and management of stroke. Current Emergency Cardiac Care 1996;7:8–9.

[8] Pepe PE, Zachariah BS, Sayre MR, et al. Ensuring the chain of recovery for stroke in your community. Acad Emerg Med 1998;5:89–95.

[9] Kidwell CS, Saver JL. Rapid clinical evaluation. In: Kasner SE, Gorelick PB, editors. Prevention and treatment of ischemic stroke. Philadelphia: Butterworth/Heinemann; 2004. p. 211–35.
[10] Acker JE, Pancioli AM, Crocco TJ, et al. Implementation strategies for emergency medical services within stroke systems of care. A policy statement from the American Heart Association/American Stroke Association expert panel on emergency medical services systems and the Stroke Council. Stroke 2007;116:3097–115.
[11] Kidwell CS, Saver JL, Eckstein M, et al. Improving paramedic recognition of stroke in the field: a Los Angeles prehospital stroke screen (LAPSS). Stroke 1998;29:313 [abstract].
[12] Cohen SN. Management of ischemic stroke. New York: McGraw-Hill; 2000.
[13] Kothari R, Hall K, Brott T, et al. Early stroke recognition: developing an out-of-hospital NIH stroke scale. Acad Emerg Med 1997;4:986–90.
[14] Kothari RU, Pancioli A, Liu T, et al. Cincinnati prehospital stroke scale: validity and reproducibility. Ann Emerg Med 1999 Apr;33(4):373–8.
[15] Harbison J, Houssain O, Jenkinson D, et al. Diagnostic accuracy of stroke referrals from primary care, emergency room physicians, and ambulance staff using the face, arm, speech test. Stroke 2003;34:71–6.
[16] Chalela JA, Kasner SE, Jauch ED, et al. Safety of air medical transportation after tissue plasminogen activator administration in acute ischemic stroke. Stroke 1999;30:2366–8.
[17] Hess DC, Wang S, Gross H, et al. Telestroke: extending stroke expertise into underserved areas. Lancet Neurol 2006;5:275–8.
[18] Saver JL, Kidwell CS, Leary MC, et al. Results of the field administration of stroke treatment—magnesium (fast-mag) pilot trial: a study of prehospital neuroprotective therapy. Stroke 2002;33:363–4.
[19] Alberts MA, Hademenos G, Latchaw RL, et al. Recommendations for the establishment of primary stroke centers. JAMA 2000;283:3102–9.
[20] Bock BF. Response system for patients presenting with acute stroke. In: Marler JR, Jones PM, Emr M, editors. Proceeding of a National Symposium on rapid identification and treatment of acute stroke: 1997. Bethesda (MD): National Institute of Neurological Disorders and Stroke, National Institutes of Health; 1997.
[21] Albers GW, Amarenco P, Easton JD, et al. Antothrombotic and thrombolytic therapy for ischemic stroke: the seventh ACCP conference on antithrombotic and thrombolytic therapy. Chest 2004;126:483S–512S.
[22] Gorelick PB, Weber MA. Handbook of stroke prevention and treatment. London: Current Medicine Group; 2007.
[23] Morgenstern L, Luna-Gonzales H, Huber JC, et al. Worst headache and subarachnoid hemorrhage: prospective, modern computed tomography and spinal fluid analysis. Ann Emerg Med 1998;32:297.
[24] Tarr RW, Hecht ST, Horton JA. Nontraumatic intracranial hemorrhage. In: LRE, editor. Magnetic resononance and computerized tomography imaging of the head, neck, and spine. St. Louis (MO): Mosby Year Book; 1991. p. 267–99.
[25] The National Institute of Neurological Disorders and Stroke rt-PA Stroke Study Group: tissue plasminogen activator for acute ischemic stroke. NEJM 1995;333:1581–8.
[26] Wardlaw JM, Farrall AJ, Perry D. Factors influencing the detection of early CT signs of cerebral ischemia. Stroke 2007;38:1250–6.
[27] Khaja AM, Grotta J. Established treatments for acute ischemic stroke. Lancet 2007;369: 319–30.
[28] Johnston K, Haley EC. Emergency imaging of the acute stroke patient. J Neuroimaging 1997;7:111–7.
[29] Chalela JA, Kidwell CS, Nentwich LM, et al. Magnetic resonance imaging and computed tomography in emergency assessment of patients with suspected acute stroke: a prospective comparison. Lancet 2007;369:203–98.

[30] Adams HP, del Zoppo G, Alberts M, et al. Guidelines for the early management of adults with ischemic stroke. Stroke 2007;38:1655–711.
[31] Strandgaard S. Autoregualtion of cerebral blood flow in hypertensive patients: the modifying influence of prolonged antihypertensive treatment on the tolerance to acute, drug-induced hypotension. Circulation 1976;53:720–7.
[32] Broderick J, Connolly S, Feldmann E, et al. Guidelines for the management of spontaneous intracerebral hemorrhage in adults. 2007 update. Stroke 2007;38:2006–7.
[33] Gray CS, Hildreth A, Sandercock PA, et al. Glucose-potassium-insulin infusions in management of post-stroke hyperglycemia: the UK glucose insulin trial (GIST-UK). Lancet Neurol 2007;6:397–406.
[34] Ginsberg M, Busto R. Combating hyperthermia in acute stroke: a significant clinical concern. Stroke 1998;29:529–34.
[35] Demaerschalk BM. Thrombolytic therapy for acute ischemic stroke. The likelihood of being helped versus harmed. Stroke 2007;38:2215–6.
[36] Wahlgren N, Ahmed N, Davalos A, et al. Thrombolysis with alteplase for acute ischemic stroke in the safe implementation of thrombolysis in stroke-monitoring study (SITS-MOST): an observational study. Lancet 2007;369:275–82.
[37] Al-Senani FM, Grotta JC. Thrombolytic therapies. In: Kasner SE, Gorelick PB, editors. Prevention and treatment of ischemic stroke. Philadelphia: Butterworth Heinemann; 2004. p. 267–81.
[38] Barber PA, Zhang J, Demchuk AM, et al. Why are stroke patients excluded from TPA therapy?: an analysis of patient eligibility. Neurology 2001;56:1015–20.
[39] Baumann CR, Baumgartner RW, Gandjour J, et al. Good outcomes in ischemic stroke patients treated with intravenous thrombolysis despite regressing neurological symptoms. Stroke 2006;37:1332–3.
[40] O'Connor RE, McGraw P, Edelsohn L. Thrombolytic therapy for acute ischemic stroke: why the majority of patients remain ineligible for treatment. Ann Emerg Med 1999;33: 9–14.
[41] Cocho D, Belvis R, Marti-Fabregas J, et al. Reasons for exclusion from thrombolytic therapy following acute ischemic stroke. Neurology 2005;64:719–20.
[42] Furlan A, Higashita RT, Wechsler L, et al. Intra-arterial pro-urokinase for acute ischemic stroke. The PROACT II study: a randomized controlled trial. Prolyse in acute cerebral thromboembolism. JAMA 1999;282:2003–11.
[43] Mandava P, Kent TA. Intra-arterial therapies for acute ischemic stroke. Neurology 2007;68: 2132–9.
[44] Smith WS, Sung G, Starkman S, et al. Safety and efficacy of mechanical embolectomy in acute ischemic stroke: results of the MERCI trial. Stroke 2005;36:1432–40.
[45] McDougall C, Clark W, Mayer T, et al. The Penumbra Stroke Trial: safety and effectiveness of a new generation of mechanical devices for clot removal in acute ischemic stroke. Presented at the International Stroke Conference 2008, Late Breakers Session. New Orleans, LA, February 22, 2008.
[46] Coull BM, Williams LS, Goldstein LB, et al. Anticoagulants and antiplatelet agents in acute ischemic stroke: report of the Joint Stroke Guideline Development Committee of the American Academy of Neurology and the American Stroke Association (a division of the American Heart Association). Stroke 2002;33:1934–42.
[47] Edlow JA, Kim S, Pelletier AJ. National study on emergency department visits for transient ischemic attack, 1992–2001. Acad Emerg Med 2006;13:666–72.
[48] Bos MJ, van Rijn MJ, Witteman JC, et al. Incidence and prognosis of transient neurological attacks. JAMA 2007;298(24):2877–85.
[49] Rothwell PM, Giles MF, Chandratheva A, et al. Effect of urgent treatment of transient ischemic attack and minor stroke on early recurrent stroke (EXPRESS study): a prospective population-based sequential comparison. Lancet 2007;370:1432–42.

[50] Ross MA, Compton S, Medado P, et al. An emergency department diagnostic protocol for patients with transient ischemic attack: a randomized controlled trial. Ann Emerg Med 2007; 50:109–19.

[51] Johnston SC, Nguyen-Huynh MN, Schwarz ME, et al. National Stroke Association guidelines for the management of transient ischemic attacks. Ann Neurol 2006;60(3):301–13.

[52] Ovbiagele B. The emergency department: first line of defense in preventing secondary stroke. Acad Emerg Med 2006;13:215–22.

[53] Collins R, Armitage J, Parish S, et al, Heart Protection Study Collaborative Group. Effects of cholesterol-lowering with simvastatin on stroke and other major vascular events in 20536 people with cerebrovascular disease or other high-risk conditions. Lancet 2004;363:757–67.

[54] Sacco RL, Adams R, Albers G, et al. Guidelines for prevention of stroke in patients with ischemic stroke of transient ischemic attack. Stroke 2006;37:577–617.

[55] Adams RJ, Albers G, Alberts MJ, et al. Update to the AHA/ASA recommendations for the prevention of stroke in patients with stroke and transient ischemic attack. Stroke; 39, in press.

ELSEVIER
SAUNDERS

NEUROLOGIC
CLINICS

Neurol Clin 26 (2008) 943–961

Acute Ischemic Stroke Management: Administration of Thrombolytics, Neuroprotectants, and General Principles of Medical Management

Aslam M. Khaja, MD

Department of Neurology and Rehabilitation, University of Illinois at Chicago, 912 South Wood Street, MC 796, Chicago, IL 60612, USA

Acute ischemic stroke (AIS) care has undergone a revolution since the approval of intravenous (IV) recombinant tissue plasminogen activator (rt-PA) for acute ischemic stroke by the US Food and Drug Administration (FDA) in 1995. Previously, ischemic stroke was a devastating disease with limited effective therapies. Although IV rt-PA remains the only approved therapy, numerous clinical trials are ongoing to expand treatment windows, increase the number of patients eligible for therapy, and evaluate new and innovative therapies, particularly for neuroprotection and intra-arterial (IA) reperfusion therapy.

Pathophysiology

In ischemic stroke, decreased or absent circulating blood flow deprives neurons of necessary metabolic substrates. Because the brain does not store glucose, ischemia is tolerated poorly [1]. Cerebral blood flow usually is compromised because of occlusion of a cerebral artery by a clot. The ischemic cascade begins with ATP depletion, which results in failure of the Na^+/K^+ pump. Subsequently, the activation of voltage-sensitive calcium channels results in calcium influx. The calcium influx results in glutamate release. Glutamate release leads to neuronal activation and further calcium influx, which perpetuates the ischemic cascade [2]. Calcium influx also activates intracellular enzymes, leading to further destruction of cell membranes.

E-mail address: aslam.m.khaja@uic.edu

doi:10.1016/j.ncl.2008.07.002 **_neurologic.theclinics.com_**

This process results in free radicals and nitrous oxide. All of these processes result in continued neuronal damage and cell death. The extent of damage depends upon various factors. Acute ischemia is not tolerated as well as progressive ischemia over time. The amount of collateral flow can influence the size of the infarct and ischemic penumbra. Temperature and glucose metabolism also have effects on cell death and tissue injury [3,4].

An important concept in AIS is the penumbra. When an artery occludes, neurons are affected differently, depending upon the amount of residual blood flow. Normal cerebral blood flow is greater than 50 mL/100 mg/min [1]. Once blood flow decreases to less than 20 mL/100 mg/min, infarction occurs. If blood flow decreases to less than 10 mL/100 mg/min, irreversible neuronal death occurs rapidly. Blood flow between 11 and 20 mL/100 mg/min is thought to represent the ischemic penumbra [5], an area where the cells are functionally silent because of ischemia, but are still able to recover if blood flow is restored. Many acute stroke therapies are targeted toward restoring flow or function to the ischemic penumbra.

Thrombolysis

The first method to restore cerebral perfusion is clot lysis, with the goal of re-establishing blood flow to the affected tissue. IV thrombolysis rt-PA is the only FDA- approved treatment for AIS. Endogenous tissue-plasminogen activator converts circulation plasminogen to plasmin, an enzyme responsible for fibrin dissolution and maintaining coagulation homeostasis. Fibrinolysis is enhanced powerfully by rt-PA. The pivotal United States trial was the National Institute for Neurologic Disorders and Stroke (NINDS) rt-PA Stroke Study. In this randomized, double-blind placebo-controlled trial, 624 patients received either rt-PA (0.9 mg/kg IV) or placebo. Favorable outcomes were reported in 31% to 50% of rt-PA-treated subjects, compared with 20% to 38% in the placebo group. Patient who received rt-PA were 30% more likely to have minimal or no disability at 3 months (odds ratio [OR] 1.7, 95% CI 1.2 to 2.6) [6]. As the major adverse affect is bleeding, only selected patients are eligible for thrombolysis; inclusion and exclusion criteria are listed in Box 1.

The treatment protocol for IV rt-PA administration is outlined in Box 2. The most serious complication of IV rt-PA treatment is symptomatic intracranial hemorrhage primarily from hemorrhagic transformation (HT) of the infarct. Factors associated with HT are increased blood pressure (BP), early ischemic changes on CT, and high National Institute of Health Stroke Scale (NIHSS) score [7]. In addition, increasing age and hyperglycemia may play a role [8]. The symptomatic intracranial hemorrhage rate in the NINDS trial was 6.4% [6]. The optimal methods to limit complications from HT are careful patient selection, scrupulous ancillary care, close monitoring, and strict adherence to BP limits [2]. There are no approved measures to control

Box 1. Criteria for thrombolysis with recombinant tissue plasminogen activator in acute ischemic stroke

Inclusion criteria

Clinical signs and symptoms consistent with ischemic stroke
Patient last seen normal within 3 hours
Measurable neurologic deficit

Exclusion criteria

Any hemorrhage on neuroimaging (CT or MRI)
Symptoms suggestive of subarachnoid hemorrhage
Seizure at stroke onset that is thought to contribute to neurologic deficit
Hypodensity greater than one third cerebral hemisphere on CT
Systolic blood pressure (SBP) greater than 185 mm Hg or diastolic blood pressure (DBP) greater than 110 mm Hg
Serum glucose less than 50 mg/dL
Platelet count less than 100 K/mm^3
International normalized ratio (INR) greater than 1.7
Elevated partial thromboplastin time (PTT)
Any history of intracranial hemorrhage
Arterial puncture at a noncompressible site in past 7 days
Major surgery in past 14 days
Gastrointestinal (GI) bleed or hematuria in past 21 days
Ischemic stroke, myocardial infarction, or serious head trauma in past 3 months

Adapted from Khaja AM, Grotta JC. Established treatments for acute ischaemic stroke. Lancet 2007;369(9558):323; with permission.

HT after IV rt-PA; published recommendations are 6 to 8 U of platelets and cryoprecipitate-containing factor 8 [9]. Carefully selecting patients for thrombolysis is critical, because deviations from criteria have been shown to increase the risk of adverse events [10–12]. These criteria only are intended to serve as a guide for selecting patients. Patients younger than 75 years of age and with mild-to-moderate strokes respond best to IV rt-PA [6].

Some controversy exists regarding the appropriate selection of patients. Most thrombolysis trials excluded patients over the age of 80, with the exception of the NINDS trial [13]. Although never fully studied in clinical trials, in clinical practice, IV rt-PA in the elderly has been reported safe without an increased risk of HT [14,15]. The outcome of elderly patients is generally worse than those younger, but this may be because of other comorbid conditions rather than age alone [16,17]. The effectiveness of thrombolysis in the elderly requires further examination, but the evidence does not support excluding patients based on age alone.

Box 2. Intravenous recombinant tissue plasminogen activator administration protocol.

Total dose of rt-PA: 0.9 mg/kg (maximum dose 90 mg)
Give 10% as initial IV bolus
Infuse remainder over 1 hour
Admit patient to an ICU or stroke unit for monitoring
Neurologic assessments: every 15 minutes during infusion, then every 30 minutes for next 6 hours, then every hour until 24 hours after treatment
BP monitoring: every 15 minutes for 2 hours, then every 30 minutes for next 6 hours, then every hour until 24 hours after treatment
Administer antihypertensive medication to maintain systolic BP less than or equal to180 mm Hg and diastolic BP less than or equal to 105 mm Hg
Delay placement of nasogastric tubes, indwelling bladder catheters, or IA pressure catheters
Follow-up CT or MRI scan at approximately 24 hours after rt-PA, before starting anticoagulation or antiplatelet agents
Delay antithrombotic agents for 24 hours after rt-PA

Data from Adams HP Jr, del Zoppo G, Alberts MJ, et al. Guidelines for the early management of adults with ischemic stroke: a guideline from the American Heart Association/American Stroke Association Stroke Council, and the Atherosclerotic Peripheral Vascular Disease and Quality of Care Outcomes in Research Interdisciplinary Groups. Stroke 2007;38(5):1676; with permission.)

Another controversy concerns patients who have minor neurologic deficits or spontaneously improving symptoms. Minor deficits have been documented as justification to exclude up to 30% of otherwise rt-PA-eligible patients from receiving thrombolytic therapy [18]. Patients who have minor neurologic deficits, however, may not have favorable outcomes at discharge [19]. Treating patients who have mild neurologic deficits may improve their outcomes at discharge [20]. A similar controversy exists regarding patients with major neurologic deficits, who have a poor prognosis in general. Such patients have an increased chance of complete recovery after thrombolysis, but overall success remains low [6]. As mentioned previously, patients who have high NIHSS scores have an increased risk of HT [7]. The decision to treat or not treat in these patients is a carefully weighed clinical decision.

CT changes on initial neuroimaging are another controversy (Fig. 1). Early ischemic changes on initial CT are associated with more severe symptoms and a longer time from symptom onset [21]. Patients who have early

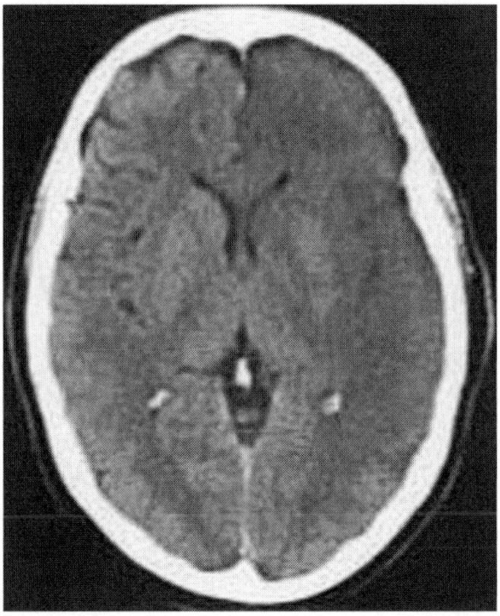

Fig. 1. Early ischemic changes on CT scan. Note the subtle loss of gray–white differentiation and sulcal effacement in the middle and anterior cerebral artery distributions on the left hemisphere.

signs of ischemia on head CT may be at increased risk of HT after IV rt-PA therapy [22,23]. Published studies, however, also report that patients who have early ischemic changes on CT should not be excluded from thrombolysis, and may have greater benefit from rt-PA [24]. Many risk factors for early ischemic CT changes, such as severe symptoms and longer duration of symptoms, also are associated with poorer outcomes [21]. The impact of early ischemic changes on CT scan on outcomes after thrombolysis remains unclear.

Another area of concern regarding thrombolytic therapy for AIS is consent. IV rt-PA is an FDA-approved therapy for AIS for patients meeting criteria. As with any medical intervention, a full discussion of risks and benefits of IV rt-PA treatment with the patient and/or legally authorized surrogate is recommended, if possible. Treatment should not be withheld, however, if the patient is incapable of decision-making, and the legally authorized surrogate is unavailable. Written consent is not necessary [2].

Emerging and experimental therapies

Numerous strategies are being evaluated for treating AIS. These include IA thrombolysis (IAT), augmentation of rt-PA with other medications, lengthening of the therapeutic window, and neuroprotection.

IAT may be a treatment option for selected patients. Possible selection criteria include presentation between 3 and 6 hours from symptom onset, major cerebral artery occlusion, severe neurologic deficits, and high risk of systemic hemorrhage with IV rt-PA (eg, recent surgery). In most circumstances, the availability of IAT should not preclude the use of IV rt-PA in patients meeting criteria. IAT requires access to emergent cerebral angiography, experienced stroke physicians, and neurointerventionalists; it should be performed only at an experienced center [2].

The MERCI (Mechanical Embolus Removal in Cerebral Ischemia) retrieval system (Concentric Medical, Inc., Mountain View, California) has been FDA-approved for recanalizing acutely occluded cerebral arteries. In the Multi-MERCI study, patients who did not improve immediately after IV rt-PA underwent mechanical embolectomy within 8 hours of symptom onset. Partial or complete recanalization occurred in 74% of patients, with a symptomatic intracerebral hemorrhage (sICH) rate of 6.7% [25]. Mechanical embolectomy with the MERCI retriever may be a feasible and safe option for patients after IV rt-PA. Further research, however, is needed to assess the effect on clinical outcomes.

Another newer FDA approved device for AIS is the Penumbra stroke system (Penumbra, Inc., Alameda, California). This device combines two methods of clot extraction, aspiration and mechanical extraction. First the clot is aspirated; then a thrombus removal ring can be used if necessary to remove remaining clot. In 125 patients who had AIS, the Penumbra system was successful recanalizing 82% [26]. This study was not designed to assess clinical outcomes, and this needs to be addressed in future trials. Other recanalization devices also are being tested for improving cerebral artery recanalization rates (Fig. 2).

IV rt-PA followed by local IAT is known as bridging therapy. The Emergency Management of Stroke Bridging Trial showed that patients randomized to treatment with 0.6 mg/kg IV rt-PA followed by IAT with IA rt-PA (up to 20 mg) achieved a higher recanalization rate (54%) compared with those treated with IA rt-PA alone (10%) ($P = .03$) [27]. Bridging therapy also has been evaluated in the Interventional Management of Stroke (IMS) phase 1 and 2 trials. All patients received 0.6 mg/kg IV rt-PA followed by IA rt-PA. Partial or complete recanalization was achieved in 56% of patients. The risk of sICH (6.3%) was similar to patients treated with IV rt-PA in the NINDS trial. When this group of patients was compared with the placebo arm of the NINDS trial, the odds of a good outcome, defined as a modified Rankin scale of 0 to 2, was higher (OR 2.18, 95% CI 1.20 to 3.99) [28]. The IMS III trial is comparing 0.9 mg/kg IV rt-PA to 0.6 mg/kg IV rt-PA followed by IAT. IAT includes the MERCI retriever, EKOS ultrasound catheter (EKOS Corporation, Bothell, Washington), or local IA rt-PA. In other series, IAT after 0.9 mg/kg IV rt-PA has been reported to be safe and may achieve higher rates of recanalization compared with IV alone [29].

There are limited published data for emergent angioplasty and stenting of intracranial and extracranial vessels after AIS. IAT in conjunction with angioplasty and stenting for acute stroke may increase the chance of sustained

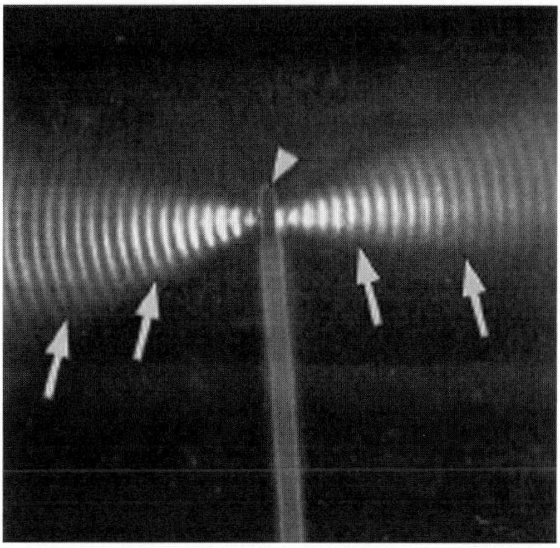

Fig. 2. EkoSonic SV Endovascular Device which uses intravascular ultrasound technology to enhance clot lysis. (*Courtesy of* EKOS Corporation, Bothell, Washington; with permission.)

recanalization and favorable outcome [30]. Endovascular interventions for AIS are a popular area of development, and hopefully will provide additional tools to aid patients in the future.

Adjunctive medications to complement the fibrinolytic action of rt-PA are being studied. Platelet aggregation is critical step for clot formation, and the final common step in platelet aggregation is the binding of fibrinogen between two platelets at the glycoprotein IIb/IIIa receptor. Glycoprotein IIb/IIIa inhibitors such as eptifibatide, abciximab, and tirofiban have garnered interest in AIS. Eptifibatide is being studied in conjunction with IV rt-PA treatment in the CLEAR trial (Combined approach to Lysis using Eptifibatide AND Rt-PA in acute ischemic stroke). Abciximab showed promise in phase 1 and 2 trials; however, a phase 3 trial was stopped early because of increased hemorrhage rates. Tirofiban is the newest member in this class, and has been studied in one phase 2 trial [31]. Further research is necessary before these agents can be recommended for treating AIS.

Argatroban, a direct thrombin inhibitor, combined with IV rt-PA, may improve clot dissolution and recanalization and decrease reocclusion rates. Early results of this paradigm suggest safety and potential efficacy [32].

Other thrombolytic agents continue to be developed and tested. Streptokinase use for AIS is not recommended because of high rates of intracerebral hemorrhage in previous trials [33]. Tenecteplase, a derivative of rt-PA, has a longer half-life and is more fibrin-specific than rt-PA and has been reported safe in a phase 2 study, with no cases of sICH in 88 treated patients who had AIS [34]. A phase 2b trial is underway to evaluate IV tenecteplase versus IV rt-PA for patients who have AIS within 3 hours from symptom onset [35].

Fibrinogen-depleting agents, such as ancrod and batroxobin, may have a more favorable safety profile than thrombolytic drugs. A meta-analysis revealed a 10% relative risk reduction for death and disability in patients who had AIS treated with fibrinogen-depleting agents compared with thrombolytic treatment [36]. Ancrod, however, derived from pit viper venom, did not show clinical benefit in one trial when used within 6 hours of AIS, and additional studies are ongoing [37].

Despite favorable prepivotal studies, desmoteplase, derived from vampire bat saliva, failed to show efficacy in a large phase 3 study of AIS patients who had MRI diffusion–perfusion mismatch presenting between 3 and 9 hours from symptom onset [38]. The future of desmoteplase is uncertain.

Transcranial Doppler ultrasound (TCD) is a novel technique to enhance rt-PA activity. Possible mechanisms include improved drug transport and enhanced binding between rt-PA and fibrin [39]. In the CLOTBUST study (Combined Lysis of Thrombus in Brain Ischemia Using Transcranial Ultrasound and Systemic t-PA) patients who had AIS received IV rt-PA within 3 hours of symptom onset and were randomized to continuous 2 MHz TCD or sham TCD procedure. TCD significantly increased the chance of complete recanalization or dramatic clinical recovery, 49% compared with 30%, ($p = .03$). The study was not powered to show efficacy [40]. TCD may have adverse effects. Midrange TCD frequency (300 MHz) in conjunction with IV rt-PA has been associated with an increased risk of intracerebral hemorrhage [41]. Studies are underway to evaluate IV rt-PA, continuous TCD, and microbubbles in combination after AIS [35]. Ultrasound technology also is being used in IA catheters to enhance thrombolysis (see Fig. 2).

The most frequently cited reason for excluding patients from IV rt-PA is presentation outside the 3-hour window [18]. Most studies using IV rt-PA and other IV thrombolytics beyond 3 hours have failed to show a benefit. However, a pooled analysis of IV rt-PA studies showed a potential benefit of IV rt-PA up to 4.5 hours after symptom onset [42] (Fig. 3). Recently, a European study is the first to show a significant improvement in clinical outcomes when AIS patients were treated with IV rt-PA 3 to 4.5 hours after symptom onset. Furthermore, there was not an increased risk of hemorrhagic transformation when compared to other rt-PA studies, despite the longer time to treatment [43]. Studies of IV rt-PA within 6 hours of symptom onset are ongoing. A this time, routine use of IV rt-PA beyond 3 hours has not yet been recommended.

Because trials of IV thrombolysis beyond 3 hours have been largely unsuccessful, attention has been focused on better ways of selecting patients beyond 3 hours who might benefit from reperfusion therapies. Acute MRI scanning with diffusion-weighted-imaging (DWI) is capable of approximating infarct size, and perfusion-weighted-imaging (PWI) may provide information about the ischemic penumbra and tissue at risk when compared

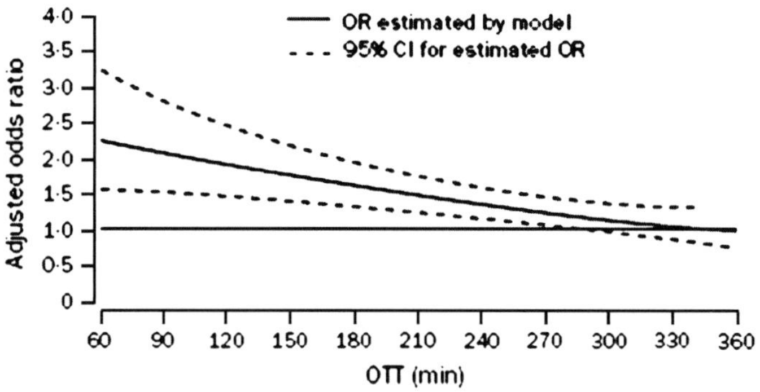

Fig. 3. Model estimating the odds ratio for a favorable outcome at 3 months in intravenous rt-PA treated patients compared with controls. Adjusted for age, baseline glucose, baseline National Institutes of Health (NIH) stroke scale score, baseline diastolic blood pressure, previous hypertension, and interaction between age and baseline NIH stroke scale score. (*From* Hacke W, Donnan G, Fieschi C, et al. Association of outcome with early stroke treatment: pooled analysis of ATLANTIS, ECASS, and NINDS rt-PA stroke trials. Lancet 2004;363(9411):772; with permission.)

with the DWI lesion (ie, mismatch) [35]. The mismatch hypothesis was tested in the DEFUSE (Diffusion-weighted imaging Evolution for Understanding Stroke Etiology) study. In DEFUSE, patients presenting within 3 to 6 hours after stroke symptom onset received an MRI scan, and those who had ischemic stroke then were treated with IV rt-PA 0.9 mg/kg. The pretreatment MRI scans then were analyzed retrospectively to identify subgroups of patients who might have benefited from treatment. Early reperfusion on PWI occurred in 49% of patients treated with IV rt-PA. A favorable clinical response occurred in 45% of patients with early reperfusion, compared with 35% in patients without early reperfusion ($P = .55$). Patients without a mismatch were not observed to benefit. In addition, a malignant profile was identified. Patients who had a DWI or a PWI lesion volume of greater than 100 mL were at higher risk of severe intracranial hemorrhage and poor outcome [44]. Further research is needed to confirm if patients who have a mismatch can benefit from IV thrombolysis beyond the 3-hour window.

Although the absolute effect is small, aspirin has been shown in clinical trials to reduce death and disability when initiated within 48 hours of symptom onset [45,46]. More recently, clopidogrel loading with an initial 300 mg dose and then 75 mg/d has been shown to be effective for reducing myocardial infarction risk during acute coronary syndrome [47]. One small study evaluated a one-time loading dose of clopidogrel 375 mg and aspirin 325 mg within 36 hours of stroke onset in patients not eligible for thrombolysis. Patients receiving clopidogrel loading were less likely to suffer neurologic deterioration compared with patients who were not loaded, without an increased risk of hemorrhage [48].

Research in AIS therapy is following a course similar to that of acute coronary syndrome (ACS), with an increasing emphasis on multiple pharmacologic agents in combination with percutaneous intervention. The current approach in ACS is antiplatelet therapy with aspirin, clopidogrel, and glycoprotein IIb/IIIa inhibitors; antithrombotic therapy with heparin; and direct percutaneous coronary intervention. Because the brain may be less tolerant of ischemia and at greater risk for devastating intracerebral hemorrhage from reperfusion than the myocardium, novel approaches first should be thoroughly evaluated for safety.

Neuroprotection

The term neuroprotectant refers to medications and other therapies designed to interrupt the process of cellular death within the brain itself, not directed toward improving vascular flow. This includes many medications and other therapies such as hypothermia and magnesium. Neuroprotection trials have a poor history of success, but past failures may have been caused in part to trial design. Suboptimal dosages, uncertain durations of therapy, and lengthy time windows may have contributed to past failures in neuroprotection [49].

Magnesium functions as an N-methyl-D-aspartic acid (NMDA) receptor blocker and voltage-gated calcium channel blocker. Magnesium is widely available, crosses the blood–brain barrier easily, and generally is tolerated well. As there are few acute adverse effects of used doses, Magnesium is a hyperacute intervention, being tested by paramedic administration in the field to patients who have acute focal neurologic symptoms. Field administration of magnesium sulfate has been reported to be feasible and safe in acute stroke patients [50]. The dose being studied is a 4 mg load in the field, followed by 16 g over 24 hours in the hospital. Further study is needed, but hyperacute prehospital therapies for AIS similar to myocardial infarction are desirable.

Another novel neuroprotectant is a combination of caffeine and ethanol, known as caffeinol. Low doses, the equivalent of 2 to 3 cups of coffee and one cocktail, have reduced infarct volume is up to 83% in animal models. Caffeinol may be more beneficial in cortical tissue compared with white matter, based on animal studies. Additionally, animals pretreated with daily ethanol have a diminished caffeinol effect, but not those pretreated with daily caffeine [51].

Hypothermia may have neuroprotective effects through multiple mechanisms of action. Hypothermia reduces cerebral oxygen demand, excitotoxicity, and inflammation. Moderate hypothermia (32 to 34° C) improves neurologic outcomes in adult cardiac arrest patients and reduces mortality [52,53]. In neonates who have perinatal asphyxia, hypothermia reduces mortality and severe disability [54,55].

Early trials suggest that both intravascular and surface cooling methods are feasible [56,57]. Surface cooling methods include simple measures like cooling blankets and ice packing, and adherent cooling jackets, pads, and head wraps [58]. Endovascular cooling can be accomplished by administering large amounts of chilled saline [59]. Newer cooling catheters, however, exchange heat by means of transduction, eliminating many of the problems associated with high-volume infusions [60] (Fig. 4).

Hypothermia, in a conscious stroke patient, carries additional risks and complications. After cardiac arrest, patients are treated with neuromuscular blockers and sedating medications to ameliorate the shivering response. In stroke patients, early detection of clinical deterioration may be critical; therefore, induced hypothermia without sedation and paralysis is desirable. The shivering response may be managed with a meperidine patient-controlled analgesia pump [61] in conjunction [44] with buspirone [62]. Induced hypothermia is labor-intensive and requires intensive care monitoring. Hypothermia is being tested both alone and in combination with thrombolysis and caffeinol [58].

Experimental evidence and clinical evidence suggest that the hydroxymethylglutaryl coenzyme A reductase inhibitors or statins have effects beyond

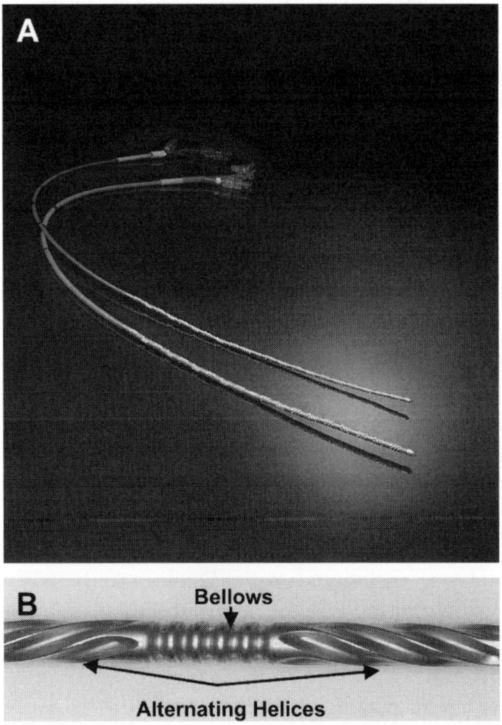

Fig. 4. Celsius Control Catheter. Intravascular cooling devices circulate fluid internally and cool via transduction. The Celsius Control catheter (*A*). Helices and bellows along the catheter (*B*) improve the cooling of circulating blood. (*Courtesy of* Innercool Therapies, Incorporated, San Diego, California; with permission.)

lowering cholesterol. Statins also have beneficial effects on endothelial function, coronary and cerebral blood flow, inflammation, and hemostasis [63,64]. Atorvastatin initiated within 24 hours after ischemic stroke has been reported to improve functional and neurologic recovery, despite no effect on infarct volume [65]. Further research will determine if statins can reduce infarct burden and disability after ischemic stroke.

The future of neuroprotection is promising. Trial design, however, is critical for success, and principles have been outlined to guide future trials [66]. Furthermore, combinations of multiple neuroprotection strategies may be more effective than individual therapies alone [49,67–69].

General medical management

As with any acute disease process, airway maintenance and adequate oxygenation are crucial to therapeutic success. Stroke patients who have reduced consciousness or brainstem involvement are at increased risk of airway compromise [70]. Endotracheal intubation may be required for these patients if they are unable to protect the airway or maintain adequate gas exchange [71]. The recommended target oxygen saturation in an acute stroke patient is greater than or equal to 95% [2]. The use of supplemental oxygen is of unproven benefit [72,73], and should be used only if required to maintain adequate oxygen saturation.

Hypothermia has been discussed as a potential strategy for neuroprotection. Hyperthermia has been associated with unfavorable neurologic outcome and increased mortality [74,75]. Even a simple 1° C reduction in body temperature almost doubles the chance of a favorable outcome [76]. Patients with fever should be evaluated thoroughly for the underlying etiology, and fever should be controlled. Measures to control fever include antipyretic medications, such as acetaminophen or ibuprofen, and cooling devices.

Hypoglycemia commonly presents with symptoms suggestive of AIS [2], and correcting the hypoglycemia should lead to a rapid resolution of the neurologic deficits. Hyperglycemia is present in up to one third of patients who have AIS [77] and is associated with worse outcomes than those with euglycemia [78], even in patients treated with thrombolytics [79]. Hyperglycemia has widespread negative effects during anaerobic glycolysis including regional lactic acidosis and free radical production. In addition, increased serum glucose may be associated with development of brain edema after stroke [80], and an increased risk of hemorrhagic transformation [81].

Despite being a well-known predictor of poor outcome, the effect of hyperglycemia treatment on outcomes is unclear. Intensive insulin protocols have been shown to be beneficial in critically ill patients, with goal blood glucose 70 to 110 mg/dL [82]. Additional clinical trial results are needed to determine the effectiveness of insulin protocols after AIS for improving outcomes [83]. In lieu of further data, the recommended approach is to treat hyperglycemia if the blood glucose level is greater than 200 mg/dL [2].

Hypotension is rare in AIS patients. When present, however, it is another predictor of an unfavorable outcome [84]. Potential causes for hypotension in patients who have AIS include aortic dissection, dehydration, blood loss, sepsis, and decreased cardiac output [2]. If hypotension is noted, immediate treatment should be initiated and an underlying cause sought.

Hypertension at presentation is found in most patients who have AIS [85]. Possible etiologies include acute stress, pain, hypoxia, or increased intracranial pressure. A U-shaped relationship between admission BP and mortality has been observed (Fig. 5) [86,87].

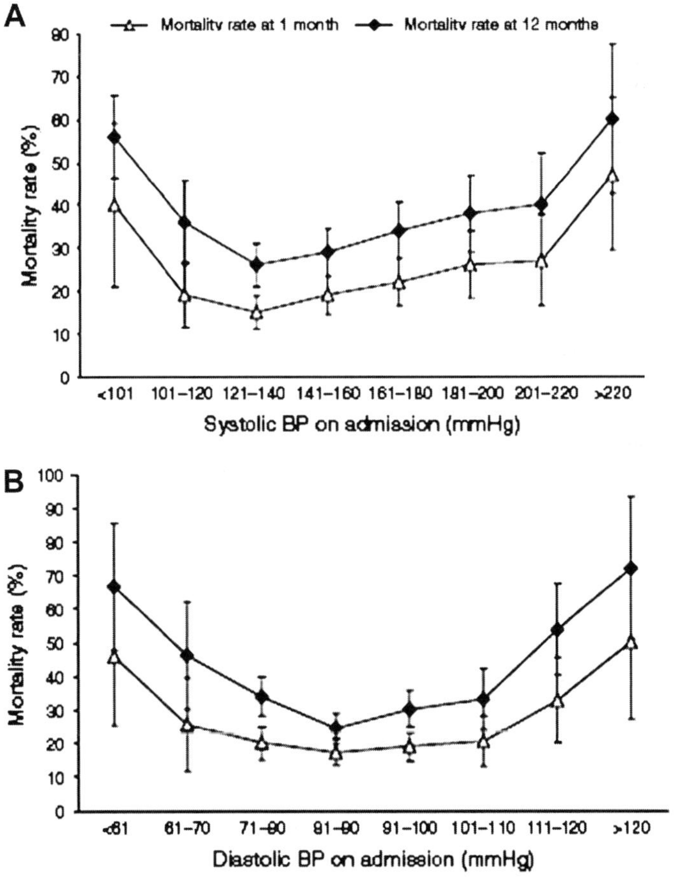

Fig. 5. Blood pressure on presentation and mortality. Line graphs showing the relationship between blood pressure on presentation and stroke mortality at 1 and 12 months. (*A*) Systolic blood pressure and (*B*) Diastolic blood pressure. Triangles and squares indicate early and late stroke mortality, respectively. 95% confidence intervals are indicated by T-bars. (*From* Vemmos KN, Tsivgoulis G, Spengos K, et al. U-shaped relationship between mortality and admission blood pressure in patients with acute stroke. J Intern Med 2004;255(2):260; with permission).

Possible advantages of inducing hypertension include improving collateral perfusion and blood flow through high-grade vascular stenoses. Animal models and small clinical studies suggest that drug-induced hypertension with phenylephrine may be beneficial in AIS [88–90]. Potential adverse effects of vasopressor infusions, however, are serious and include myocardial infarction, pulmonary edema, and systemic end organ ischemia. Furthermore, the safety and benefit of induced hypertension in people remain unproven, and it is not recommended in AIS outside of clinical trials [2].

Despite the observational data, optimal BP management after AIS remains unclear. Acutely lowering BP may decrease the risk of hemorrhagic transformation and cerebral edema. Actively lowering BP, however may lead to neurologic worsening by increasing ischemia in the penumbra [91].

The data so far are inconclusive. Spontaneous or iatrogenic reductions in BP greater than 20 mmHg have been associated with neurologic worsening, larger infarctions, and increased mortality [85]. Also, early administration (within 24 hours of admission) of antihypertensive agents in patients who have AIS with systolic blood pressure (SBP) greater than 180 mm Hg has been associated with neurologic deterioration, poor outcome, and mortality [85]. Conversely, reductions in BP in the first week after AIS also have been associated with improved short-term outcomes [92]. Large, well-designed trials are needed to clarify the most appropriate management of BP after AIS. BP greater than 185/110 mm Hg after thrombolysis has been associated with an increased risk of hemorrhagic transformation [7,22].

Recommendations for BP lowering after AIS are summarized in Table 1. The consensus is that antihypertensive medication should be withheld unless the SBP is greater than 220 mm Hg or the DBP is greater than 120 mm Hg

Table 1
Blood pressure management acute ischemic stroke

Blood pressure (mm Hg)	Treatment
In patients not eligible for thrombolysis or other acute reperfusion therapies	
SBP ≤220 or DBP ≤120	Observation
SBP >220 or DBP 121–140	Enalaprilat (intravenous [IV]) or Hydralazine (IV) or Labetalol (IV) or Clonidine (IV or subcutaneous) or Nicardipine infusion (IV)
DBP >140	Nicardipine infusion (IV) or Nitroprusside infusion (IV)
B. In patients eligible for thrombolysis or other acute reperfusion therapies	
SBP ≤185 or DBP ≤110	Observation
SBP >185 or DBP >110	Labetalol (IV) or Hydralazine (IV) or Clonidine (IV or Subcutaneous) or Nicardipine Infusion (IV)
DBP >140	Nicardipine infusion (IV) or Nitroprusside infusion (IV)

in patients who have AIS but are not eligible for IV rt-PA. Patients eligible for thrombolysis should have a goal SBP of less than 185 mm Hg and DBP of less than 110 mm Hg [2]. Angiotensin converting enzyme inhibitors are not recommended for BP lowering in patients eligible for thrombolysis. This is because of concern over orolingual angioedema, a rare but potentially serious allergic reaction that is reported to occur more commonly when this class of medications is used with IV rt-PA [93].

Summary

Thrombolysis with IV rt-PA within 3 hours of symptom onset remains the only FDA- approved medical therapy for AIS. The MERCI concentric retriever and Penumbra device, however, also have been approved for mechanical embolectomy in cerebral arteries, but the effect on outcomes remains uncertain. Multiple other acute reperfusion strategies are being tested that hopefully have improve reperfusion efficiency and extend the treatment window.

Despite earlier disappointments, there is renewed enthusiasm for neuroprotection therapies. Improved trial designs and combining various neuroprotective strategies may help achieve success.

With the increasing emphasis on thrombolysis and neuroprotection, the importance of good general medical management cannot be forgotten. Defining optimal management of serum glucose, temperature, and BP is vital to achieving favorable outcomes in ischemic stroke.

References

[1] Jones TH, Morawetz RB, Crowell RM, et al. Thresholds of focal cerebral ischemia in awake monkeys. J Neurosurg 1981;54(6):773–82.

[2] Adams HP Jr, del Zoppo G, Alberts MJ, et al. Guidelines for the early management of adults with ischemic stroke: a guideline from the American Heart Association/American Stroke Association Stroke Council, Clinical Cardiology Council, Cardiovascular Radiology and Intervention Council, and the Atherosclerotic Peripheral Vascular Disease and Quality of Care Outcomes in Research Interdisciplinary Working Groups. The American Academy of Neurology affirms the value of this guideline as an educational tool for neurologists. Stroke 2007; 38(5):1655–711.

[3] Bruno A, Biller J, Adams HP Jr, et al. Acute blood glucose level and outcome from ischemic stroke. Trial of ORG 10172 in Acute Stroke Treatment (TOAST) investigators. Neurology 1999;52(2):280–4.

[4] Reith J, Jorgensen HS, Pedersen PM, et al. Body temperature in acute stroke: relation to stroke severity, infarct size, mortality, and outcome. Lancet 1996;347(8999):422–5.

[5] Baron JC. Mapping the ischaemic penumbra with PET: implications for acute stroke treatment. Cerebrovasc Dis 1999;9(4):193–201.

[6] The National Institute of Neurological Disorders and Stroke rt-PA Stroke Study Group. Tissue plasminogen activator for acute ischemic stroke. N Engl J Med 1995;333(24):1581–7.

[7] The NINDS t-PA Stroke Study Group. Intracerebral hemorrhage after intravenous t-PA therapy for ischemic stroke. Stroke 1997;28(11):2109–18.

[8] Khatri P, Wechsler LR, Broderick JP. Intracranial hemorrhage associated with revascularization therapies. Stroke 2007;38(2):431–40.

[9] Broderick J, Connolly S, Feldmann E, et al. Guidelines for the management of spontaneous intracerebral hemorrhage in adults: 2007 update. A guideline from the American Heart Association/American Stroke Association Stroke Council, High Blood Pressure Research Council, and the Quality of Care and Outcomes in Research Interdisciplinary Working Group. Stroke 2007;38(6):2001–23.

[10] Katzan IL, Furlan AJ, Lloyd LE, et al. Use of tissue-type plasminogen activator for acute ischemic stroke: the Cleveland area experience. JAMA 2000;283(9):1151–8.

[11] Katzan IL, Hammer MD, Hixson ED, et al. Utilization of intravenous tissue plasminogen activator for acute ischemic stroke. Arch Neurol 2004;61(3):346–50.

[12] Graham GD. Tissue plasminogen activator for acute ischemic stroke in clinical practice: a meta-analysis of safety data. Stroke 2003;34(12):2847–50.

[13] Khaja AM, Grotta JC. Established treatments for acute ischaemic stroke. Lancet 2007; 369(9558):319–30.

[14] Tanne D, Kasner SE, Demchuk AM, et al. Markers of increased risk of intracerebral hemorrhage after intravenous recombinant tissue plasminogen activator therapy for acute ischemic stroke in clinical practice: the Multicenter rt-PA Stroke Survey. Circulation 2002; 105(14):1679–85.

[15] van Oostenbrugge RJ, Hupperts RM, Lodder J. Thrombolysis for acute stroke with special emphasis on the very old: experience from a single Dutch centre. J Neurol Neurosurg Psychiatry 2006;77(3):375–7.

[16] Engelter ST, Reichhart M, Sekoranja L, et al. Thrombolysis in stroke patients aged 80 years and older: Swiss survey of IV thrombolysis. Neurology 2005;65(11):1795–8.

[17] Sylaja PN, Cote R, Buchan AM, et al. Thrombolysis in patients older than 80 years with acute ischaemic stroke: Canadian Alteplase for Stroke Effectiveness Study. J Neurol Neurosurg Psychiatry 2006;77(7):826–9.

[18] Barber PA, Zhang J, Demchuk AM, et al. Why are stroke patients excluded from TPA therapy? An analysis of patient eligibility. Neurology 2001;56(8):1015–20.

[19] Smith EE, Abdullah AR, Petkovska I, et al. Poor outcomes in patients who do not receive intravenous tissue plasminogen activator because of mild or improving ischemic stroke. Stroke 2005;36(11):2497–9.

[20] Gonzales N, Albright K, Noser E, et al. Mild stroke should not exclude patients from thrombolytic therapy. Stroke 2006;37(2):621.

[21] Patel SC, Levine SR, Tilley BC, et al. Lack of clinical significance of early ischemic changes on computed tomography in acute stroke. JAMA 2001;286(22):2830–8.

[22] Larrue V, von Kummer R, del Zoppo G, et al. Hemorrhagic transformation in acute ischemic stroke. Potential contributing factors in the European Cooperative Acute Stroke Study. Stroke 1997;28(5):957–60.

[23] Larrue V, von Kummer RR, Muller A, et al. Risk factors for severe hemorrhagic transformation in ischemic stroke patients treated with recombinant tissue plasminogen activator: a secondary analysis of the European–Australasian Acute Stroke Study (ECASS II). Stroke 2001;32(2):438–41.

[24] Demchuk AM, Hill MD, Barber PA, et al. Importance of early ischemic computed tomography changes using ASPECTS in NINDS rtPA Stroke Study. Stroke 2005;36(10):2110–5.

[25] Smith WS. Safety of mechanical thrombectomy and intravenous tissue plasminogen activator in acute ischemic stroke. Results of the Multimechanical Embolus Removal in Cerebral Ischemia (MERCI) trial, part I. AJNR Am J Neuroradiol 2006;27(6):1177–82.

[26] The Penumbra Stroke Trial Investigators. The penumbra stroke trial: safety and effectiveness of a new generation of mechanical devices for clot removal in acute ischemic stroke. Stroke 2008;39(2):527–729.

[27] Lewandowski CA, Frankel M, Tomsick TA, et al. Combined intravenous and intra-arterial r-TPA versus intra-arterial therapy of acute ischemic stroke: emergency management of stroke (EMS) bridging trial. Stroke 1999;30(12):2598–605.
[28] The IMS Study Investigators. Combined intravenous and intra-arterial recanalization for acute ischemic stroke: the Interventional Management of Stroke Study. Stroke 2004;35(4): 904–11.
[29] Shaltoni HM, Albright KC, Gonzales NR, et al. Is intra-arterial thrombolysis safe after full-dose intravenous recombinant tissue plasminogen activator for acute ischemic stroke? Stroke 2007;38(1):80–4.
[30] Nedeltchev K, Brekenfeld C, Remonda L, et al. Internal carotid artery stent implantation in 25 patients with acute stroke: preliminary results. Radiology 2005;237(3):1029–37.
[31] Bukow SC, Daffertshofer M, Hennerici MG. Tirofiban for the treatment of ischaemic stroke. Expert Opin Pharmacother 2006;7(1):73–9.
[32] Sugg RM, Pary JK, Uchino K, et al. Argatroban TPA Stroke Study: study design and results in the first-treated cohort. Arch Neurol 2006;63(8):1057–62.
[33] The Multicenter Acute Stroke Trial—Europe Study Group. Thrombolytic therapy with streptokinase in acute ischemic stroke. N Engl J Med 1996;335(3):145–50.
[34] Haley EC Jr, Lyden PD, Johnston KC, et al. A pilot dose-escalation safety study of tenecteplase in acute ischemic stroke. Stroke 2005;36(3):607–12.
[35] Sacco RL, Chong JY, Prabhakaran S, et al. Experimental treatments for acute ischaemic stroke. Lancet 2007;369(9558):331–41.
[36] Liu M, Counsell C, Zhao XL, et al. Fibrinogen-depleting agents for acute ischaemic stroke. Cochrane Database Syst Rev 2003;3:CD000091.
[37] Hennerici MG, Kay R, Bogousslavsky J, et al. Intravenous ancrod for acute ischaemic stroke in the European stroke treatment with ancrod trial: a randomised–controlled trial. Lancet 2006;368(9550):1871–8.
[38] Hacke W, Albers G, Al-Rawi Y, et al. The desmoteplase in acute ischemic stroke trial (DIAS): a phase II MRI-based 9-hour window acute stroke thrombolysis trial with intravenous desmoteplase. Stroke 2005;36(1):66–73.
[39] Lauer CG, Burge R, Tang DB, et al. Effect of ultrasound on tissue-type plasminogen activator-induced thrombolysis. Circulation 1992;86(4):1257–64.
[40] Alexandrov AV, Molina CA, Grotta JC, et al. Ultrasound-enhanced systemic thrombolysis for acute ischemic stroke. N Engl J Med 2004;351(21):2170–8.
[41] Daffertshofer M, Gass A, Ringleb P, et al. Transcranial low-frequency ultrasound-mediated thrombolysis in brain ischemia: increased risk of hemorrhage with combined ultrasound and tissue plasminogen activator: results of a phase II clinical trial. Stroke 2005; 36(7):1441–6.
[42] Hacke W, Donnan G, Fieschi C, et al. Association of outcome with early stroke treatment: pooled analysis of ATLANTIS, ECASS, and NINDS rt-PA stroke trials. Lancet 2004; 363(9411):768–74.
[43] Hacke W, Kaste M, Bluhmki E, et al. Thrombolysis with Alteplase 3 to 4.5 hours after acute ischemic stroke. N Eng J Med 2008;359(13):1317–29.
[44] Albers GW, Thijs VN, Wechsler L, et al. Magnetic resonance imaging profiles predict clinical response to early reperfusion: the diffusion and perfusion imaging evaluation for understanding stroke evolution (DEFUSE) study. Ann Neurol 2006;60(5):508–17.
[45] CAST (Chinese Acute Stroke Trial) Collaborative Group. CAST: randomised placebo-controlled trial of early aspirin use in 20,000 patients with acute ischaemic stroke. Lancet 1997; 349(9066):1641–9.
[46] International Stroke Trial Collaborative Group. The International Stroke Trial (IST): a randomised trial of aspirin, subcutaneous heparin, both, or neither among 19435 patients with acute ischaemic stroke. Lancet 1997;349(9065):1569–81.

[47] Harrington RA, Becker RC, Ezekowitz M, et al. Antithrombotic therapy for coronary artery disease: the Seventh ACCP Conference on Antithrombotic and Thrombolytic Therapy. Chest 2004;126(3 Suppl):513S–48S.
[48] Meyer DM, Albright KC, Allison TA, et al. LOAD: a pilot study of the safety of loading of aspirin and clopidogrel in acute ischemic stroke and transient ischemic attack. J Stroke Cerebrovasc Dis 2008;17(1):26–9.
[49] Stroke Therapy Academic Industry Roundtable II. Recommendations for clinical trial evaluation of acute stroke therapies. Stroke 2001;32(7):1598–606.
[50] Saver JL, Kidwell C, Eckstein M, et al. Prehospital neuroprotective therapy for acute stroke: results of the Field Administration of Stroke Therapy—Magnesium (FAST-MAG) pilot trial. Stroke 2004;35(5):e106–8.
[51] Aronowski J, Strong R, Shirzadi A, et al. Ethanol plus caffeine (caffeinol) for treatment of ischemic stroke: preclinical experience. Stroke 2003;34(5):1246–51.
[52] The Hypothermia after Cardiac Arrest Study Group. Mild therapeutic hypothermia to improve the neurologic outcome after cardiac arrest. N Engl J Med 2002;346(8):549–56.
[53] Bernard SA, Gray TW, Buist MD, et al. Treatment of comatose survivors of out-of-hospital cardiac arrest with induced hypothermia. N Engl J Med 2002;346(8):557–63.
[54] Gluckman PD, Wyatt JS, Azzopardi D, et al. Selective head cooling with mild systemic hypothermia after neonatal encephalopathy: multicentre randomised trial. Lancet 2005; 365(9460):663–70.
[55] Shankaran S, Laptook AR, Ehrenkranz RA, et al. Whole-body hypothermia for neonates with hypoxic–ischemic encephalopathy. N Engl J Med 2005;353(15):1574–84.
[56] Krieger DW, De Georgia MA, Abou-Chebl A, et al. Cooling for acute ischemic brain damage (COOL AID): an open pilot study of induced hypothermia in acute ischemic stroke. Stroke 2001;32(8):1847–54.
[57] De Georgia MA, Krieger DW, Abou-Chebl A, et al. Cooling for Acute Ischemic Brain Damage (COOL AID): a feasibility trial of endovascular cooling. Neurology 2004;63(2):312–7.
[58] Hemmen TM, Lyden PD. Induced hypothermia for acute stroke. Stroke 2007;38(2 Suppl): 794–9.
[59] Baumgardner JE, Baranov D, Smith DS, et al. The effectiveness of rapidly infused intravenous fluids for inducing moderate hypothermia in neurosurgical patients. Anesth Analg 1999;89(1):163–9.
[60] Mack WJ, Huang J, Winfree C, et al. Ultrarapid, convection-enhanced intravascular hypothermia: a feasibility study in nonhuman primate stroke. Stroke 2003;34(8):1994–9.
[61] Alfonsi P, Sessler DI, Du Manoir B, et al. The effects of meperidine and sufentanil on the shivering threshold in postoperative patients. Anesthesiology 1998;89(1):43–8.
[62] Mokhtarani M, Mahgoub AN, Morioka N, et al. Buspirone and meperidine synergistically reduce the shivering threshold. Anesth Analg 2001;93(5):1233–9.
[63] Amarenco P, Labreuche J, Lavallee P, et al. Statins in stroke prevention and carotid atherosclerosis: systematic review and up-to-date meta-analysis. Stroke 2004;35(12):2902–9.
[64] Ballantyne CM. Current and future aims of lipid-lowering therapy: changing paradigms and lessons from the Heart Protection Study on standards of efficacy and safety. Am J Cardiol 2003;92(4B):3K–9K.
[65] Chen J, Zhang ZG, Li Y, et al. Statins induce angiogenesis, neurogenesis, and synaptogenesis after stroke. Ann Neurol 2003;53(6):743–51.
[66] Hickenbottom SL, Grotta J. Neuroprotective therapy. Semin Neurol 1998;18(4):485–92.
[67] Stroke Therapy Academic Industry Roundtable. Recommendations for standards regarding preclinical neuroprotective and restorative drug development. Stroke 1999;30(12):2752–8.
[68] Fisher M. Recommendations for advancing development of acute stroke therapies: stroke therapy academic industry roundtable 3. Stroke 2003;34(6):1539–46.
[69] Fisher M, Albers GW, Donnan GA, et al. Enhancing the development and approval of acute stroke therapies: stroke therapy academic industry roundtable. Stroke 2005;36(8):1808–13.

[70] Grotta J, Pasteur W, Khwaja G, et al. Elective intubation for neurologic deterioration after stroke. Neurology 1995;45(4):640–4.
[71] Hacke W, Krieger D, Hirschberg M. General principles in the treatment of acute ishemic stroke. Cerebrovasc Dis 1991;1(Suppl 1):93–9.
[72] Ronning OM, Guldvog B. Should stroke victims routinely receive supplemental oxygen? A quasi-randomized controlled trial. Stroke 1999;30(10):2033–7.
[73] Treib J, Grauer MT, Woessner R, et al. Treatment of stroke on an intensive stroke unit: a novel concept. Intensive Care Med 2000;26(11):1598–611.
[74] Azzimondi G, Bassein L, Nonino F, et al. Fever in acute stroke worsens prognosis. A prospective study. Stroke 1995;26(11):2040–3.
[75] Ginsberg MD, Busto R. Combating hyperthermia in acute stroke: a significant clinical concern. Stroke 1998;29(2):529–34.
[76] Jorgensen HS, Reith J, Nakayama H, et al. What determines good recovery in patients with the most severe strokes? The Copenhagen Stroke Study. Stroke 1999;30(10):2008–12.
[77] Scott JF, Robinson GM, French JM, et al. Prevalence of admission hyperglycaemia across clinical subtypes of acute stroke. Lancet 1999;353(9150):376–7.
[78] Bruno A, Levine SR, Frankel MR, et al. Admission glucose level and clinical outcomes in the NINDS r-TPA stroke trial. Neurology 2002;59(5):669–74.
[79] Alvarez-Sabin J, Molina CA, Ribo M, et al. Impact of admission hyperglycemia on stroke outcome after thrombolysis: risk stratification in relation to time to reperfusion. Stroke 2004;35(11):2493–8.
[80] Lindsberg PJ, Roine RO. Hyperglycemia in acute stroke. Stroke 2004;35(2):363–4.
[81] Kase CS, Furlan AJ, Wechsler LR, et al. Cerebral hemorrhage after intra-arterial thrombolysis for ischemic stroke: the PROACT II trial. Neurology 2001;57(9):1603–10.
[82] Van den Berghe G, Wouters PJ, Bouillon R, et al. Outcome benefit of intensive insulin therapy in the critically ill: insulin dose versus glycemic control. Crit Care Med 2003;31(2): 359–66.
[83] Gray CS, Hildreth AJ, Alberti GK, et al. Poststroke hyperglycemia: natural history and immediate management. Stroke 2004;35(1):122–6.
[84] Leonardi-Bee J, Bath PM, Phillips SJ, et al. Blood pressure and clinical outcomes in the International Stroke Trial. Stroke 2002;33(5):1315–20.
[85] Castillo J, Leira R, Garcia MM, et al. Blood pressure decrease during the acute phase of ischemic stroke is associated with brain injury and poor stroke outcome. Stroke 2004; 35(2):520–6.
[86] Vemmos KN, Spengos K, Tsivgoulis G, et al. Factors influencing acute blood pressure values in stroke subtypes. J Hum Hypertens 2004;18(4):253–9.
[87] Vemmos KN, Tsivgoulis G, Spengos K, et al. U-shaped relationship between mortality and admission blood pressure in patients with acute stroke. J Intern Med 2004;255(2):257–65.
[88] Rordorf G, Cramer SC, Efird JT, et al. Pharmacological elevation of blood pressure in acute stroke. Clinical effects and safety. Stroke 1997;28(11):2133–8.
[89] Rordorf G, Koroshetz WJ, Ezzeddine MA, et al. A pilot study of drug-induced hypertension for treatment of acute stroke. Neurology 2001;56(9):1210–3.
[90] Wityk RJ, Restrepo L. Hypoperfusion and its augmentation in patients with brain ischemia. Curr Treat Options Cardiovasc Med 2003;5(3):193–9.
[91] Johnston KC, Mayer SA. Blood pressure reduction in ischemic stroke: a two-edged sword? Neurology 2003;61(8):1030–1.
[92] Rodriguez-Garcia JL, Botia E, de La Sierra A, et al. Significance of elevated blood pressure and its management on the short-term outcome of patients with acute ischemic stroke. Am J Hypertens 2005;18(3):379–84.
[93] Hill MD, Lye T, Moss H, et al. Hemi-orolingual angioedema and ACE inhibition after alteplase treatment of stroke. Neurology 2003;60(9):1525–7.

ELSEVIER
SAUNDERS

NEUROLOGIC CLINICS

Neurol Clin 26 (2008) 963–985

Acute Hemorrhagic Stroke Pathophysiology and Medical Interventions: Blood Pressure Control, Management of Anticoagulant-Associated Brain Hemorrhage and General Management Principles

Fernando D. Testai, MD, PhD*, Venkatesh Aiyagari, MBBS, DM

Department of Neurology and Rehabilitation, Section of Cerebrovascular Disease and Neurological Critical Care, University of Illinois College of Medicine at Chicago, 912 South Wood Street, Room 855N, Chicago, IL 60612, USA

Spontaneous intracerebral hemorrhage (ICH) is a neurologic emergency that accounts for about 10% to 20% of all strokes and has a 30-day mortality rate of 35% to 52% [1,2]. Furthermore, only 21% of patients suffering ICH are expected to be independent at 6 months [3]. Despite advances in our understanding of the pathophysiology and complications associated with ICH, in-hospital mortality from ICH decreased by a mere 6% between 1990 and 2000, compared with 36% and 10% mortality reductions achieved for ischemic stroke and subarachnoid hemorrhage, respectively [4].

This article reviews the pathophysiology and general medical management principles of ICH, including the acute management of elevated blood pressure and management of anticoagulant-associated intracerebral hemorrhage.

Pathophysiology

Causes of intracerebral hemorrhage

Chronic hypertension (HTN) is the most important risk factor for ICH and is responsible for almost 60% of cases [2,5–7]. Sustained hypertension

* Corresponding author.
E-mail address: testai@uic.edu (F.D. Testai).

doi:10.1016/j.ncl.2008.06.001

induces smooth muscle cell proliferation in the arterioles. This process is termed hyperplastic arteriolosclerosis [8]. Over time, smooth muscle cells die and the tunica media is replaced by collagen, resulting in vessels with decreased tone and poor compliance. The arterioles ultimately undergo ectasia and aneurysmal dilation (Fig. 1) [8]. These microaneurysms, called Charcot-Bouchard aneurysms, are susceptible to rupture leading to cerebral hemorrhage and were proposed by Charcot and Bouchard in 1868 as a key element of deep ICH [9–11].

The second most common cause of ICH, cerebral amyloid angiopathy (CAA), accounts for almost 20% of cases in patients older than 70 years of age [12]. CAA is characterized by the deposition of β-amyloid protein in the tunica media and adventitia of the leptomeningeal and cortical arteries, arterioles, and capillaries (Fig. 2) [13,14]. These amyloid-laden vessels can undergo fibrinoid degeneration, necrosis, segmental dilation, or aneurysm formation, rendering them prone to rupture [13]. The apolipoprotein E alleles $\epsilon 2$ and $\epsilon 4$ have been associated with degenerative changes of the vessel wall and increased deposition of β-amyloid protein, respectively [15]. Carriers of the $\epsilon 2/\epsilon 2$ and $\epsilon 4/\epsilon 4$ genotype have a 28% 2-year recurrent ICH rate, compared with 10% for patients with the $\epsilon 3/\epsilon 3$ genotype [15]. The association between apolipoprotein E genotype and ICH varies among different ethnicities. It has been reported that the risk of ICH in patients carrying an $\epsilon 2$ or $\epsilon 4$ allele is 1.48 times for Europeans (95% confidence interval or CI = 0.76 to 2.87) and 2.11 times for Asians (95% CI = 1.28 to 3.47), compared with those with the $\epsilon 3/\epsilon 3$ genotype [16].

Another common cause of parenchymal bleeding is anticoagulant-associated ICH (AAICH). This is the most feared complication of anticoagulant use. Over the years, the continuing increase in the elderly population in the United States has lead to a higher prevalence of medical conditions that require the administration of anticoagulants and a consequent increase

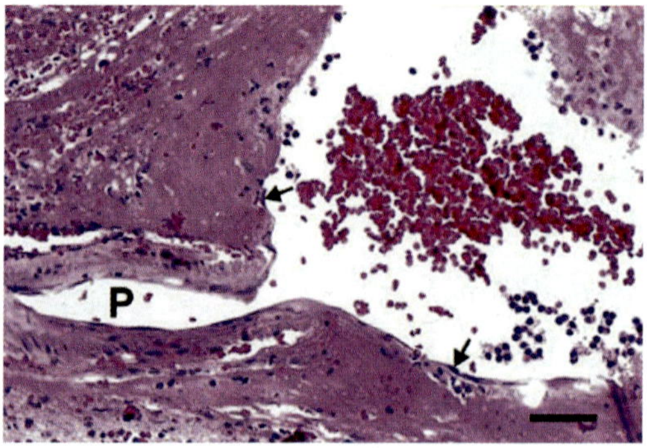

Fig. 1. Charcot-Bouchard aneurysm as seen in neurosurgical material from evacuation of an intracerebral hematoma. Endothelial cells (*arrows*) lining the cavity attest to its vascular origin. Parent vessel (P) of Charcot- Bouchard aneurysm is indicated. Bar = 100 mm. (*From* Sutherland GR, Auer RN. Primary intracerebral hemorrhage. J Clin Neurosci 2006;13:511–7; with permission.)

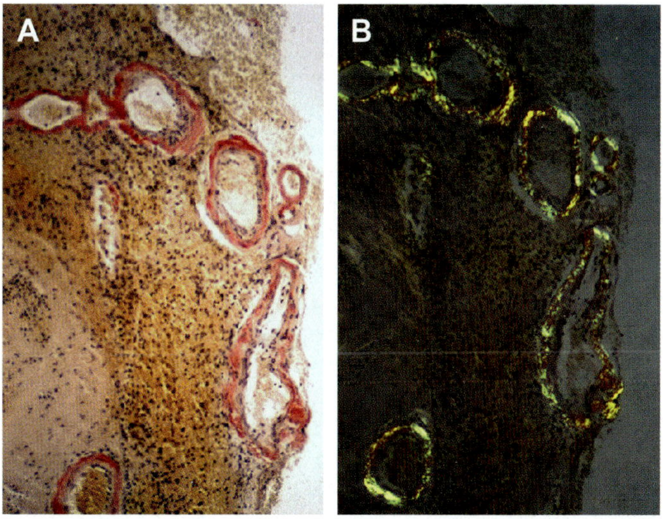

Fig. 2. Surgical specimens from the matrix of a hematoma associated with amyloid angiopathy. Specimens stained with Congo red. (*A*) Shows deposits of amyloid seen through ordinary transmitted light as a dense red staining hyaline material within the vessel walls (× 100). (*B*) Shows in the same field the characteristic green-yellow birefringence of amyloid evidenced under polarized light (× 100). (*Courtesy of* Dr. Peter Ostrow, Department of Pathology, State University of New York, Buffalo.)

in AAICH [17]. Anticoagulants have been shown to be effective for prevention of venous thromboembolism and systemic embolism in patients with atrial fibrillation or prosthetic valves [18]. Warfarin is the most commonly used anticoagulant worldwide. It inhibits the conversion of vitamin K epoxide to reduced vitamin K, a cofactor necessary for the γ-carboxylation and activation of the coagulation factors II, VII, IX, and X [18]. It is estimated that warfarin use is associated with 5% to 24% of ICH cases [19–21]. The annual frequency of ICH in patients undergoing chronic anticoagulation with warfarin is 0.3% to 0.6% [22]. Although the intensity of anticoagulation proportionally increases the risk of AAICH, almost 70% of the cases occur with an international normalized ratio (INR) of 3 or less [21]. In addition, the degree of INR elevation is associated with hematoma expansion and mortality [21,23,24]. Other risk factors for AAICH include advanced age, history of hypertension, simultaneous use of antiplatelet agents, CAA, apolipoprotein genotype $\epsilon 2$, and presence of leukoaraiosis on neuroimaging [21,22,25–27].

Antiplatelet agents, such as aspirin and clopidrogel, are commonly used in patients with coronary artery and cerebrovascular disease and have been implicated in the causation of ICH, although this association is less well established [28]. Several studies have reported larger hematomas and higher ICH-related mortality rate in patients using antiplatelet agents [28–30]. However, other reports contradict these observations [31–33].

Thrombolytic agents are proteases that convert plasminogen to plasmin, which subsequently lyses clot by breaking down fibrinogen and fibrin. The available agents today are tissue-type plasminogen activator or alteplase (tPA), reteplase, tenecteplase, urokinase, anisoylated purified streptokinase activator complex, and streptokinase. Intravenous tPA has been approved by the Food and Drug Administration for the treatment of acute ischemic stroke in patients who present within 3 hours of onset of symptoms. The risk of developing symptomatic ICH is 6% in patients treated with intravenous tPA [34]. Thrombolytic therapy is also used in the treatment of acute myocardial infarction; in this setting, the incidence of ICH is about 0.7% [35]. Symptomatic thrombolytic-associated ICH has a 30-day mortality rate of almost 60% [34]. Other less frequent causes of ICH are included in Box 1.

Location of intracerebral hemorrhage

A biracial population study of 1,038 ICH cases showed that 49% were located deep in hemisphere, 35% lobar, 10% cerebellar, and 6% in the brain stem [36]. The hematoma location may be suggestive of the underlying etiology. Hematomas in the thalamus, basal ganglia, cerebellum, or pons are commonly associated with HTN. On the other hand, lobar ICH in an elderly patient is highly suggestive of CAA [37].

Consequences of intracerebral hemorrhage

Hematoma expansion

It is well established that hematoma expansion in spontaneous ICH occurs within the first 24 hours after ictus in about one third of patients [38,39]. Hematoma volume and hematoma expansion are predictors of 30-day functional outcome and mortality [38,40,41]. A direct relationship between blood pressure and risk of hematoma enlargement has been shown in some studies, but others do not support this association [42–44]. It is also unclear if high blood pressure is the cause or a hemodynamic response to the growing hematoma [44].

Hydrocephalus

Initially, extravasation of blood into the ventricular system impairs cerebrospinal fluid (CSF) circulation, causing obstructive hydrocephalus; later, blood and debris obstruct the arachnoid villi, impairing CSF reabsortion and causing communicating hydrocephalus. Hydrocephalus is an independent 30-day mortality predictor after ICH [45]. In particular, dilation of the third and fourth ventricles has been noted to carry a worse prognosis [46,47].

Cerebral edema

Traditionally, ICH was believed to cause permanent brain injury directly by mass effect. However, the importance of hematoma-induced

Box 1. Causes of nontraumatic intracerebral hemorrhage

- Hypertension
- Cerebral amyloid angiopathy
- Inherited bleeding diathesis
- Antithrombotic use
  - Anticoagulants
  - Fibrinolytics
  - Antiplatelets
- Vascular malformations
  - Arteriorvenous malformations
  - Dural arteriovenous fistulas
  - Cavernous malformations
  - Venous angioma
- Aneurysms
  - Saccular
  - Infective
  - Fusiform
- Tumors
  - Primary brain tumors
    - Pituitary adenoma
    - Glioblastoma multiforme
  - Metastastatic tumor
    - Breast cancer
    - Melanoma
    - Choriocarcinoma
    - Renal cell
    - Bronchogenic carcinoma
- Hemorrhagic transformation of a cerebral infarction
- Dural venous sinus thrombosis with secondary venous infarction and hemorrhage
- Moyamoya disease
- Vasculitis
- Illicit drug use
  - Amphetamines
  - Cocaine
  - Other

inflammatory response and edema as contributors to secondary neuronal damage has since been recognized [48].

At least three stages of edema development occur after ICH (Table 1). In the first stage, the hemorrhage dissects along the white matter tissue planes, infiltrating areas of intact brain. Within several hours, edema forms after clot retraction by consequent extrusion of osmotically active plasma proteins

Table 1
Stages of edema after ICH

First stage (hours)	Second stage (within first 2 days)	Third stage (after first 2 days)
Clot retraction and extrusion of osmotically active proteins	Activation of the coagulation cascade and thrombin synthesis Complement activation Perihematomal inflammation and leukocyte infiltration	Hemoglobin induced neuronal toxicity

into the underlying white matter [49,50]. The second stage occurs during the first 2 days and is characterized by a robust inflammatory response. In this stage, ongoing thrombin production activates by the coagulation cascade, complement system, and microglia. This attracts polymorphonuclear leukocytes and monocyte/macrophage cells, leading to up-regulation of numerous immunomediators that disrupt the blood-brain barrier and worsen the edema [51,52]. A delayed third stage occurs subsequently, when red blood cell lysis leads to hemoglobin-induced neuronal toxicity [53]. Perihematomal edema volume increases by approximately 75% during the first 24 hours after spontaneous ICH and has been implicated in the delayed mass effect that occurs in the second and third weeks after ICH [54,55].

Ischemia

Normal cerebral blood flow (CBF) in an adult brain is approximately 50 mL per 100 g^{-1} per $minute^{-1}$ [56]. CBF is determined by the relationship between cerebral perfusion pressure (CPP) and cerebrovascular resistance [56]. CPP represents the difference between the mean arterial pressure (MAP) and the intracranial pressure (ICP) [57,58]. Under normal circumstances, cerebral arterioles dilate in response to a decrease in CPP and constrict in response to an increase in blood pressure. This dynamic regulation of cerebrovascular resistance maintains a constant CBF in the CPP range between 50 mm Hg to 150 mm Hg and is called autoregulation (Fig. 3) [59,60]. A decrease in the CPP below the lower limit of autoregulation leads to a decrease in CBF and an increase in oxygen extraction [59]. However, when CBF falls below 20 mL per 100 g^{-1} per $minute^{-1}$, the increase in oxygen extraction is no longer able to meet the demand and ischemia occurs [56,57,61]. In chronic HTN, the cerebral vasculature is adapted to higher blood pressure and the autoregulation curve is shifted to the right (see Fig. 3) [59]. Precipitous blood pressure lowering in chronically hypertensive patients may cause cerebral ischemia even at normotensive levels. Prolonged control of hypertension can return the autoregulatory range to normal limits [59].

Patients with ICH can have elevated ICP because of hematoma-related mass effect, cerebral edema, and hydrocephalus. Furthermore, the regional increase in pressure around the hematoma can compress the

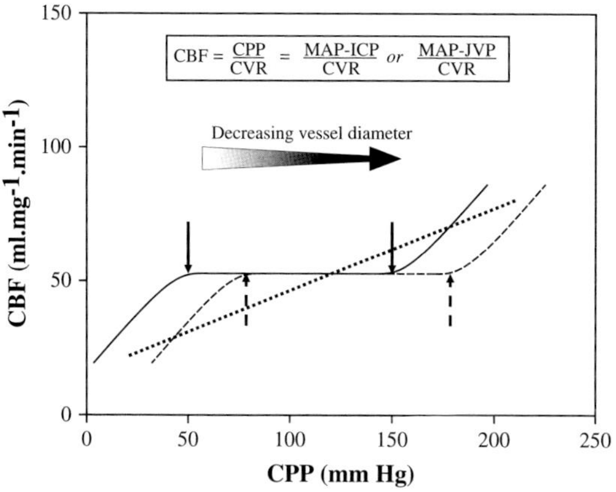

Fig. 3. Cerebral autoregulation curve. In the normal state (*solid line*), the CBF is held constant across a wide range of CPPs (50 mm Hg–150 mm Hg). In chronic hypertension (*dashed line*), the autoregulation curve shifts to the right. In intracranial hypertension (*dotted line*) the cerebral autoregulation may be impaired, and the CBF becomes dependent on the CPP. *Abbreviations:* CBF, cerebral blood flow; CPP, cerebral perfusion pressure; CVR, cerebral venous resistance; ICP, intracranial pressure; JVP, jugular venous pressure; MAP, mean arterial pressure.

microvasculature, increasing resistance and causing ischemia in the periphery of the clot [62–64]. In this scenario, an elevated MAP might be necessary to preserve adequate regional CBF. These issues raise the theoretic concern that aggressive blood pressure lowering after ICH could cause regional hypoperfusion. However, the concept of perihematomal ischemia has been challenged. Positron emission tomography studies suggest that the perihematomal area has low cerebral metabolic rate for oxygen and reduced CBF, suggesting metabolic suppression rather than ischemia. Furthermore, reduction in the MAP by 15% (143 ± 10 mm Hg to 119 ± 11 mm Hg) in patients with ICH volume less than 45 mL had no effect on periclot CBF or oxygen extraction fraction [65,66].

Apoptosis and necrosis

Mechanical forces that occur during hematoma formation and the chemical toxicity induced by the perihematomal inflammatory reaction may cause necrosis in the adjacent brain tissue [53]. In addition, in a rat model TUNEL-positive stained astrocytes and neurons with morphologies suggesting apoptosis were observed not only in the center but also in the periphery of the hemorrhage, suggesting that programmed cell-death mediates some of the brain injury after ICH [67].

Biochemical mediators of brain injury

Several biochemical mediators have been implicated in secondary brain damage after ICH (Fig. 4).

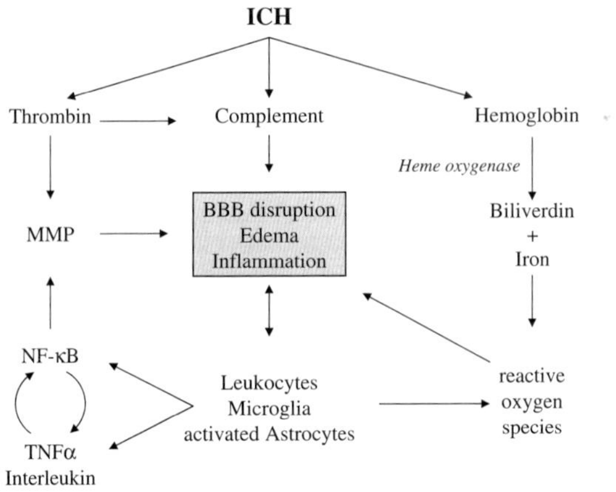

Fig. 4. Simplified mechanism of the underlying inflammation and brain edema formation after ICH. *Abbreviations*: BBB, blood brain barrier; MMP, matrix metalloproteinases; TNFα, tumor necrosis factor alpha.

Thrombin is an essential component of the coagulation cascade, which is activated in ICH. In low concentrations thrombin is necessary to achieve hemostasis. However, in high concentrations, thrombin induces apoptosis and early cytotoxic edema by a direct effect. Furthermore, it can activate the complement cascade and matrix metalloproteinases (MMP) which increase the permeability of the blood brain barrier [52,53].

Delayed brain edema has been attributed, at least in part, to iron and hemoglobin degradation. Hemoglobin is metabolized into iron, carbon monoxide, and biliverdin by heme oxygenase. Studies in animal models show that heme oxygenase inhibition attenuates perihematomal edema and reduces neuronal loss [53]. Furthermore, intracerebral infusion of iron causes brain edema and aggravates thrombin-induced brain edema. In addition, iron induces lipid peroxidation generating reactive oxygen species (ROS), and deferoxamine, an iron chelator, has been shown to reduce edema after experimental ICH [53].

Inflammatory mediators of secondary brain damage

A robust inflammatory reaction occurs in the perihematomal area, contributing to secondary brain damage. Several cellular and molecular inflammatory mediators have been identified.

Cellular mediators

Leukocytes infiltrate the perihematomal area in the first 24 hours. This process peaks on day two or three and disappears by days three to seven. Infiltrating leukocytes secrete proinflammatory mediators and generate ROS [68,69]. Reactive microglia in the perihematomal area has been demonstrated in a rat model as early as 4 hours after induction of ICH. Active microglia can express heme oxygenase, release cytokines (TNFα and interleukins), generate ROS, and contribute significantly to leukocyte recruitment and astrocyte activation in the perihematomal area [51,69,70].

In experimental models of ICH, an initial loss of astrocytes followed by strong astroglial activation in the core and in the perihematomal area has been observed [71,72]. Reactive astrocytes can contribute to local inflammation by secreting metalloproteinases and cytokines (TNFα, interleukins, and INFγ) and by expressing inducible nitric oxide synthase [73]. Astrocytes can also modulate glutamate excitotoxicity and brain inflammation by decreasing the expression of microglial inflammatory mediators [74]. In addition, neurons become more resistant to oxidative stress in the presence of astrocytes, suggesting that astrocytes may influence neuronal survival in the post-ICH period [73].

Molecular mediators

The transcription factor NF-κB and its downstream inflammatory mediators, including TNFα and IL-1β, are activated in the perihematomal area within hours of ICH [75,76]. TNFα and IL-1β are also potent activators of NF-κB, leading to self-perpetuation of the inflammatory response. TNFα and IL-6 have been found to increase in the peripheral blood of patients with spontaneous ICH admitted within 24 hours of onset, and this rise is associated with the magnitude of subsequent perihematomal edema [51]. NF-κB may also contribute to local inflammation by activating heme-oxygenase and thus worsening iron- and ROS-induced toxicity.

MMP are a family of endopeptidases involved in extracellular matrix remodeling. MMP are proposed to have a role in ICH-induced brain blood barrier disruption, thereby contributing to secondary brain damage by increasing vascular permeability and brain edema [68,77]. In a small series of patients with ICH, serum level of MMP-9 correlated with edema, and increased MMP-3 with 30-day mortality [78]. Deletion of the MMP-9 gene was shown to ameliorate edema formation in mouse ICH, supporting the role of this enzyme in secondary brain damage [79].

After an acute ICH, there is a surge of ROS released by neutrophils, vascular endothelium, and activated microglia and macrophages. Iron and iron-containing molecules, such as hemoglobin, can initiate oxidative stress within minutes after ICH. In animal models, other markers of ROS production (such as protein carbonyl and oxidized hydroethidine formation) are elevated in the perihemathomal area [69]. In addition to the direct toxic effect, ROS trigger an inflammatory response by activating NF-κB [51]. Peeling and colleagues [80] showed a significant reduction of the perihematomal neutrophil infiltration 48 hours after ictus using the free-radical-trapping agent NXY-059 in a rat ICH model, suggesting that ROS have an important role in the physiopathology of the inflammatory response.

Although much has been learned about the molecular and cellular mechanisms implicated in ICH, additional work is necessary to determine if pharmacologic manipulation of these mediators can improve outcome after ICH.

Medical management of intracerebral hemorrhage

Airway protection and mechanical ventilation

Patients with large ICH, upper brain stem involvement, or hydrocephalus may have depressed consciousness and are at risk of airway obstruction and aspiration pneumonia. Patients with a Glasgow Coma Scale (GCS) score of less than or equal to 8 are usually intubated and mechanically ventilated. Before intubation, intravenous lidocaine (1 mg/kg–2 mg/kg) may be administered to prevent ICP elevation. Intravenous etomidate (0.1 mg/kg–0.3 mg/kg) or short-acting barbiturates, such as thiopental (1.0 mg/kg–1.5 mg/kg) or propofol (10 mg–20 mg in incremental doses every 10 seconds) may be used for induction. Neuromuscular paralysis, if needed, may be accomplished with short-acting intravenous nondepolarizing agents, such as atracurium besylate (0.3 mg/kg–0.5 mg/kg) and vecuronium bromide 0.01 mg–0.015 mg/kg [81]. Depolarizing agents may increase the ICP in those at risk and should therefore be avoided. Once the airway is secured, mechanical ventilation should be adjusted to ensure adequate ventilation and oxygenation. The role of hyperventilation to treat elevated ICP is discussed below.

Blood pressure control

Elevated blood pressure is common acutely after ICH, even in patients without a prior history of HTN [60,82,83]. In most cases, blood pressure spontaneously declines over 7 to 10 days, and the maximal decline occurs over the first 24 hours [83]. Lowering blood pressure after ICH decreases long-term morbidity and mortality [60]; however, the management of hypertension immediately after ICH is a matter of debate. Issues such as the timing and magnitude of blood pressure lowering are still unsettled.

Proponents of early blood pressure lowering argue that this practice may decrease the risk of hematoma expansion, cerebral edema, and systemic complications. On the other hand, opponents argue that lowering blood pressure may worsen secondary brain damage by causing cerebral ischemia, especially in the perihematomal area.

At the time of this writing, several initiatives are underway in an effort to settle this controversy. The Antihypertensive Treatment in Acute Cerebral Hemorrhage (ATACH), funded by The National Institute of Neurologic Disorders and Stroke, is a multicenter open-labeled pilot trial that plans to recruit a total of 60 subjects with acute supratentorial ICH who will be treated with intravenous nicardipine infusion to achieve the blood pressure goal of 110 mm Hg to 140 mm Hg, 140 mm Hg to 170 mm Hg, or 170 mm Hg to 200 mm Hg. The goal of this trial is to determine tolerability and safety of aggressive pharmacologic reduction of acutely elevated blood pressure after ICH [84]. An interim analysis of 58 patients showed that aggressive systolic blood pressure (SBP) reduction to 110 mm Hg to 140 mm Hg in the first 24 hours after ICH is well tolerated, with a low risk of hematoma expansion ($n = 2$; 3.5%), neurologic deterioration ($n = 3$; 5%), or in-hospital mortality ($n = 2$; 10%); however, the incidence of hematoma expansion was not statistically different among tiers [85].

The multinational phase III open-labeled pilot trial Intensive Blood Reduction in Acute Cerebral Hemorrhage (INTERACT), sponsored by the National Health and Medical Research Council of Australia, is also underway. This study is designed to establish whether lowering acutely elevated high blood pressure in ICH will reduce mortality or dependency at 3 months [86]. In its vanguard phase, subjects with ICH ($n = 404$), presenting within 6 hours of stroke symptoms and SBP between 150 mm Hg and 220 mm Hg, were randomized to receive either intensive antihypertensive treatment (SBP goal of < 140 mm Hg) or a more conservative treatment (SBP goal of < 180 mm Hg). The systolic blood pressure after the first hour of treatment was an average of 14-mm Hg lower in the intensive treatment arm. The average hematoma growth and the frequency of significant hematoma growth (more than one-third the initial volume) were respectively 22.6% (95% CI = −0.6 to −44.6) and 36% (95% CI = 0 to 59) lower in the intensive group than in those patients treated conservatively [87].

Finally, the randomized double-blinded United Kingdom's Control of Hypertension and Hypotension Immediately Post-Stroke trial (CHHIPS) seeks to investigate whether hypertension and relative hypotension, manipulated therapeutically in the first 24 hours following acute stroke, affects short-term outcome [88]. Subjects with an acute ischemic or hemorrhagic stroke within the previous 36 hours and SBP greater than 160 mm Hg are being randomized to receive either antihypertensive drugs (lisinopril or labetalol) or placebo at increasing doses for 14 days to achieve the target SBP of 145 mm Hg to 155 mm Hg or greater than or equal to 15 mm Hg reduction in SBP from baseline values. This trial plans to recruit a total of 1,650 subjects with stroke and hypertension; the interim analysis of 179 subjects showed that the 30-day mortality in the placebo group was 2.2 times higher than in the antihypertensive arm (95% CI = 1.0 to 5.0) [89].

The final results of these clinical trials will help to define optimal hemodynamic parameters for the management of acute ICH. In the interim, the American Heart Association Guidelines for the Management of Spontaneous Intracerebral Hemorrhage in Adults should be consulted for suggested management recommendations (Box 2). If blood pressure lowering is elected, short-acting intravenous medications are preferred (Table 2).

Box 2. American Heart Association guidelines for treating elevated blood pressure after ICH

SBP greater than 200 mm Hg or MAP greater than 150 mm Hg: consider continuous intravenous antihypertensive infusion, with frequent blood pressure monitoring.

SBP greater than 180 mm Hg or MAP greater than 130 mm Hg and evidence of or suspicion of elevated ICP: consider monitoring ICP and intermittent or continuous intravenous antihypertensive medications to maintain cerebral perfusion pressure greater than 60 mm Hg to 80 mm Hg.

SBP greater than 180 mm Hg or MAP greater than 130 mm Hg and no evidence of or suspicion of elevated ICP: consider modest reduction of blood pressure (eg, MAP of 110 mm Hg or target blood pressure of 160/90 mm Hg) using intermittent or continuous antihypertensive intravenous medications and clinically reexamine the patient every 15 minutes

From Broderick J, Connolly S, Feldmann E, et al. American Heart Association; American Stroke Association Stroke Council; High Blood Pressure Research Council; Quality of Care and Outcomes in Research Interdisciplinary Working Group. Guidelines for the management of spontaneous intracerebral hemorrhage in adults: 2007 update: a guideline from the American Heart Association/American Stroke Association Stroke Council, High Blood Pressure Research Council, and the Quality of Care and Outcomes in Research Interdisciplinary Working Group. Stroke 2007;38:2010; with permission.

Intracranial hypertension

The incidence of elevated ICP after ICH is unknown. ICP may be elevated because of increased intracranial content caused by the hematoma mass, cerebral edema, or hydrocephalus. As previously discussed, increased ICP can lower the CPP and, consequently, the CBF causing hypoperfusion (see Fig. 3). Hypoperfusion can trigger reflex vasodilatation, increasing the cerebral blood volume and the ICP in a vicious cycle that can have devastating consequences. Different approaches are available to measure the ICP. The pros and cons of each of these techniques have been reviewed previously and are beyond the scope of this article [57].

In practice, ICP monitoring is often employed in comatose patients (GCS ≤ 8) using a fiberoptic parenchymal probe or an intraventricular catheter. The goal of ICP management is to assure an adequate CBF by targeting an ICP below 20 mm Hg and CPP above 70 mm Hg [57]. This can be achieved by using different approaches. The simplest one is elevating the head of the bed to 30° and keeping the head midline. This may lower the ICP by improving jugular venous outflow without significantly lowering

Table 2
Intravenous medications that may be considered for blood pressure control in patients with ICH

Drug	Intravenous bolus dose	Continuous infusion rate
Labetalol	5 mg–20 mg every 15 min	2 mg/min (max 300 mg/d)
Nicardipine	NA	5 mg–15 mg per hour
Esmolol	250 µg/kg IVP loading dose	25 $\mu g\ kg^{-1}\ min^{-1}$ –300 $\mu g\ kg^{-1}\ min^{-1}$
Enalapril	1.25 mg–5 mg IVP every 6 h[a]	NA
Hydralazine	5 mg–20 mg IVP every 30 min	1.5 $\mu g\ kg^{-1}\ min^{-1}$ –5 $\mu g\ kg^{-1}\ min^{-1}$
Na nitroprusside	NA	0.1 $\mu g\ kg^{-1}\ min^{-1}$ –10 $\mu g\ kg^{-1}\ min^{-1}$

Abbreviations: IVP, intravenous push; NA, not applicable.

[a] Because of the risk of precipitous blood pressure drop, the enalapril first dose should be 0.625 mg.

From Broderick J, Connolly S, Feldmann E, et al. American Heart Association; American Stroke Association Stroke Council; High Blood Pressure Research Council; Quality of Care and Outcomes in Research Interdisciplinary Working Group. Guidelines for the management of spontaneous intracerebral hemorrhage in adults: 2007 update: a guideline from the American Heart Association/American Stroke Association Stroke Council, High Blood Pressure Research Council, and the Quality of Care and Outcomes in Research Interdisciplinary Working Group. Stroke 2007;38:2001–23; with permission.

CPP, CBF, or cardiac output [90,91]. In cases of hypovolemia, this approach can lower the cardiac output and the CBF and should therefore be avoided [90]. In patients with reduced intracranial compliance, agitation and pain can cause ICP elevation. Analgesics, such as morphine or alfentanil, and sedatives, such as propofol, etomidate or midazolam, may lower ICP [92]. However, these medications can also lower the MAP and increase the ICP because of autoregulatory dilation of cerebral vessels; thus, they should only be used with caution.

Hyperventilation, targeting a CO_2 level of 30 mm Hg to 35 mm Hg, is one of the most effective and immediate methods to reduce ICP [93]. However, hypocarbia can lower CBF and has a short-lived effect [93]; furthermore, prolonged severe hyperventilation ($pCO_2 < 25$ mmHg) can cause vasoconstriction and ischemia [90]. Osmotic agents, such as mannitol and hypertonic saline (3%–23.4%) are often used to treat elevated ICP. Mannitol is an osmotically active agent that increases diuresis and lowers the ICP by drawing fluid from edematous and nonedematous brain tissue; however, single-photon emission computed tomography studies did not show evidence of regional CBF changes after mannitol infusion in ICH patients [94]. It has been proposed that by decreasing the blood viscosity, mannitol may cause reflex vasoconstriction and lower the cerebral blood volume [95]. The initial recommended dose of mannitol 20% solution is 0.25 g/kg to 1 g/kg, with repeat doses of 0.25 g/kg to 0.50 g/kg every 3 to 6 hours [90]. The main adverse effects are hypovolemia, worsening of congestive heart failure because of the initial intravascular volume expansion, acute tubular necrosis, and hypokalemia [90]. Intraventricular catheters can be used for CSF drainage. This can effectively lower the ICP, particularly in patients with obstructive hydrocephalus. However, it carries the risk of cerebral hemorrhage and infection and has not been shown to improve outcome [96,97]. In refractory cases of intracranial hypertension, barbiturates in high doses can be effective. Barbiturates decrease cerebral metabolic activity, cerebral blood flow, and ICP [98]. This method requires continuous electroencephalography. The dose of barbiturate (usually pentobarbital) is titrated with the goal of achieving burst suppression activity. Complications of barbiturate administration include decreased systemic vascular resistance and myocardial contractility, arrhythmia, and predisposition to infection [90].

Antithrombotic- and anticoagulant-associated brain hemorrhage

Anticoagulants

The treatment of AAICH begins with rapidly reversing the coagulopathic state to minimize the risk of hematoma expansion. Warfarin has a half-life of 36 to 42 hours and, therefore, its withdrawal alone is not sufficient. Intravenous vitamin K 10 mg takes at least 6 hours to normalize the INR, carries the risk of hypotension and anaphylaxis, and should be infused slowly [99]. Fresh frozen plasma (FFP) can be used to replace vitamin K-dependent coagulation factors. However, FFP requires compatibility and thawing before transfusion; in addition, it can cause allergic reactions and has a variable and unpredictable concentration of individual coagulation factors [100]. Furthermore, at the recommended dose of 15 mL/kg to 20 mL/kg, the large infused volume may cause fluid overload and is time-consuming, making FFP an impractical approach. Prothrombin complex concentrate (PPC) contains factors II, VII, IX, and X. The recommended dose of PPC is calculated according to body weight, degree of INR prolongation, and desired level of correction; typically, dosages are 15 units/kg to 50 units/kg. Unlike FFP, it does not require compatibility or thawing before transfusion, and only small infusion volumes are necessary [100]. Several limited studies suggest that prothrombin complex concentrate corrects a prolonged INR faster than FFP [101–103]; however, an improvement in clinic outcome has not been demonstrated. The main concerns with prothrombin complex concentrate are the potential to induce thrombosis and disseminated intravascular coagulation [57]. Recombinant activated factor VII (rFVIIa) also can correct the INR within minutes of its infusion without the risk of fluid overload and incompatibility seen with FFP [104]. However, it is not clear if INR correction translates to correction of coagulopathy.

Parenteral anticoagulants, such as unfractionated heparin (UH), low molecular weight heparin (LMWH), hirudin derivatives, and argatroban may also cause ICH. The incidence, associated risk factors, and prognosis have not been reported. Intravenous heparin has a half-life of 60 minutes and its effect can be reversed with protamine sulfate (PS). The dose of PS needs to be adjusted according to the time elapsed since the last dose of heparin. The recommended dose of PS is 1 mg per 100 units of UH if the heparin was stopped within the last 30 minutes, 0.5 mg to 0.75 mg per 100 units of UH if stopped for 30 to 60 minutes, 0.375 mg to 0.5 mg per 100 units of UH if stopped for 60 to 120 minutes, and 0.25 mg to 0.375 mg per 100 units of UH if stopped for more than 120 minutes [105]. PS is infused slowly, not exceeding 5 mg per minute because of its risk of causing severe hypotension. Reversal of LMWH with PS is poorly documented or variable in human beings [105,106]. The dose recommended is 1 mg of PS for each millegram of LMWH administered in the last 4 to 8 hours [106]. Hirudin-derived anticoagulants and argatroban are potent thrombin inhibitors. Antidotes are not available; suggested approaches include using desmopressin acetate 0.3 μg/kg, plasma concentrates containing von Willebrand factor, rFVIIa, and dialysis [106].

Antiplatelets

In the acute phase, it is common practice to transfuse five units of platelets to counterbalance the effect of antiplatelet agents [1,106,107]. However, controlled trials addressing the management of ICH in this setting are lacking.

Thrombolytics

The treatment of thrombolytic associated ICH is empiric and includes infusion of six to eight units of platelets and ten units of cryoprecipitate [1,106].

Reinitiating anticoagulant therapy

Whether or not antithrombotic therapy should be restarted and when it is considered safe after ICH is controversial. Published guidelines state that the decision should be individualized [1]. In patients with an expected low risk of cerebral infarction and high risk of CAA, or with poor neurologic function, the possibility of using an antiplatelet agent instead of anticoagulants may be considered [1]. In those patients with high risk of thromboembolism in whom reinitiating anticoagulation is deemed necessary, warfarin may be restarted 7 to 10 days after ICH [1].

Antiepileptic drugs

Seizures are common after ICH. In a large clinical series, the overall 30-day seizure incidence was 8.1% [108]. However, seizure risk may vary by ICH location. In the Northern Manhattan Stroke Study, seizures were seen in 14% of subjects with lobar and 4% of subjects with deep ICH in the first 7 days [109]. Studies using continuous electrographic monitoring have reported a much higher (28%–31%) incidence of seizures. Over half were clinically unrecognized [110,111]. Electrographic seizures have been associated with expanding hematoma and lobar ICH [110,112]. Seizures increase the cerebral metabolic rate that can increase CBF and ICP, even in patients who are sedated or paralyzed [91]. Pharmacologic seizure management commonly includes the use of intravenous antiepileptic medications. The most commonly used medications are benzodiazepines, such as lorazepam or diazepam, followed by phenytoin or fos-phenytoin. Valproic acid and phenobarbital are used less often. Levetiracetam is a newer anticonvulsant that is also increasingly being used in the management of critically ill patients [113]. It has a more benign adverse effect profile and fewer drug interactions than older anticonvulsants.

Hemostatic therapy

A phase II clinical trial in spontaneous ICH suggested that rFVIIa might limit hematoma growth, reduce mortality, and improve functional outcomes at 90 days with a small increased frequency of thromboembolic adverse events [48]. Unfortunately, the survival benefit and improved functional outcome were not reproduced in a larger phase III trial [114]. A post hoc exploratory analysis showed that with an earlier treatment window and exclusion of known determinants of poor outcome at baseline (age and magnitude of ICH and intraventricular hemorrhage), a subgroup of ICH patients may still benefit from rFVIIa [115]. Although promising, the role of this drug in ICH management is still uncertain.

General medical management

Glucose

Hyperglycemia (> 140 mg/dL) is common after ICH in diabetic and nondiabetic patients, and elevated glucose level has been associated with increased mortality [116–118]. Thus, there is general consensus that hyperglycemia should be treated in these patients [1]. Of note, a significant association has been observed between admission blood glucose and higher MAP, larger hematoma volume, greater lateral shift of cerebral midline structures, intraventricular and subarachnoid extension, hydrocephalus, and disturbed consciousness, which are all markers of ICH severity [118]. This suggests that hyperglycemia may be a stress reaction to ICH rather than the direct cause of increased brain damage and higher mortality. Clinical trials to define the optimal approach to hyperglycemia in acute ICH are needed. In lieu of additional data, published guidelines recommend treatment with insulin for glucose of greater than 185 (and possibly > 140) [1].

Temperature management

The incidence of hyperthermia in ICH is high, especially in patients with intraventricular hemorrhage. One study reported elevated temperature on admission in 19% of patients with ICH, and in almost 91% of the patients during the first 72 hours after hospitalization [119]. Fever is associated with early neurologic deterioration and is a poor outcome risk factor in ICH [68,119]. Fever should trigger aggressive assessment for an infectious source, which should be promptly treated with an appropriate antibiotic regimen. Elevated temperature may be treated pharmacologically using antipyretics, or mechanically, using surface or intravascular cooling devices. The role of hypothermia as a possible neuroprotectant strategy is under investigation [120–122].

Fluids

Hypovolemia can decrease cerebral and systemic organ perfusion and should be avoided. Hypo-osmolarity may lead to fluid shifts that can worsen cerebral edema and increase secondary brain damage. Additionally, the blood-brain barrier in ICH is disrupted and allows molecules, such as glucose, to extravasate from the intravascular to the extracellular space. Glucose is an osmotically active molecule that can draw water into the interstitium, further worsening cerebral edema; thus, glucose-containing fluids should be avoided except in patients with hypoglycemia. Isotonic intravenous saline should be infused to maintain an euvolemic state.

Deep venous thrombosis prophylaxis

ICH patients are at risk of developing deep venous thrombosis (DVT) and pulmonary embolism (PE) because of prolonged immobilization. A retrospective study of 1,926 consecutive patients with ICH reported the incidence of DVT to be 1.9% [123]. In another study, asymptomatic DVT was detected by lower extremity Doppler at day 10 in about 16% of the ICH patients wearing elastic stockings alone, and in 4.7% of those using elastic stockings and intermittent pneumatic compression devices [124]. DVT prophylaxis initiated on day two after ICH with 5,000 units of heparin subcutaneously three times daily has been reported to be safe without increasing the risk of rebleeding [125]. However, the safety of more aggressive anticoagulation in patients with ICH who develop DVT or PE is unclear. Until further study, immediately after ICH, patients with DVT or PE should be considered for inferior vena cava filter placement.

Nutrition

Dysphagia is common after ICH. Because of increased aspiration risk, patients with stroke are usually kept on a nothing-by-mouth regimen over the first few days after admission. It is during the first week that a hypermetabolic state with increased catabolism of protein and fat occurs [126]. Measuring biochemical and anthropometric parameters during the first week after admission, a small study observed that almost 62% of consecutive ICH patients are malnourished or undernourished [127]. In the large multicenter Feed or Ordinary Food trial, the initiation of tube feeding within the first 7 days after stroke showed a 5.8% (95% CI = −0.8 to 12.5) absolute reduction in case fatality compared with those in whom tube feeding initiation was delayed for more than 7 days [128]. The caloric and nutritional requirements of ICH patient should be monitored closely and enteral feeding should be initiated as early as possible to avoid undernourishment and reduce stress gastritis risk.

Summary

Knowledge of the underlying mechanisms of neural injury after ICH, as well as its associated complications, has markedly increased over the last 10 years. However, further research is needed to answer key questions regarding the management of ICH patients.

References

[1] Broderick J, Connolly S, Feldmann E, et al. American Heart Association; American Stroke Association Stroke Council High Blood Pressure Research Council; Quality of Care and Outcomes in Research Interdisciplinary Working Group. Guidelines for the management of spontaneous intracerebral hemorrhage in adults: 2007 update: a guideline from the American Heart Association/American Stroke Association Stroke Council, High Blood Pressure Research Council, and the Quality of Care and Outcomes in Research Interdisciplinary Working Group. Stroke 2007;38:2001–23.

[2] Kissela B, Schneider A, Kleindorfer D, et al. Stroke in a biracial population: the excess burden of stroke among blacks. Stroke 2004;35:426–31.

[3] Counsell C, Boonyakarnkul S, Dennis M, et al. Primary intracerebral haemorrhage in the Oxfordshire Community Stroke Project. Cerebrovasc Dis 1995;5:26–34.

[4] Qureshi AI, Suri MF, Nasar A, et al. Changes in cost and outcome among US patients with stroke hospitalized in 1990 to 1991 and those hospitalized in 2000 to 2001. Stroke 2007;38:2180–4.

[5] Foulkes MA, Wolf PA, Price TR, et al. The stroke data bank: design, methods, and baseline characteristics. Stroke 1988;19:547–54.

[6] Brott T, Thalinger K, Hertzberg V. Hypertension as a risk factor for spontaneous intracerebral hemorrhage. Stroke 1986;17:1078–83.

[7] Woo D, Haverbusch M, Sekar P, et al. Effect of untreated hypertension on hemorrhagic stroke. Stroke 2004;35:1703–8.

[8] Sutherland GR, Auer RN. Primary intracerebral hemorrhage. J Clin Neurosci 2006;13: 511–7.

[9] Fisher CM. Hypertensive cerebral hemorrhage. Demonstration of the source of bleeding. J Neuropathol Exp Neurol 2003;62:104–7.

[10] Cole FM, Yates P. Intracerebral microaneurysms and small cerebrovascular lesions. Brain 1967;90:759–68.

[11] Takebayashi S, Kaneko M. Electron microscopic studies of ruptured arteries in hypertensive intracerebral hemorrhage. Stroke 1983;14:28–36.

[12] Manno EM, Atkinson JL, Fulgham JR, et al. Emerging medical and surgical management strategies in the evaluation and treatment of intracerebral hemorrhage. Mayo Clin Proc 2005;80:420–33.

[13] Vinters HV. Cerebral amyloid angiopathy. A critical review. Stroke 1987;18:311–24.

[14] Vinters HV. Imaging cerebral microvascular amyloid. Ann Neurol 2007;62:209–12.

[15] O'Donnell HC, Rosand J, Knudsen KA, et al. Apolipoprotein E genotype and the risk of recurrent lobar intracerebral hemorrhage. N Engl J Med 2000;342:240–5.

[16] Tzourio C, Arima H, Harrap S, et al. APOE genotype, ethnicity, and the risk of cerebral hemorrhage. Neurology 2008 [epub ahead of print].

[17] Flaherty ML, Kissela B, Woo D, et al. The increasing incidence of anticoagulant-associated intracerebral hemorrhage. Neurology 2007;68:116–21.
[18] Hirsh J. Oral anticoagulants: mechanism of action, clinical effectiveness, and optimal therapeutic range. Chest 2001;119:8S–21S.
[19] Punthakee X, Doobay J, Anand SS. Oral-anticoagulant-related intracerebral hemorrhage. Thromb Res 2002;108:31–6.
[20] Nilsson OG, Lindgren A, Ståhl N, et al. Incidence of intracerebral and subarachnoid haemorrhage in southern Sweden. J Neurol Neurosurg Psychiatry 2000;69:601–7.
[21] Rosand J, Eckman MH, Knudsen KA, et al. The effect of warfarin and intensity of anticoagulation on outcome of intracerebral hemorrhage. Arch Intern Med 2004;164:880–4.
[22] Hart RG, Tonarelli SB, Pearce LA. Avoiding central nervous system bleeding during antithrombotic therapy: recent data and ideas. Stroke 2005;36:1588–93.
[23] Flibotte JJ, Hagan N, O'Donnell J, et al. Warfarin, hematoma expansion, and outcome of intracerebral hemorrhage. Neurology 2004;63:1059–64.
[24] Yasaka M, Minematsu K, Naritomi H, et al. Predisposing factors for enlargement of intracerebral hemorrhage in patients treated with warfarin. Thromb Haemost 2003;89:278–83.
[25] Rosand J, Hylek EM, O'Donnell HC, et al. Warfarin-associated hemorrhage and cerebral amyloid angiopathy: a genetic and pathologic study. Neurology 2000;55:947–51.
[26] Smith EE, Rosand J, Knudsen KA, et al. Leukoaraiosis is associated with warfarin-related hemorrhage following ischemic stroke. Neurology 2002;59:193–7.
[27] Fang MC, Chang Y, Hylek EM, et al. Anticoagulation intensity, and risk for intracranial hemorrhage among patients taking warfarin for atrial fibrillation. Ann Intern Med 2004; 141:745–52.
[28] Lacut K, Le Gal G, Seizeur R, et al. Antiplatelet drug use preceding the onset of intracerebral hemorrhage is associated with increased mortality. Fundam Clin Pharmacol 2007;21: 327–33.
[29] Roquer J, Rodríguez Campello A, Gomis M, et al. Previous antiplatelet therapy is an independent predictor of 30-day mortality after spontaneous supratentorial intracerebral hemorrhage. J Neurol 2005;252:412–6.
[30] Saloheimo P, Ahonen M, Juvela S, et al. Regular aspirin-use preceding the onset of primary intracerebral hemorrhage is an independent predictor for death. Stroke 2006;37:129–33.
[31] Choi NK, Park BJ, Jeong SW, et al. Nonaspirin nonsteroidal anti-inflammatory drugs and hemorrhagic stroke risk: the Acute Brain Bleeding Analysis study. Stroke 2008;39: 845–9.
[32] Viswanathan A, Rakich SM, Engel C, et al. Antiplatelet use after intracerebral hemorrhage. Neurology 2006;66:206–9.
[33] Sansing LH, Messe SR, Cucchiara BL, et al. For the CHANT Investigators. Antiplatelet medications and hemorrhage growth after intracerebral hemorrhage. 2008 International Stroke Conference Poster Presentation. Stroke 2008;39(2):529.
[34] The NINDS t-PA Stroke Study Group. Intracerebral hemorrhage after intravenous t-PA therapy for ischemic stroke. Stroke 1997;28:2109–18.
[35] Cabañas JG. Thrombolytic therapy. Available at: http://www.emedicine.com/emerg/TOPIC831.HTM. Accessed online on May 6, 2008.
[36] Flaherty ML, Woo D, Haverbusch M, et al. Racial variations in location and risk of intracerebral hemorrhage. Stroke 2005;36:934–7.
[37] Maia LF, Mackenzie IR, Feldman HH. Clinical phenotypes of cerebral amyloid angiopathy. J Neurol Sci 2007;257:23–30.
[38] Brott T, Broderick J, Kothari R, et al. Early hemorrhage growth in patients with intracerebral hemorrhage. Stroke 1997;28:1–5.
[39] Kazui S, Naritomi H, Yamamoto H, et al. Enlargement of spontaneous intracerebral hemorrhage. Incidence and time course. Stroke 1996;27:1783–7.
[40] Broderick JP, Brott TG, Duldner JE, et al. Volume of intracerebral hemorrhage. A powerful and easy-to-use predictor of 30-day mortality. Stroke 1993;24:987–93.

[41] Davis SM, Broderick J, Hennerici M, et al. Recombinant Activated Factor VII Intracerebral Hemorrhage Trial Investigators. Hematoma growth is a determinant of mortality and poor outcome after intracerebral hemorrhage. Neurology 2006;66:1175–81.
[42] Jauch EC, Lindsell CJ, Adeoye O, et al. Lack of evidence for an association between hemodynamic variables and hematoma growth in spontaneous intracerebral hemorrhage. Stroke 2006;37:2061–5.
[43] Kazui S, Minematsu K, Yamamoto H, et al. Predisposing factors to enlargement of spontaneous intracerebral hematoma. Stroke 1997;28:2370–5.
[44] Ohwaki K, Yano E, Nagashima H, et al. Blood pressure management in acute intracerebral hemorrhage: relationship between elevated blood pressure and hematoma enlargement. Stroke 2004;35:1364–7.
[45] Diringer MN, Edwards DF, Zazulia AR. Hydrocephalus: a previously unrecognized predictor of poor outcome from supratentorial intracerebral hemorrhage. Stroke 1998;7:1352–7.
[46] Ozdemir O, Calisaneller T, Hastürk A, et al. Prognostic significance of third ventricle dilation in spontaneous intracerebral hemorrhage: a preliminary clinical study. Neurol Res 2008 [epub ahead of print].
[47] Shapiro SA, Campbell RL, Scully T. Hemorrhagic dilation of the fourth ventricle: an ominous predictor. J Neurosurg 1994;80:805–9.
[48] Mayer SA, Brun NC, Begtrup K, et al. Recombinant Activated Factor VII Intracerebral Hemorrhage Trial Investigators. Recombinant activated factor VII for acute intracerebral hemorrhage. N Engl J Med 2005;352:777–85.
[49] Xi G, Keep RF, Hoff JT. Pathophysiology of brain edema formation. Neurosurg Clin N Am 2002;13:371–83.
[50] Butcher KS, Baird T, MacGregor L, et al. Perihematomal edema in primary intracerebral hemorrhage is plasma derived. Stroke 2004;35:1879–85.
[51] Aronowski J, Hall CE. New horizons for primary intracerebral hemorrhage treatment: experience from preclinical studies. Neurol Res 2005;27:268–79.
[52] Hua Y, Keep RF, Hoff JT, et al. Brain injury after intracerebral hemorrhage: the role of thrombin and iron. Stroke 2007;38:759–62.
[53] Xi G, Keep R, Hoff J. Mechanisms of brain injury after intracerebral haemorrhage. Lancet Neurol 2006;5:53–63.
[54] Gebel JM Jr, Jauch EC, Brott TG, et al. Natural history of perihematomal edema in patients with hyperacute spontaneous intracerebral hemorrhage. Stroke 2002;33:2631–5.
[55] Zazulia AR, Diringer MN, Derdeyn CP, et al. Progression of mass effect after intracerebral hemorrhage. Stroke 1999;30:1167–73.
[56] Powers WJ. Hemodynamics and metabolism in ischemic cerebrovascular disease. Neurol Clin 1992;10:31–48.
[57] Steiner LA, Andrews PJ. Monitoring the injured brain: ICP and CBF. Br J Anaesth 2006;97:26–38.
[58] Andrews PJ, Citerio G. Intracranial pressure. Part one: historical overview and basic concepts. Intensive Care Med 2004;30:1730–3.
[59] Strandgaard S, Paulson OB. Cerebral autoregulation. Stroke 1984;15:413–6.
[60] Shah QA, Ezzeddine MA, Qureshi AI. Acute hypertension in intracerebral hemorrhage: pathophysiology and treatment. J Neurol Sci 2007;261:74–9.
[61] Paulson OB, Strandgaard S, Edvinsson L. Cerebral autoregulation. Cerebrovasc Brain Metab Rev 1990;2:161–92.
[62] Kidwell CS, Saver JL, Mattiello J, et al. Diffusion-perfusion MR evaluation of perihematomal injury in hyperacute intracerebral hemorrhage. Neurology 2001;57:1611–7.
[63] Schellinger PD, Fiebach JB, Hoffmann K, et al. Stroke MRI in intracerebral hemorrhage: is there a perihemorrhagic penumbra? Stroke 2003;34:1674–9.

[64] Warach S. Is there a perihematomal ischemic penumbra? More questions and an overlooked clue. Stroke 2003;34:1680.
[65] Powers WJ, Zazulia AR, Videen TO, et al. Autoregulation of cerebral blood flow surrounding acute (6 to 22 hours) intracerebral hemorrhage. Neurology 2001;57:18–24.
[66] Zazulia AR, Diringer MN, Videen TO, et al. Hypoperfusion without ischemia surrounding acute intracerebral hemorrhage. J Cereb Blood Flow Metab 2001;21: 804–10.
[67] Matsushita K, Meng W, Wang X, et al. Evidence for apoptosis after intercerebral hemorrhage in rat striatum. J Cereb Blood Flow Metab 2000;20:396–404.
[68] Leira R, Dávalos A, Silva Y, et al. Stroke Project, Cerebrovascular Diseases Group of the Spanish Neurological Society. Early neurologic deterioration in intracerebral hemorrhage: predictors and associated factors. Neurology 2004;63:461–7.
[69] Wang J, Doré S. Inflammation after intracerebral hemorrhage. J Cereb Blood Flow Metab 2007;27:894–908.
[70] Hanisch UK. Microglia as a source and target of cytokines. Glia 2002;40:140–55.
[71] Koeppen AH, Dickson AC, McEvoy JA. The cellular reactions to experimental intracerebral hemorrhage. J Neurol Sci 1995;134(Suppl):102–12.
[72] Kowiański P, Karwacki Z, Dziewiatkowski J, et al. Evolution of microglial and astroglial response during experimental intracerebral haemorrhage in the rat. Folia Neuropathol 2003;41:123–30.
[73] Swanson RA, Ying W, Kauppinen TM. Astrocyte influences on ischemic neuronal death. Curr Mol Med 2004;4:193–205.
[74] Pyo H, Yang MS, Jou I, et al. Wortmannin enhances lipopolysaccharide-induced inducible nitric oxide synthase expression in microglia in the presence of astrocytes in rats. Neurosci Lett 2003;346:141–4.
[75] Hickenbottom SL, Grotta JC, Strong R, et al. Nuclear factor-kappaB and cell death after experimental intracerebral hemorrhage in rats. Stroke 30:2472–7.
[76] Zhou J, Ando H, Macova M, et al. Angiotensin II AT1 receptor blockade abolishes brain microvascular inflammation and heat shock protein responses in hypertensive rats. J Cereb Blood Flow Metab 2005;25:878–86.
[77] Rosengerg GA, Navratil M. Metalloproteinase inhibition blocks edema in intracerebral hemorrhage in the rat. Neurology 1997;48:921–6.
[78] Alvarez-Sabín J, Delgado P, Abilleira S, et al. Temporal profile of matrix metalloproteinases and their inhibitors after spontaneous intracerebral hemorrhage: relationship to clinical and radiological outcome. Stroke 2004;35:1316–22.
[79] Tejima E, Zhao BQ, Tsuji K, et al. Astrocytic induction of matrix metalloproteinase-9 and edema in brain hemorrhage. J Cereb Blood Flow Metab 2007;27:460–8.
[80] Peeling J, Del Bigio MR, Corbett D, et al. Efficacy of disodium 4-[(tert-butylimino)methyl]-benzene-1,3-disulfonate N-oxide (NXY-059), a free radical trapping agent, in a rat model of hemorrhagic stroke. Neuropharmacology 2001;40:433–9.
[81] Diringer MN. Intracerebral hemorrhage: pathophysiology and management. Crit Care Med 1993;21:1591–603.
[82] Carlberg B, Asplund K, Hägg E. Factors influencing admission blood pressure levels in patients with acute stroke. Stroke 1991;22:527–30.
[83] Rasool AH, Rahman AR, Choudhury SR, et al. Blood pressure in acute intracerebral haemorrhage. J Hum Hypertens 2004;18:187–92.
[84] Qureshi AI. Antihypertensive treatment of acute cerebral hemorrhage (ATACH): rationale and design. Neurocrit Care 2007;6:56–66.
[85] Qureshi AI. Antihypertensive treatment of acute cerebral hemorrhage (ATACH). 2008 International Stroke Conference. Scientific e-posters. Available at: http://asa.scientificposters.com/epsView.cfm?pid=LBP1&yr=2008. Accessed April 08, 2008.

[86] Stroke trials registry. Available at: http://www.strokecenter.org/trials/TrialDetail.aspx?tid=569. Accessed April 08, 2008.
[87] Anderson CS, Huang Y, Wang JG, et al. For the INTERACT Investigators. Intensive blood pressure reduction in acute cerebral haemorrhage trial (INTERACT): a randomised pilot trial. Lancet Neurol 2008;7:391–9.
[88] Potter J, Robinson T, Ford G, et al. The CHHIPS Trial Group. CHHIPS (Controlling hypertension and hypotension immediately post-stroke) pilot trial: rationale and design. J Hypertens 2005;23:649–55.
[89] Potter JF. Controlling hypertension and hypotension immediately post-stroke (CHHIPS). 2008 International Stroke Conference. Late-breaking science news. Available at: http://www.scienceondemand.org/stroke2008/sessions/player.html?sid=080201100.4626. Accessed May 04, 2008.
[90] Mayer SA, Chong JY. Critical care management of increased intracranial pressure. J Intensive Care Med 2002;17:55–67.
[91] Ng I, Lim J, Wong HB. Effects of head posture on cerebral hemodynamics: its influences on intracranial pressure, cerebral perfusion pressure, and cerebral oxygenation. Neurosurgery 2004;54:593–7.
[92] Citerio G, Cormio M. Sedation in neurointensive care: advances in understanding and practice. Curr Opin Crit Care 2003;9:120–6.
[93] Stocchetti N, Maas AI, Chieregato A, et al. Hyperventilation in head injury: a review. Chest 2005;127:1812–27.
[94] Kalita J, Misra UK, Ranjan P, et al. Effect of mannitol on regional cerebral blood flow in patients with intracerebral hemorrhage. J Neurol Sci 2004;224:19–22.
[95] Andrews RJ, Bringas JR, Muto RP. Effects of mannitol on cerebral blood flow, blood pressure, blood viscosity, hematocrit, sodium, and potassium. Surg Neurol 1993;39:218–22.
[96] Adams RE, Diringer MN. Response to external ventricular drainage in spontaneous intracerebral hemorrhage with hydrocephalus. Neurology 1998;50:519–23.
[97] Dasic D, Hanna SJ, Bojanic S, et al. External ventricular drain infection: the effect of a strict protocol on infection rates and a review of the literature. Br J Neurosurg 2006;20:296–300.
[98] Sacco S, Marini C, Carolei A. Medical treatment of intracerebral hemorrhage. Neurol Sci 2004;25(Suppl 1):S6–9.
[99] Raj G, Kumar R, McKinney WP. Time course of reversal of anticoagulant effect of warfarin by intravenous and subcutaneous phytonadione. Arch Intern Med 1999;159:2721–4.
[100] Steiner T, Rosand J, Diringer M. Intracerebral hemorrhage associated with oral anticoagulant therapy: current practices and unresolved questions. Stroke 2006;37:256–62.
[101] Siddiq F, Jalil A, McDaniel C, et al. Effectiveness of factor IX complex concentrate in reversing warfarin associated coagulopathy for intracerebral hemorrhage. Neurocrit Care 2008;8:36–41.
[102] Boulis NM, Bobek MP, Schmaier A, et al. Use of factor IX complex in warfarin-related intracranial hemorrhage. Neurosurgery 1999;45:1113–8.
[103] Evans G, Luddington R, Baglin T. Beriplex P/N reverses severe warfarin-induced overanticoagulation immediately and completely in patients presenting with major bleeding. Br J Haematol 2001;115:998–1001.
[104] Aguilar MI, Hart RG, Kase CS, et al. Treatment of warfarin-associated intracerebral hemorrhage: literature review and expert opinion. Mayo Clin Proc 2007;82:82–92.
[105] Schulman S, Bijsterveld NR. Anticoagulants and their reversal. Transfus Med Rev 2007;21:37–48.
[106] Powner DJ, Hartwell EA, Hoots WK. Counteracting the effects of anticoagulants and antiplatelet agents during neurosurgical emergencies. Neurosurgery 2005;57:823–31.
[107] Vilahur G, Choi BG, Zafar MU, et al. Normalization of platelet reactivity in clopidogrel-treated subjects. J Thromb Haemost 2007;5:82–90.
[108] Passero S, Rocchi R, Rossi S, et al. Seizures after spontaneous supratentorial intracerebral hemorrhage. Epilepsia 2002;43:1175–80.

[109] Labovitz DL, Hauser WA, Sacco RL. Prevalence and predictors of early seizure and status epilepticus after first stroke. Neurology 2001;57:200–6.

[110] Claassen J, Jetté N, Chum F, et al. Electrographic seizures and periodic discharges after intracerebral hemorrhage. Neurology 2007;69:1356–65.

[111] Vespa PM, O'Phelan K, Shah M, et al. Acute seizures after intracerebral hemorrhage: a factor in progressive midline shift and outcome. Neurology 2003;60:1441–6.

[112] De Reuck J, Hemelsoet D, Van Maele G. Seizures and epilepsy in patients with a spontaneous intracerebral haematoma. Clin Neurol Neurosurg 2007;109:501–4.

[113] Szaflarski JP, Meckler JM, Szaflarski M, et al. Levetiracetam use in critically ill patients. Neurocrit Care 2007;7:140–7.

[114] Mayer SA, Brun NC, Begtrup K, et al. FAST Trial Investigators. Efficacy and safety of recombinant activated factor VII for acute intracerebral hemorrhage. N Engl J Med 2008;358:2127–37.

[115] Mayer SA, Davis SM, Begtrup K, et al. Subgroup analysis in the fast trial: a subset of intracerebral hemorrhage patients that benefit from recombinant activated Factor VII? 2008 International Stroke Conference poster presentation. Stroke 2008;39(2):528.

[116] Kimura K, Iguchi Y, Inoue T, et al. Hyperglycemia independently increases the risk of early death in acute spontaneous intracerebral hemorrhage. J Neurol Sci 2007;255:90–4.

[117] Godoy DA, Di Napoli M. Hyperglycemia in acute phase of spontaneous intracerebral hemorrhage (sICH). J Neurol Sci 2007;263:228–9.

[118] Fogelholm R, Murros K, Rissanen A, et al. Admission blood glucose and short term survival in primary intracerebral haemorrhage: a population based study. J Neurol Neurosurg Psychiatry 2005;76:349–53.

[119] Schwarz S, Häfner K, Aschoff A, et al. Incidence and prognostic significance of fever following intracerebral hemorrhage. Neurology 2000;54:354–61.

[120] Diringer MN, Neurocritical Care Fever Reduction Trial Group. Treatment of fever in the neurologic intensive care unit with a catheter-based heat exchange system. Crit Care Med 2004;32:559–64.

[121] Gupta R, Jovin TG, Krieger DW. Therapeutic hypothermia for stroke: do new outfits change an old friend? Expert Rev Neurother 2005;5:235–46.

[122] Fingas M, Clark DL, Colbourne F. The effects of selective brain hypothermia on intracerebral hemorrhage in rats. Exp Neurol 2007;208:277–84.

[123] Gregory PC, Kuhlemeier KV. Prevalence of venous thromboembolism in acute hemorrhagic and thromboembolic stroke. Am J Phys Med Rehabil 2003;82:364–9.

[124] Lacut K, Bressollette L, Le Gal G, et al. VICTORIAh(Venous Intermittent Compression and Thrombosis Occurrence Related to Intra-cerebral Acute hemorrhage) Investigators. Prevention of venous thrombosis in patients with acute intracerebral hemorrhage. Neurology 2005;65:865–9.

[125] Boeer A, Voth E, Henze T, et al. Early heparin therapy in patients with spontaneous intracerebral haemorrhage. J Neurol Neurosurg Psychiatry 1991;54:466–7.

[126] Touho H, Karasawa J, Shishido H, et al. Hypermetabolism in the acute stage of hemorrhagic cerebrovascular disease. J Neurosurg 1990;72:710–4.

[127] Choi-Kwon S, Yang YH, Kim EK, et al. Nutritional status in acute stroke: undernutrition versus overnutrition in different stroke subtypes. Acta Neurol Scand 1998;98:187–92.

[128] Dennis MS, Lewis SC, Warlow C et al. FOOD Trial Collaboration. Effect of timing and method of enteral tube feeding for dysphagic stroke patients (FOOD): a multicentre randomised controlled trial. Lancet 2005;365:764–72.

ELSEVIER
SAUNDERS

Neurol Clin 26 (2008) 987–1005

NEUROLOGIC
CLINICS

Surgical Management of Acute Intracranial Hemorrhage, Surgical Aneurysmal and Arteriovenous Malformation Ablation, and Other Surgical Principles

William W. Ashley, Jr, MD, PhD, MBA,
Fady T. Charbel, MD,
Sepideh Amin-Hanjani, MD*

Department of Neurosurgery, University of Illinois at Chicago, 912 South Wood Street (MC 799), Chicago, IL 60612, USA

As discussed earlier in this issue, strokes can be broadly classified into ischemic and hemorrhagic variants, with hemorrhagic strokes accounting for approximately 13% of all strokes [1]. Although hemorrhagic strokes are much less common, they carry a disproportionate burden of the mortality. Hemorrhagic stroke has a 30-day mortality rate of 37% to 38% compared with only 8% to 12% for ischemic stroke [1]. For hemorrhagic stroke due to aneurysmal subarachnoid hemorrhage (SAH) or arteriovenous malformation (AVM), surgery is often the first-line approach. The benefit of surgical treatment for spontaneous hemorrhagic stroke is still controversial.

In light of the potentially devastating effects of hemorrhagic stroke, it is critical that an effective treatment paradigm be defined. This report briefly reviews the various subtypes of hemorrhagic stroke, considers the indications for surgery, and discusses specific surgical treatment options.

Hemorrhagic stroke subtypes

There are a variety of stroke classification systems and multiple subtypes. For the purposes of this article, hemorrhagic stroke is subdivided into three

* Corresponding author.
E-mail address: hanjani@uic.edu (S. Amin-Hanjani).

0733-8619/08/$ - see front matter
doi:10.1016/j.ncl.2008.06.006

groups based on the underlying pathophysiology—spontaneous, vascular lesional, and treatment related. These groupings are practical for conceptualizing the role of surgery in the overall treatment strategy.

Spontaneous hemorrhagic stroke, also known as primary intracerebral hemorrhage (ICH), comprises 87% of hemorrhagic strokes and is generally attributable to hypertension or amyloid angiopathy [2–4] but may also be related to inherited bleeding disorders or hepatic failure [5,6]. Hypertensive hemorrhages are often associated with chronic hypertensive microvascular degeneration and subsequent lipohyalinosis or possible formation of fragile Charcot-Bouchard microaneuryms that may rupture [2–4]. In general, this disease occurs more commonly in men than women and at a younger age than ischemic stroke. It often causes large deep hemorrhages predominantly in the basal ganglia, thalamus, pons, and cerebellum [3,7,8]. Amyloid angiopathy tends to form fluffy lobar hemorrhages in older persons secondary to the accumulation of amyloid protein in microvessel walls. The outcome of a spontaneous hemorrhagic stroke can be predicted by the patient's age, condition at presentation, and medical comorbidities, the time to treatment initiation, the location of the hemorrhage, and, most importantly, the hematoma volume [5,7].

Vascular and other secondary causes account for approximately 13% of ICHs. SAH is a relatively common form of hemorrhagic stroke and is usually caused by a ruptured cerebral aneurysm or, less commonly, an AVM rupture. Other causes include cavernomas, dural arteriovenous fistulae (AVF), telangiectasias, and other vasculopathic conditions including moyamoya syndrome and drug-induced vasculopathy. The initial clinical condition of the patient, the size and location of the vascular lesion, the volume and location of the blood, and the time to treatment are predictors of outcomes for this group [3,5,6,8]. A detailed discussion of each vascular lesion is beyond the scope of this report.

Iatrogenic ICH is the result of medical therapy and includes hemorrhage after thrombolysis or anticoagulation, reperfusion hemorrhage after carotid revascularization, breakthrough hemorrhage after AVM resection, and bleeding secondary to endovascular intervention.

Spontaneous hemorrhagic stroke

In 1961 McKissock and colleagues [9] reported the first randomized, prospective, controlled trial which suggested that surgical evacuation was not beneficial for treating ICH. In total, 12 prospective randomized trials have investigated the role of surgical evacuation in the treatment of ICH [10–19]. In summary, these results have shown that surgery does not significantly improve outcomes when compared with medical therapy alone. In 2005 the landmark Surgical Trial in Intracerebral Hemorrhage (STICH) study prospectively examined the role of surgery in 1033 patients. Surgical clot removal within 24 hours of spontaneous supratentorial ICH was of no significant benefit [10]; however, the STICH results must be interpreted with caution because high crossover from the medical group to surgery (140 out of 530 patients) and the lack of clinical equipoise regarding surgical evacuation of large lobar hematomas and nondominant hemisphere hematomas leading to nonrandomization into STICH may have resulted in bias favoring medical treatment [19]. A meta-analysis examining mortality in these 12 studies [18,19] reported 392 of 1182 (33%) deaths in the medical group versus 346 of 1183 (29%) in the surgical group. Although no statistically significant benefit can be attributed to surgical treatment, the trend favoring surgery is seen despite imminently herniating and deteriorating patients being excluded from the trials.

Although the preponderance of evidence suggests that routine surgical evacuation of supratentorial hematomas is not superior to medical treatment alone, surgery may be beneficial in a subset of patients. Post hoc analyses of the aforementioned studies suggest that surgery via craniotomy shows a trend toward benefit in patients with superficial clots located less than 1 cm from the surface and those with moderate initial impairment (Glasgow coma score [GCS], 9–12) and subsequent deterioration [18]. Despite a paucity of class I data regarding cerebellar hematomas, retrospective data suggest that surgical evacuation for patients with clots larger than 3 cm, hydrocephalus, or evidence of brainstem compression leads to improved outcomes [19–25]. Both the American Heart Association [20] (AHA) and European Stroke Initiative writing committee [19] (EUSI) guidelines recommend considering surgery in these limited situations. The AHA recommends, "For patients presenting with lobar clots within 1 cm of the surface, evacuation of supratentorial ICH by standard craniotomy might be considered" (Fig. 1). "Patients with cerebellar hemorrhage >3 cm who are deteriorating neurologically or who have brainstem compression and/or hydrocephalus from ventricular obstruction should have surgical removal of the hemorrhage as soon as possible (Class I, Level of Evidence B)" (Fig. 2). Likewise the EUSI states, "Consider craniotomy if there is deterioration in consciousness (from a GCS level of between 12 and 9 to <8), if the ICH is superficial (the clot is subcortical <1 cm from the surface and does not reach the deep basal ganglia), or if it is located in the cerebellum."

Otherwise, the AHA and EUSI guidelines agree on several points. Deep hemorrhages do not benefit from craniotomy (Fig. 3), and there is limited evidence suggesting that minimally invasive treatment may be beneficial in patients with significant mass effect. Also, deeply comatose and very old patients have not been shown to benefit from surgery. Certainly, more studies are needed. Completion of the STICH II [26] and Minimally Invasive Surgery plus t-PA for Intracerebral Hemorrhage Evacuation (MISTIE) [27] trials may help clarify some of these issues (Box 1).

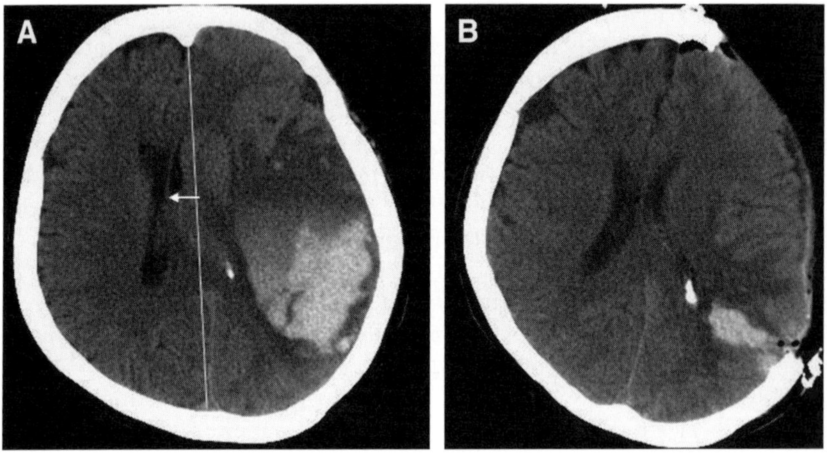

Fig. 1. Noncontrast CT of the brain showing a large hypertensive acute left temporoparietal hemorrhagic stroke in a 60-year-old man who presented with aphasia, right hemiparesis, and declining mental status. Initial imaging (*A*) reveals a superficial lobar hematoma with midline shift but no intraventricular involvement or hydrocephalus. A hemicraniectomy and clot evacuation were performed (*B*) with good results.

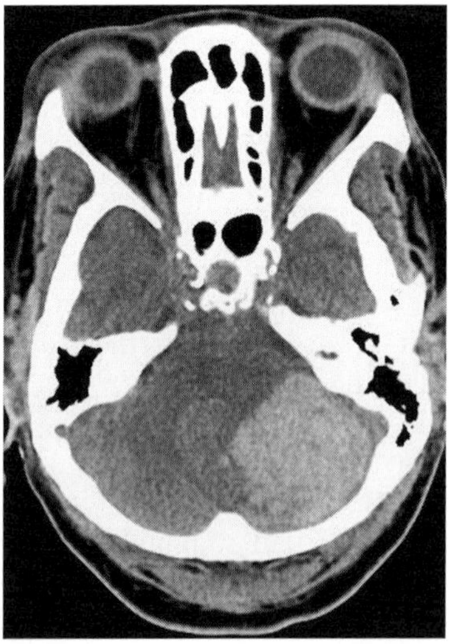

Fig. 2. Noncontrast CT of the brain shows a large acute hypertensive cerebellar hemorrhage in a 54-year-old woman with end-stage renal disease. The fourth ventricle is obliterated, and there was acute hydrocephalus (not shown). She was sleepy and showed early signs of lower cranial nerve dysfunction. She was admitted for craniectomy and evacuation of hematoma.

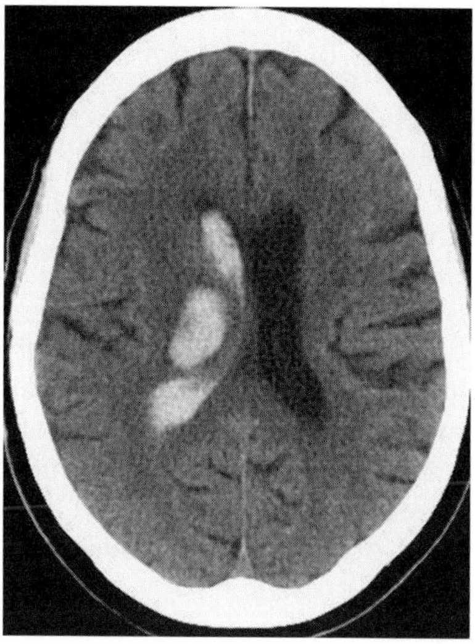

Fig. 3. Noncontrast CT of the brain showing a hypertensive acute hemorrhagic stroke in the right thalamus with intraventricular extension in a 61-year-old woman. The patient was managed without any surgical intervention.

Timing

Several studies have investigated the timing of surgery, with the rationale that earlier surgery may decrease the morbidity associated with rebleeding, mass effect, and prolonged exposure of the brain to toxic hematoma breakdown products [5]. Morgenstern and colleagues [28] compared patients having surgery within 4 hours with historical controls having surgery beyond 12 hours or medical therapy alone in a small study published in 2001. Due to safety concerns, the study was stopped after a planned interim analysis of 11 patients. They reported 36% mortality in the ultra early group versus 18% in the 12-hour surgery group and 29% in the medical therapy group ($P = .58$). Rebleeding occurred in 40% of the patients treated within 4 hours as compared with 12% of the patients treated beyond 12 hours. In the 4-hour group, 75% of patients with rebleeding died. Although this was a limited study due to its open treatment pilot design and small sample size, the data suggest more bleeding complications and death with early surgery.

The natural history of ICH is that clinical deterioration secondary to hematoma expansion or rebleeding occurs within the first 20 hours in almost 40% of patients [29]. Furthermore, 26% of patients have hematoma growth within 1 hour after the initial CT scan, and approximately 38% of patients increase the volume of clot by one third within 3 hours of ictus [29]. Despite preliminary data that suggested that recombinant factor VII may be of some benefit in reducing hematoma growth [30], phase III data show that the use of

Box 1. Brief descriptions of two major ongoing surgical ICH treatment trials

MISTIE (http://mistietrial.com/default.aspx)
- **Name**: Minimally Invasive Surgery plus t-PA for Intracerebral Hemorrhage Evacuation
- **Design**: multicenter, randomized, prospective
- **Purpose**: to establish that a combination of minimally invasive surgery and clot lysis with rt-PA safely achieves more rapid and complete recovery of function and decreased mortality from ICH when compared with conventional medical management without subjecting the patient to craniotomy
- **Enrollment**: planned 110 patients (phase I–60; phase II–50)
- **Status**: recruitment opened in late 2005

STICH II (http://www.ncl.ac.uk/stich/)
- **Name**: Surgical Trial in Intracerebral Hemorrhage II
- **Design**: multicenter, randomized, prospective
- **Purpose**: to establish whether earlier surgical evacuation of hematomas in selected patients with spontaneous isolated, superficial, lobar ICH will improve outcome when compared with a policy of initial conservative treatment
- **Enrollment**: planned 600 patients
- **Status**: recruitment opened late 2006

recombinant factor VII increases the risk of serious arterial thromboembolic events and does not improve survival or functional outcome after ICH [31].

The outcome of surgery has been investigated at 12, 25, 48, and 96 hours after ICH [10,19,20,32] and has not been reported to have a significant benefit at any time point. The timing of surgery should be guided by the clinical situation and not routinely employed in lieu of additional data.

Goals and techniques

The goals of surgical treatment are the preservation of life and neurologic function. Human and animal data suggest that the deleterious effects of spontaneous ICH are due to primary injury from compression, obstruction, or intracranial hypertension caused by the expanding hematoma mass and secondary injury caused by perihematomal hypoperfusion, edema, and toxic hematoma breakdown products [3,5,8]. To achieve the goals of surgical treatment, the specific aims may include decompression to reduce or prevent elevated intracranial pressure and removal of the acute hematoma to reduce mass effect and toxicity to the surrounding brain. Several surgical options exist that vary in the degree of invasiveness and associated morbidity. These options include ventriculostomy, stereotactic aspiration of hematoma with or without rt-PA, endoscopic hematoma evacuation, craniotomy for evacuation of hematoma, and hemicraniectomy for decompression with or without evacuation of hematoma.

Ventriculostomy can decompress the ventricular system and has low procedural morbidity and mortality. A frontal approach through a burr hole 2 to 3 cm from the midline and 1 cm anterior to the coronal suture is the standard technique and can be performed at the bedside. Most complications are related to infection or bleeding, which may be higher in ICH patients with a known or occult coagulopathy. The role of ventriculostomy is clear in patients with elevated intracranial pressure due to obstructive hydrocephalus, but no studies have directly evaluated the effect of ventriculostomy alone on the outcome of ICH patients. It may be useful in patients requiring control of intracranial pressure and cerebrospinal fluid diversion or as a temporizing measure while preparing the operating room for more aggressive modalities.

Minimally invasive techniques such as endoscopic aspiration, stereotactic infusion of lytic agents, and clot aspiration [12,33] usually require image-guided placement of a cannula within the hematoma and infusion of fluid to facilitate aspiration of blood products. These procedures are less invasive and allow access to deep hemorrhages without destruction of eloquent tissue [12]; however, they prevent direct visualization and control of bleeding, often require the instillation of agents that increase the risk of hemorrhage (eg, rt-PA), and have an increased infection risk with prolonged indwelling catheter use. These techniques have shown modest benefit in small studies, but further study is required before routine use can be recommended. The STITCH trial showed that patients treated with minimally invasive techniques tended to have worse outcomes [10], although this result may have been influenced by selection bias.

Craniotomy is the most studied modality. A complete evacuation under direct vision can be performed, which facilitates exploration for vascular lesions and control of bleeding sources. There is a higher procedural morbidity that is positively associated with invasiveness, hematoma volume and location, and the patient's clinical status [3,5,34].

Decompressive hemicraniectomy can be performed alone or in combination with clot evacuation. Limited data are available on the use of hemicraniectomy alone after ICH [20,35]. It is reasonable to control intracranial pressure and mass effect, but more studies need to be done to investigate its impact on outcome. In combination with clot evacuation, hemicraniectomy offers the potential benefits of craniotomy with additional decompression. The drawbacks of hemicraniectomy are additional time in surgery, persistent hydrocephalus [36] due to disturbed cerebrospinal fluid dynamics that may require shunting [36,37], the syndrome of the trephined (headache, dizziness, seizures, discomfort at site, apprehension, irritability or other psychiatric symptoms) [38], possible secondary injury from trauma at the craniectomy site, and the need for a second surgery to replace the bone flap.

Vascular lesional hemorrhagic stroke

Unlike in spontaneous hemorrhagic stroke, the role of surgery in the treatment of hemorrhagic stroke secondary to vascular lesions has been well defined [39,40].

Aneurysmal rupture

Aneurysmal rupture leading to SAH is a devastating problem. It has an associated initial mortality rate of 10% to 15%. Of patients who are able to reach medical care, 25% die within the first 2 weeks, and 20% to 30% of the survivors are severely and permanently disabled. Overall, the mortality rate associated with aneurysmal SAH is 32% to 67%, which makes it the most lethal type of hemorrhagic stroke [41–46]. Approximately 20% of aneurysmal ruptures have associated intracerebral hematomas [47], which carries an even more dismal prognosis [47–49] (Fig. 4). Rebleeding is the most serious

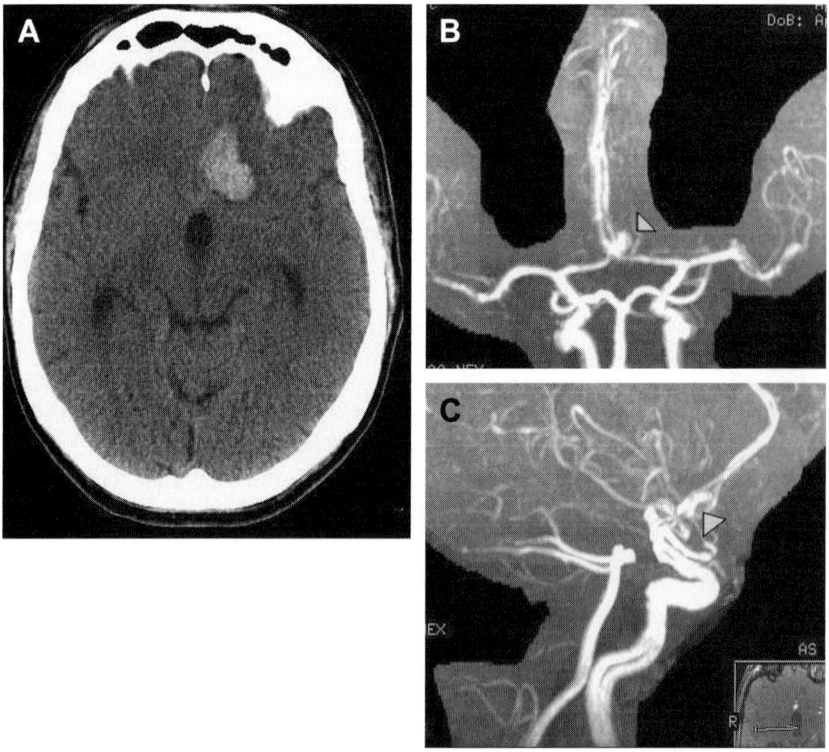

Fig. 4. Noncontrast head CT (*A*) and magnetic resonance angiogram (*B*, anteroposterior; *C*, lateral) show an acute left frontal intraparenchymal hemorrhage in a 66-year-old man in the setting of a ruptured anterior communicating aneurysm (*arrowhead*). He was treated with surgical clipping and hematoma evacuation.

and deadly complication of aneurysm rupture, with a mortality rate of over 70%. Consequently, rapid treatment of a ruptured aneurysm through surgical or endovascular means is imperative.

Historically, the optimal timing of surgery for a ruptured aneurysm has been debated. In the past, surgeons preferred to wait at least 2 weeks, because earlier surgery was associated with higher procedure morbidity than late surgery [50]. Additionally, patients with worse clinical grades and higher surgical risk may have died or deteriorated from rebleeding, delayed cerebral ischemia, and other complications such that a Darwinian selection bias favored late surgery for long-term outcome. It has since been shown that the risk of rebleeding from an unprotected aneurysm is approximately 20% within the first 2 weeks and up to 40% within a month [39,46], supporting early aneurysm obliteration [51,52] for most cases within 24 hours of presentation. Even patients who present with symptomatic or radiographic vasospasm can be successfully treated with surgery and then aggressively treated for vasospasm [52] with medical and endovascular strategies.

Securing the aneurysm to prevent rebleeding and enable treatment of delayed cerebral ischemia with hypertensive therapy is the primary goal of surgery. Cerebral infarction due to vasospasm and hydrocephalus are the most common sequelae of SAH [44–46]. Secondary surgical goals may include cisternal lavage, thrombolysis [53], and placement of prolonged-release nicardipine capsules [54,55], which have been reported to mitigate vasospasm.

Acute hydrocephalus is present in 19% to 46% of SAH patients [56] and requires placement of an external ventricular drain. Shunt-dependent chronic hydrocephalus occurs in 14% to 19% [56]. Although controversial [57], some studies have shown that opening the lamina terminalis during surgery for aneurysm clipping may reduce the risk of shunt-dependent chronic hydrocephalus [58]. In cases of SAH due to a giant aneurysm or accompanied by a large ICH, an additional goal may be to reduce the mass effect from the aneurysm or related hematoma [59,60].

The advent of endovascular therapy has revolutionized aneurysm treatment. Endovascular aneurysm obliteration is beyond the scope of this article and is discussed elsewhere in this volume. Surgical treatment of aneurysms has also made significant progress over the last decade. More recently, it has been shown that treatment of complex aneurysms has a better outcome when performed at specialized centers [61,62]. Improved microsurgical technique including the use of the intraoperative microscope, direct vessel flow measurements via an ultrasonic flow probe [63], and the availability of intraoperative conventional [64,65] or indocyanogreen [66] angiography may increase procedural success.

Surgical options for securing cerebral aneurysms include clip obliteration, trapping with or without bypass, and wrapping. For most aneurysms requiring surgical treatment, clipping is the treatment of choice offering durable protection against rebleeding. Rerupture [67] and recurrence rates are reportedly low after complete clipping [68]. Although a meta-analysis of over 60 studies demonstrated a 2.6% mortality rate for clipping of unruptured aneurysms [69], other studies have reported mortality rates of 3% to 25% for surgical treatment of ruptured aneurysms [39,40]. These rates are strongly and positively related to the severity of initial SAH, the timing of surgery, and the presenting clinical grade [39,40].

Complex lesions such as giant or fusiform aneurysms often cannot be clipped without compromising the parent or perforating vessels. In these cases, alternative strategies are necessary. One such strategy is trapping the aneurysm between two clips. A similar strategy involves proximal ligation or distal occlusion to induce aneurysm thrombosis. These strategies often interrupt the parent vessel flow; therefore, they may require revascularization to ensure adequate blood flow to distal vascular beds. Multiple strategies exist, including use of the superficial temporal artery, occipital artery, radial artery, or saphenous vein as a graft, depending on distal flow requirements and aneurysm location. The ability to directly measure flow intraoperatively provides a means to optimize the bypass strategy by matching the supply with the demand [63]. Technologic advances such as excimer laser–assisted nonocclusive anastomosis [70] and the automated extracranial-intracranial bypass [71] eliminate the need for extended temporary clipping times and may provide potentially safer treatment of complex aneurysms.

When the aforementioned surgical treatment strategies cannot be successfully employed and endovascular treatment is not a feasible option, wrapping may protect against rupture by inducing fibrosis and scarring around the aneurysm, which provides additional wall strength. This strategy was previously more popular [72]; however, the evidence regarding wrapping is mixed, and re-operation may be made more difficult [73,74]. More recently, it has been has shown that wrapping may be an effective strategy in select cases [74].

Arteriovenous malformation rupture

AVMs are the second most common cause of SAH [75,76]. They are also a common cause of intraparenchymal hemorrhage in younger patients [76] (Fig. 5). The overall rupture rate is 2% to 4% per year [77], and the risk of subsequent rupture is 6% [76] to 18% [75] in the first year, decreasing to 2% per year after 10 years [75]. To prevent AVM rerupture and consequent neurologic disability, the consensus is that definitive treatment is indicated [77,78]. The goal of surgical resection is complete removal of the AVM nidus while preserving normal arterial flow. If the patient has chronic seizures, a secondary goal may be to improve seizure control. Nonsurgical options include stereotactic radiosurgery with or without endovascular embolization. Endovascular therapy has low procedural morbidity but is usually not an effective sole treatment modality [79]. It is usually used before treatment with surgery or radiosurgery to reduce the flow in large AVMs

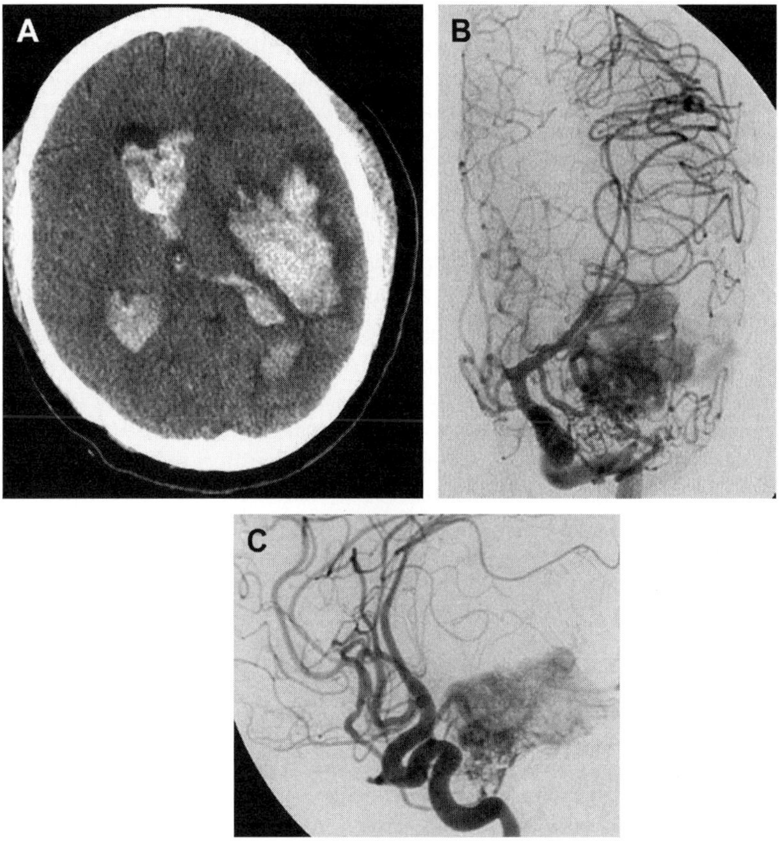

Fig. 5. Noncontrast head CT (*A*) and cerebral angiogram (*B*, *C*) showing diffuse acute left temporoparietal intraparenchymal and intraventricular hemorrhage due to a large AVM (*B*, anteroposterior; *C*, lateral) in a 42-year-old man. Due to worsening clinical examination and mass effect, he was initially treated urgently with venticulostomy and craniotomy for partial clot evacuation. Continued mass effect necessitated hemicraniectomy for further clot evacuation and resection of the AVM.

to reduce the risk of significant blood loss during open surgery or to shrink the AVM and make it more amenable to radiosurgery [79]. A detailed discussion of endovascular therapy is beyond the scope of this article and can be found elsewhere in this issue. Stereotactic radiosurgery can be used as the sole therapy for lesions less than 3 cm in size [79]. In general, it is well tolerated with less procedural risk than surgery, but it has reported obliteration rates of only 54% to 92% and can take up to 3 years to completely obliterate the AVM [79–81]. Staged multiple embolizations combined with stereotactic radiosurgery or fractionated radiosurgery for patients with high-grade lesions not amenable to surgery can be employed [82–84]. An in-depth discussion of stereotactic radiosurgery is also beyond the scope of this article.

Because AVM rerupture rates are relatively low in the acute time period following rupture, unlike the surgical treatment for aneurysms, surgical AVM resection can be performed on a subacute basis 3 to 6 weeks following the ictus. Waiting until the hematoma resolves can improve visualization of the AVM nidus with conventional angiography and MRI [85]. Moreover, clot cavity formation may simplify the resection by creating a well-defined dissection plane that is distinct from the brain parenchyma [78]. If the rupture includes a significant component of intraparenchymal hemorrhage, more acute surgery may be indicated to reduce mass effect [86].

Large or high-flow AVMs may be subject to significant bleeding during surgery. Postoperative bleeding can occur in up to 10% secondary to cerebral hyperemia, also known as perfusion pressure breakthrough, due to residual abnormal leaky surrounding vessels [87–90]. This form of hemorrhagic infarction may require separate surgical intervention. The risk of intraoperative bleeding can be reduced by maintaining the integrity of the nidus and strict blood pressure control [91]. Likewise, the risk for postoperative breakthrough bleeding may be limited by complete nidal resection and by careful postoperative blood pressure management [90]. Preoperative staged embolization may ameliorate these risks [92] by reducing the nidal arterial supply and gradually normalizing pressure within the AVM and surrounding vessels. Features such as high pressure in the nidus or feeding artery, a deep perforating artery supply, a single draining vein, deep venous drainage, and feeding artery aneurysms may increase the risk of hemorrhage and complicate resection [93–96].

Less common etiologies

Less common lesional causes of hemorrhagic stroke include cavernomas, dural AVF, moyamoya disease, and other rare vasculopathies.

Cavernomas are comprised of a grapelike cluster of abnormal thin-walled vessels without any intervening brain parenchyma. They are much less common than AVMs. They represent only 5% to 13% of central nervous system vascular malformations and have a small hemorrhage rate of 2% to 3% per year [97]. Because they lack large feeding arteries or draining veins, they are angiographically occult [97,98]. Surgery may be indicated for cavernomas causing refractory seizures or mass effect from hemorrhage. Routine surgical resection after an initial hemorrhage is controversial. Hemorrhages from cavernomas are rarely life threatening or neurologically devastating, and, although the risk of symptomatic rehemorrhage is likely low, it has not been clearly defined [97–99]. As is true for AVMs, if surgical resection following bleeding is elected, it can usually be postponed for several weeks unless symptomatic mass effect warrants otherwise. The goal of surgery is complete resection to reduce the risk of hemorrhage and refractory seizures. Cavernomas are usually treated with open surgery; there is no clear evidence to support the use of stereotactic radiosurgery. Cavernomas are often associated with venous angiomas [100], which should be preserved during surgical resection to avoid the risk of venous infarction [100].

Dural AVFs are an abnormality in which an arteriovenous shunt is contained with the leaflets of the dura. They are often classified as a subset of AVMs and comprise up to 15% of all intracranial AVMs [101,102]. Most are stable or resolve spontaneously and have minimal chance of serious complications [103,104]; however, lesions with leptomeningeal venous drainage, variceal or aneurysmal venous dilations, and galenic drainage can have significant hemorrhage risk and serious neurologic sequelae [103–105]. Overall, the hemorrhage rate for dural AVFs is 1.5% to 1.8%; however, retrograde cortical venous drainage can lead to rehemorrhage with serious neurologic consequences in 10% to 35% of patients [103–105]. Expeditious and definitive treatment should be considered for these lesions. Options include endovascular treatment or surgical ligation. Radiosurgery is a less optimal treatment for high-risk AVF due to the prolonged time for complete obliteration. Rapid and severe bleeding, especially at the time of the craniotomy, may complicate surgical treatment [106]. Dural AVFs can be preoperatively embolized endovascularly to reduce the risk of extensive bleeding [107]. Treatment consists of ligating the venous outflow at the level of the dura; complete extirpation of the fistula within the dura is not necessary [108–110].

Moyamoya disease is characterized by the formation of fragile collateral vessels in response to progressive stenotic occlusion of the distal internal carotid artery or its proximal branches [111]. It can present with ischemic symptoms or hemorrhage [111–115]. In a recent retrospective analysis of 34 adult patients with moyamoya disease who presented over a 9-year period, 71% presented with ischemia and 21% with hemorrhage [112]. Most hemorrhages occur in deep regions or are intraventricular, reflecting the location of the collateral vessels which are the presumed source of bleeding. A significant hemorrhage may require acute evacuation, as is true for other forms of ICH; however, because the risk of acute rebleeding is low, cerebral revascularization by direct bypass or indirect methods can be performed on a semi-elective basis [111–113] with the goal of leading to the regression of the fragile basal collateral network. The efficacy of revascularization in reducing the risk of bleeding has not been established and is the basis of ongoing study [116].

Hemorrhagic stroke as a consequence of treatment

Hemorrhages in this category include anticoagulant and thrombolytic associated hemorrhage, breakthrough hyperperfusion hemorrhage after cerebral revascularization, and acute hemorrhage following endovascular intervention. As anticoagulant and thrombolytic usage increase and endovascular and surgical revascularization become more frequent, this category of hemorrhage is likely to become increasingly common.

Cerebral revascularization procedures with a risk for reperfusion hemorrhage include carotid endarterectomy, endovascular carotid and intracranial angioplasty, and surgical extracranial-intracranial bypass. The surgical indications and goals are the same as for spontaneous ICH. Careful attention must be paid preoperatively to reversing anticoagulant- or thrombolytic-induced coagulopathy and maintaining normal postoperative coagulation function in these patients because they have a significant chance of rehemorrhage. In some cases, the risk of rebleeding may outweigh any potential benefit of surgical intervention.

Summary

Hemorrhagic stroke is a devastating problem. The vast majority is spontaneous ICH related to hypertension. Although controversial for routine treatment of spontaneous ICH, the role of surgery is much clearer to prevent rebleeding from lesional problems. Patients with large (>3 cm) cerebellar hemorrhages or with imminent deterioration from superficial lobar hemorrhages may benefit from surgery [19,20]. Additional trial data on alternate surgical approaches to ICH are needed. Until then, practitioners should consult published guidelines for treatment recommendations and consider each patient on a case-by-case basis [19,20].

References

[1] Rosamond W, Flegal K, Friday G, et al. Heart disease and stroke statistics–2007 update: a report from the American Heart Association Statistics Committee and Stroke Statistics Subcommittee. Circulation 2007;115:e99–106.

[2] Fisher CM. Pathological observations in hypertensive cerebral hemorrhage. J Neuropathol Exp Neurol 1971;30:536–50.

[3] Fewel ME, Thompson BG Jr, Hoff JT. Spontaneous intracerebral hemorrhage: a review. Neurosurg Focus 2003;15(4):1–16.

[4] Vinters HV. Cerebral amyloid angiopathy: a critical review. Stroke 1987;18:311–24.

[5] Hsieh PC, Awad IA, Getch CC, et al. Current updates in perioperative management of intracerebral hemorrhage. Neurol Clin 2006;24:745–64.

[6] Quinones-Hinojosa A, Gulati M, Singh V, et al. Spontaneous intracerebral hemorrhage due to coagulation disorders. Neurosurg Focus 2003;15(4):1–17.

[7] Broderick JP, Brott TG, Duldner JE, et al. Volume of intracerebral hemorrhage: a powerful and easy-to-use predictor of 30-day mortality. Stroke 1993;24:987–93.

[8] Pouratian N, Kassell NF, Dumont AS. Update on management of intracerebral hemorrhage. Neurosurg Focus 2003;15(4):1–6.

[9] McKissock W, Richardson A, Taylor J. Primary intracerebral haemorrhage: a controlled trial of surgical and conservative treatment in 180 unselected cases. Lancet 1961;2: 221–6.

[10] Mendelow AD, Gregson BA, Fernandes HM, et al. Early surgery versus initial conservative treatment in patients with spontaneous supratentorial intracerebral haematomas in the International Surgical Trial in Intracerebral Haemorrhage (STICH): a randomised trial. Lancet 2005;365:387–97.

[11] Teernstra OP, Evers SM, Lodder J, et al. Stereotactic treatment of intracerebral hematoma by means of a plasminogen activator: a multicenter randomized controlled trial (SICHPA). Stroke 2003;34:968–74.
[12] Auer LM, Deinsberger W, Niederkorn K, et al. Endoscopic surgery versus medical treatment for spontaneous intracerebral hematoma: a randomized study. J Neurosurg 1989; 70:530–5.
[13] Juvela S, Heiskanen O, Poranen A, et al. The treatment of spontaneous intracerebral hemorrhage: a prospective randomized trial of surgical and conservative treatment. J Neurosurg 1989;70:755–8.
[14] Batjer HH, Reisch JS, Allen BC, et al. Failure of surgery to improve outcome in hypertensive putaminal hemorrhage: a prospective randomized trial. Arch Neurol 1990;47:1103–6.
[15] Chen X, Yang H, Czherig Z. A prospective randomized trial of surgical and conservative treatment of hypertensive intracranial haemorrhage. Acta Academiae Medicinae Shanghai 1992;19:237–40.
[16] Zuccarello M, Brott T, Derex L, et al. Early surgical treatment for supratentorial intracerebral hemorrhage: a randomized feasibility study. Stroke 1999;30:1833–9.
[17] Morgenstern LB, Frankowski RF, Shedden P, et al. Surgical treatment for intracerebral hemorrhage (STICH): a single-center, randomized clinical trial. Neurology 1998;51: 1359–63.
[18] Mendelow AD, Unterberg A. Surgical treatment of intracerebral haemorrhage. Curr Opin Crit Care 2007;13:169–74.
[19] Steiner T, Kaste M, Forsting M, et al. Recommendations for the management of intracranial haemorrhage. Part I. Spontaneous intracerebral haemorrhage. The European Stroke Initiative Writing Committee and the Writing Committee for the EUSI Executive Committee. Cerebrovasc Dis 2006;22:294–316.
[20] Broderick J, Connolly S, Feldmann E, et al. Guidelines for the management of spontaneous intracerebral hemorrhage in adults: 2007 update. A guideline from the American Heart Association/American Stroke Association Stroke Council, High Blood Pressure Research Council, and the Quality of Care and Outcomes in Research Interdisciplinary Working Group. Circulation 2007;116:e391–413.
[21] Dunne JW, Chakera T, Kermode S. Cerebellar haemorrhage–diagnosis and treatment: a study of 75 consecutive cases. Q J Med 1987;64:739–54.
[22] Salazar J, Vaquero J, Martinez P, et al. Clinical and CT scan assessment of benign versus fatal spontaneous cerebellar haematomas. Acta Neurochir (Wien) 1986;79:80–6.
[23] Da Pian R, Bazzan A, Pasqualin A. Surgical versus medical treatment of spontaneous posterior fossa haematomas: a cooperative study on 205 cases. Neurol Res 1984;6:145–51.
[24] Firsching R, Huber M, Frowein RA. Cerebellar haemorrhage: management and prognosis. Neurosurg Rev 1991;14:191–4.
[25] van Loon J, Van Calenbergh F, Goffin J, et al. Controversies in the management of spontaneous cerebellar haemorrhage: a consecutive series of 49 cases and review of the literature. Acta Neurochir (Wien) 1993;122:187–93.
[26] Available at:http://www.ncl.ac.uk/stich/. Accessed May 12, 2008.
[27] Available at:http://mistietrial.com/default.aspx. Accessed May 12, 2008.
[28] Morgenstern LB, Demchuk AM, Kim DH, et al. Rebleeding leads to poor outcome in ultra-early craniotomy for intracerebral hemorrhage. Neurology 2001;56:1294–9.
[29] Brott T, Broderick J, Kothari R, et al. Early hemorrhage growth in patients with intracerebral hemorrhage. Stroke 1997;28:1–5.
[30] Mayer SA, Brun NC, Begtrup K, et al. Recombinant activated factor VII for acute intracerebral hemorrhage. N Engl J Med 2005;352:777–85.
[31] Mayer SA, Brun NC, Begtrup K, et al. Efficacy and safety of recombinant activated factor VII for acute intracerebral hemorrhage. N Engl J Med 2008;358:2127–37.
[32] Hanggi D, Steiger HJ. Spontaneous intracerebral haemorrhage in adults: a literature overview. Acta Neurochir (Wien) 2008;150:371–9.

[33] Cho DY, Chen CC, Chang CS, et al. Endoscopic surgery for spontaneous basal ganglia hemorrhage: comparing endoscopic surgery, stereotactic aspiration, and craniotomy in noncomatose patients. Surg Neurol 2006;65:547–55 [discussion: 55–6].
[34] Gregson BA, Mendelow AD, Fernandes H, et al. Surgery for intracerebral hemorrhage. Stroke 2000;31:791–2.
[35] Murthy JM, Chowdary GV, Murthy TV, et al. Decompressive craniectomy with clot evacuation in large hemispheric hypertensive intracerebral hemorrhage. Neurocrit Care 2005;2: 258–62.
[36] Waziri A, Fusco D, Mayer SA, et al. Postoperative hydrocephalus in patients undergoing decompressive hemicraniectomy for ischemic or hemorrhagic stroke. Neurosurgery 2007; 61:489–93 [discussion: 93–4].
[37] Carvi y Nievas MN, Hollerhage HG. Early combined cranioplasty and programmable shunt in patients with skull bone defects and CSF-circulation disorders. Neurol Res 2006;28:139–44.
[38] Dujovny M, Aviles A, Agner C, et al. Cranioplasty: cosmetic or therapeutic? Surg Neurol 1997;47:238–41.
[39] Kassell NF, Torner JC, Haley EC Jr, et al. The International Cooperative Study on the Timing of Aneurysm Surgery. Part 1. Overall management results. J Neurosurg 1990;73:18–36.
[40] Kassell NF, Torner JC, Jane JA, et al. The International Cooperative Study on the Timing of Aneurysm Surgery. Part 2. Surgical results. J Neurosurg 1990;73:37–47.
[41] Hop JW, Rinkel GJ, Algra A, et al. Changes in functional outcome and quality of life in patients and caregivers after aneurysmal subarachnoid hemorrhage. J Neurosurg 2001; 95:957–63.
[42] Hop JW, Rinkel GJ, Algra A, et al. Quality of life in patients and partners after aneurysmal subarachnoid hemorrhage. Stroke 1998;29:798–804.
[43] Hop JW, Rinkel GJ, Algra A, et al. Case-fatality rates and functional outcome after subarachnoid hemorrhage: a systematic review. Stroke 1997;28:660–4.
[44] Manno EM. Subarachnoid hemorrhage. Neurol Clin 2004;22:347–66.
[45] Al-Shahi R, White PM, Davenport RJ, et al. Subarachnoid haemorrhage. BMJ 2006;333: 235–40.
[46] Ferro JM, Canhao P, Peralta R. Update on subarachnoid haemorrhage. J Neurol 2008;255: 465–79.
[47] Abbed KM, Ogilvy CS. Intracerebral hematoma from aneurysm rupture. Neurosurg Focus 2003;15(4):1–5.
[48] Pasqualin A, Bazzan A, Cavazzani P, et al. Intracranial hematomas following aneurysmal rupture: experience with 309 cases. Surg Neurol 1986;25:6–17.
[49] Wheelock B, Weir B, Watts R, et al. Timing of surgery for intracerebral hematomas due to aneurysm rupture. J Neurosurg 1983;58:476–81.
[50] Drake CG. Intracranial aneurysms. Acta Neurol Latinoam 1939;23:43–68.
[51] Milhorat TH, Krautheim M. Results of early and delayed operations for ruptured intracranial aneurysms in two series of 100 consecutive patients. Surg Neurol 1986;26:123–8.
[52] Torner JC, Kassell NF, Haley EC Jr. The timing of surgery and vasospasm. Neurosurg Clin N Am 1990;1:335–47.
[53] Amin-Hanjani S, Ogilvy CS, Barker FG 2nd. Does intracisternal thrombolysis prevent vasospasm after aneurysmal subarachnoid hemorrhage? A meta-analysis. Neurosurgery 2004;54:326–34 [discussion: 34–5].
[54] Barth M, Capelle HH, Weidauer S, et al. Effect of nicardipine prolonged-release implants on cerebral vasospasm and clinical outcome after severe aneurysmal subarachnoid hemorrhage: a prospective, randomized, double-blind phase IIa study. Stroke 2007;38:330–6.
[55] Kasuya H, Onda H, Sasahara A, et al. Application of nicardipine prolonged-release implants: analysis of 97 consecutive patients with acute subarachnoid hemorrhage. Neurosurgery 2005;56:895–902 [discussion: 895–902].

[56] Dehdashti AR, Rilliet B, Rufenacht DA, et al. Shunt-dependent hydrocephalus after rupture of intracranial aneurysms: a prospective study of the influence of treatment modality. J Neurosurg 2004;101:402–7.
[57] Kim JM, Jeon JY, Kim JH, et al. Influence of lamina terminalis fenestration on the occurrence of the shunt-dependent hydrocephalus in anterior communicating artery aneurysmal subarachnoid hemorrhage. J Korean Med Sci 2006;21:113–8.
[58] Andaluz N, Zuccarello M. Fenestration of the lamina terminalis as a valuable adjunct in aneurysm surgery. Neurosurgery 2004;55:1050–9.
[59] Spetzler RF, Riina HA, Lemole GM Jr. Giant aneurysms. Neurosurgery 2001;49:902–8.
[60] Lawton MT, Spetzler RF. Surgical management of giant intracranial aneurysms: experience with 171 patients. Clin Neurosurg 1995;42:245–66.
[61] Cross DT 3rd, Tirschwell DL, Clark MA, et al. Mortality rates after subarachnoid hemorrhage: variations according to hospital case volume in 18 states. J Neurosurg 2003;99: 810–7.
[62] Barker FG 2nd, Amin-Hanjani S, Butler WE, et al. In-hospital mortality and morbidity after surgical treatment of unruptured intracranial aneurysms in the United States, 1996–2000: the effect of hospital and surgeon volume. Neurosurgery 2003;52:995–1007.
[63] Ashley WW, Amin-Hanjani S, Alaraj A, et al. Flow-assisted surgical cerebral revascularization. Neurosurg Focus 2008;24(2):1–12.
[64] Klopfenstein JD, Spetzler RF, Kim LJ, et al. Comparison of routine and selective use of intraoperative angiography during aneurysm surgery: a prospective assessment. J Neurosurg 2004;100:230–5.
[65] Chiang VL, Gailloud P, Murphy KJ, et al. Routine intraoperative angiography during aneurysm surgery. J Neurosurg 2002;96:988–92.
[66] Raabe A, Nakaji P, Beck J, et al. Prospective evaluation of surgical microscope-integrated intraoperative near-infrared indocyanine green videoangiography during aneurysm surgery. J Neurosurg 2005;103:982–9.
[67] Johnston SC, Dowd CF, Higashida RT, et al. Predictors of rehemorrhage after treatment of ruptured intracranial aneurysms: the Cerebral Aneurysm Rerupture After Treatment (CARAT) study. Stroke 2008;39:120–5.
[68] David CA, Vishteh AG, Spetzler RF, et al. Late angiographic follow-up review of surgically treated aneurysms. J Neurosurg 1999;91:396–401.
[69] Raaymakers TW, Rinkel GJ, Limburg M, et al. Mortality and morbidity of surgery for unruptured intracranial aneurysms: a meta-analysis. Stroke 1998;29:1531–8.
[70] Langer DJ, Van Der Zwan A, Vajkoczy P, et al. Excimer laser-assisted nonocclusive anastomosis: an emerging technology for use in the creation of intracranial-intracranial and extracranial-intracranial cerebral bypass. Neurosurg Focus 2008;24(2):1–11.
[71] Bregy A, Alfieri A, Demertzis S, et al. Automated end-to-side anastomosis to the middle cerebral artery: a feasibility study. J Neurosurg 2008;108:567–74.
[72] Gillingham FJ. The management of ruptured intracranial aneurysm. Ann R Coll Surg Engl 1958;23:89–117.
[73] Todd NV, Tocher JL, Jones PA, et al. Outcome following aneurysm wrapping: a 10-year follow-up review of clipped and wrapped aneurysms. J Neurosurg 1989;70:841–6.
[74] Deshmukh VR, Kakarla UK, Figueiredo EG, et al. Long-term clinical and angiographic follow-up of unclippable wrapped intracranial aneurysms. Neurosurgery 2006; 58:434–42.
[75] Fults D, Kelly DL Jr. Natural history of arteriovenous malformations of the brain: a clinical study. Neurosurgery 1984;15:658–62.
[76] Graf CJ, Perret GE, Torner JC. Bleeding from cerebral arteriovenous malformations as part of their natural history. J Neurosurg 1983;58:331–7.
[77] Kondziolka D, McLaughlin MR, Kestle JR. Simple risk predictions for arteriovenous malformation hemorrhage. Neurosurgery 1995;37:851–5.

[78] Sengupta R. Classification, evaluation, and general principles of treatment of arteriovenous malformations. In: Sekhar L, Fessler R, editors. Atlas of neurosurgical techniques: brain. New York: Thieme; 2006. p. 231–41.
[79] Starke RM, Komotar RJ, Hwang BY, et al. A comprehensive review of radiosurgery for cerebral arteriovenous malformations: outcomes, predictive factors, and grading scales. Stereotact Funct Neurosurg 2008;86:191–9.
[80] Nataf F, Schlienger M, Bayram M, et al. Microsurgery or radiosurgery for cerebral arteriovenous malformations? A study of two paired series. Neurosurgery 2007;61:39–49.
[81] Pikus HJ, Beach ML, Harbaugh RE. Microsurgical treatment of arteriovenous malformations: analysis and comparison with stereotactic radiosurgery. J Neurosurg 1998;88:641–6.
[82] Gobin YP, Laurent A, Merienne L, et al. Treatment of brain arteriovenous malformations by embolization and radiosurgery. J Neurosurg 1996;85:19–28.
[83] Sirin S, Kondziolka D, Niranjan A, et al. Prospective staged volume radiosurgery for large arteriovenous malformations: indications and outcomes in otherwise untreatable patients. Neurosurgery 2006;58:17–27 [discussion: 17–27].
[84] Jones J, Jang S, Getch CC, et al. Advances in the radiosurgical treatment of large inoperable arteriovenous malformations. Neurosurg Focus 2007;23(6):1–6.
[85] Ropper AH, Davis KR. Lobar cerebral hemorrhages: acute clinical syndromes in 26 cases. Ann Neurol 1980;8:141–7.
[86] Jafar JJ, Rezai AR. Acute surgical management of intracranial arteriovenous malformations. Neurosurgery 1994;34:8–12.
[87] Batjer HH, Devous MD Sr, Meyer YJ, et al. Cerebrovascular hemodynamics in arteriovenous malformation complicated by normal perfusion pressure breakthrough. Neurosurgery 1988;22:503–9.
[88] Spetzler RF, Wilson CB, Weinstein P, et al. Normal perfusion pressure breakthrough theory. Clin Neurosurg 1978;25:651–72.
[89] Young WL, Kader A, Ornstein E, et al. Cerebral hyperemia after arteriovenous malformation resection is related to "breakthrough" complications but not to feeding artery pressure: the Columbia University Arteriovenous Malformation Study Project. Neurosurgery 1996; 38:1085–93 [discussion: 1093–95].
[90] Stapf C, Connolly ES, Schumacher HC, et al. Dysplastic vessels after surgery for brain arteriovenous malformations. Stroke 2002;33:1053–6.
[91] Thompson RC, Steinberg GK, Levy RP, et al. The management of patients with arteriovenous malformations and associated intracranial aneurysms. Neurosurgery 1998;43:202–11 [discussion: 211–12].
[92] Vinuela F, Dion JE, Duckwiler G, et al. Combined endovascular embolization and surgery in the management of cerebral arteriovenous malformations: experience with 101 cases. J Neurosurg 1991;75:856–64.
[93] Du R, Keyoung HM, Dowd CF, et al. The effects of diffuseness and deep perforating artery supply on outcomes after microsurgical resection of brain arteriovenous malformations. Neurosurgery 2007;60:638–46 [discussion: 646–48].
[94] Duong DH, Young WL, Vang MC, et al. Feeding artery pressure and venous drainage pattern are primary determinants of hemorrhage from cerebral arteriovenous malformations. Stroke 1998;29:1167–76.
[95] Stapf C, Mast H, Sciacca RR, et al. Predictors of hemorrhage in patients with untreated brain arteriovenous malformation. Neurology 2006;66:1350–5.
[96] Stapf C, Mohr JP, Pile-Spellman J, et al. Concurrent arterial aneurysms in brain arteriovenous malformations with haemorrhagic presentation. J Neurol Neurosurg Psychiatry 2002; 73:294–8.
[97] Moriarity JL, Wetzel M, Clatterbuck RE, et al. The natural history of cavernous malformations: a prospective study of 68 patients. Neurosurgery 1999;44:1166–71 [discussion: 1172–73].

[98] Kondziolka D, Lunsford LD, Kestle JR. The natural history of cerebral cavernous malformations. J Neurosurg 1995;83:820–4.
[99] Simard JM, Garcia-Bengochea F, Ballinger WE Jr, et al. Cavernous angioma: a review of 126 collected and 12 new clinical cases. Neurosurgery 1986;18:162–72.
[100] Abdulrauf SI, Kaynar MY, Awad IA. A comparison of the clinical profile of cavernous malformations with and without associated venous malformations. Neurosurgery 1999; 44:41–6 [discussion: 46–7].
[101] Borden JA, Wu JK, Shucart WA. A proposed classification for spinal and cranial dural arteriovenous fistulous malformations and implications for treatment. J Neurosurg 1995;82: 166–79.
[102] Cognard C, Gobin YP, Pierot L, et al. Cerebral dural arteriovenous fistulas: clinical and angiographic correlation with a revised classification of venous drainage. Radiology 1995;194:671–80.
[103] Satomi J, van Dijk JM, Terbrugge KG, et al. Benign cranial dural arteriovenous fistulas: outcome of conservative management based on the natural history of the lesion. J Neurosurg 2002;97:767–70.
[104] van Dijk JM, TerBrugge KG. Dural arteriovenous fistulas. J Neurosurg 2002;97:1486 [author reply: 1487].
[105] Duffau H, Lopes M, Janosevic V, et al. Early rebleeding from intracranial dural arteriovenous fistulas: report of 20 cases and review of the literature. J Neurosurg 1999;90:78–84.
[106] Sundt TM Jr, Piepgras DG. The surgical approach to arteriovenous malformations of the lateral and sigmoid dural sinuses. J Neurosurg 1983;59:32–9.
[107] Barnwell SL, Halbach VV, Higashida RT, et al. Complex dural arteriovenous fistulas: results of combined endovascular and neurosurgical treatment in 16 patients. J Neurosurg 1989;71:352–8.
[108] Thompson BG, Doppman JL, Oldfield EH. Treatment of cranial dural arteriovenous fistulae by interruption of leptomeningeal venous drainage. J Neurosurg 1994;80:617–23.
[109] Ushikoshi S, Houkin K, Kuroda S, et al. Surgical treatment of intracranial dural arteriovenous fistulas. Surg Neurol 2002;57:253–61.
[110] van Dijk JM, TerBrugge KG, Willinsky RA, et al. Selective disconnection of cortical venous reflux as treatment for cranial dural arteriovenous fistulas. J Neurosurg 2004;101: 31–5.
[111] Suzuki J, Kodama N. Moyamoya disease–a review. Stroke 1983;14:104–9.
[112] Hallemeier CL, Rich KM, Grubb RL Jr, et al. Clinical features and outcome in North American adults with moyamoya phenomenon. Stroke 2006;37:1490–6.
[113] Zipfel GJ, Fox DJ Jr, Rivet DJ. Moyamoya disease in adults: the role of cerebral revascularization. Skull Base 2005;15:27–41.
[114] Ueki K, Meyer FB, Mellinger JF. Moyamoya disease: the disorder and surgical treatment. Mayo Clin Proc 1994;69:749–57.
[115] Drake CG. Cerebral arteriovenous malformations: considerations for and experience with surgical treatment in 166 cases. Clin Neurosurg 1979;26:145–208.
[116] Miyamoto S. Study design for a prospective randomized trial of extracranial-intracranial bypass surgery for adults with moyamoya disease and hemorrhagic onset–the Japan Adult Moyamoya Trial Group. Neurol Med Chir (Tokyo) 2004;44:218–9.

Section III

Stroke Prevention: What Has the Evidence Taught Us?

ELSEVIER
SAUNDERS

Neurol Clin 26 (2008) 1007–1045

NEUROLOGIC
CLINICS

Risk Factor Management to Prevent First Stroke

Tatjana Rundek, MD, PhD*,
Ralph L. Sacco, MD, MS, FAHA, FAAN

Department of Neurology, Miller School of Medicine, University of Miami, Miami, Florida, USA

Despite substantial advances for treatment of patients with acute stroke, effective primary stroke prevention remains the best means for reducing the stroke burden [1]. More than 70% of all strokes occurring each year are first strokes and therefore primary prevention of stroke is of immense public health importance [2]. High-risk or stroke-prone individuals can be identified and targeted for specific management and interventions. The ultimate public health benefit, however, depends on not only identification of stroke risk but also on assessing global vascular risk and the management and modification of these risks [3]. Many preventive strategies are available to manage a number of factors that increase the risk of a first stroke. Such successful implementation in preventive medicine remains a great challenge worldwide.

The evidence-based guidelines for the management of risk factors to prevent first stroke have been published [4]. This article provides an overview of the management of risk factors in primary stroke prevention, the gaps in successful management, and future directions for the research and management of stroke risk factors. The management of modifiable and potentially modifiable risk factors or risk markers for a first stroke is reviewed. Nonmodifiable factors, such as age, sex, race/ethnicity, and various genetic factors, are mentioned in the context of risk stratification for a first stoke. The major focus is given to the management of modifiable risk factors for stroke, including hypertension, diabetes, dyslipidemia, atrial fibrillation and other cardiac conditions, carotid artery stenosis (CAS), smoking, poor diet, physical inactivity, and obesity. A brief discussion of the management of potentially modifiable risk factors, such as alcohol and drug abuse, sleep apnea,

* Corresponding author.
E-mail address: TRundek@med.miami.edu (T. Rundek).

doi:10.1016/j.ncl.2008.09.001

and hyperhomocysteinemia, is included, as is the use of antiplatelet therapy in primary stroke prevention. The less well documented risk factors for first stroke, such as inflammation, infection, and hypercoagulable disorders, are beyond the scope of this article. Finally, prognostic scores to assess an individual risk for a first stroke are reviewed.

Management of well-documented modifiable risk factors to prevent first stroke

Evidence-based guidelines exist for the management of several modifiable risk factors of a first stroke. The modification of these risk factors clearly reduces risk of first stroke. Selected well-documented modifiable risk factors are discussed below.

Hypertension

Hypertension is one of the most important modifiable risk factors for prevention of a first stroke. The control of high blood pressure contributes to the prevention of a first stroke but also to the prevention or reduction of other end-organ damage, such as renal or heart failure [5]. A comprehensive evidence-based approach to treatment of hypertension is provided in the document published by the Seventh Report of the Joint National Committee on Prevention, Detection, Evaluation, and Treatment of High Blood Pressure (JNC 7) [6].

The JNC 7 guidelines (Table 1) recommend lowering blood pressure to less than 140/90 mm Hg (or <130/80 mm Hg in individuals with diabetes). The optimal blood pressure target levels are still being explored in ongoing trials [6]. Overall, antihypertensive therapy is associated with a 35% to 44% reduction in the incidence of stroke [7]. Several categories of antihypertensive medications, such as thiazide diuretics, angiotensin-converting enzyme inhibitors (ACEIs), angiotensin receptor blockers (ARBs), β-adrenergic receptor blockers, and calcium channel blockers, reduce the risk of stroke in patients with hypertension [8–11].

Thiazide-type diuretics were recommended as the preferred initial drugs for treatment of hypertension in most patients [6]. Several other classes of blood pressure–lowering agents, such as ACEIs and ARBs, are recommended as next in priority. β-Blockers seem to have a lesser role in the management of uncomplicated hypertension [6,12].

The Systolic Hypertension in the Elderly Program (SHEP) trial found a 36% reduction in the incidence of stroke with treatment with a thiazide diuretic with or without a β-blocker in patients over age of 60 with isolated systolic hypertension [13]. The results from the Antihypertensive and Lipid-Lowering Treatment to Prevent Heart Attack Trial (ALLHAT), a randomized, double-blind, active, controlled clinical trial of 24,316 participants, showed the superiority of diuretic-based over α-blocker–based antihypertensive treatment for the prevention of stroke and cardiovascular disease.

Table 1
Classification and treatment of blood pressure according to the JNC 7

Classification	Blood pressure	Without convincing antihypertensive indication[a]	With convincing antihypertensive indication[a]
Normal	<120/80 mm Hg	No drug	No drug
Prehypertension	<139/90 mm Hg	No drug	Drugs for the compelling indication
Stage 1 hypertension	<159/99 mm Hg	Thiazide-type diuretics; may consider ACEIs, ARBs, β-blockers, calcium channel blockers, or combination	Drugs for the compelling indication; other drugs (diuretics, ACEIs, ARBs, β-blockers, calcium channel blockers) as needed
Stage 2 hypertension	≥160/100 mm Hg	Two-drug combination for most[b] (usually thiazide-type diuretic and ACEI or ARB or β-blocker or calcium channel blocker)	Drugs for the compelling indication and other drugs as needed

[a] Lifestyle modifications are encouraged for all and include (1) weight reduction if overweight, (2) limitation of ethyl alcohol intake, (3) increased aerobic physical activity (30–45 min/d), (4) reduction of sodium intake (<2.34 g), (5) maintenance of adequate dietary potassium (>120 mmol/d), (6) smoking cessation, and (7) Dietary Approaches to Stop Hypertension diet (rich in fruit, vegetables, and low-fat dairy products and reduced saturated and total fat). Compelling indications include (1) congestive heart failure, (2) myocardial infarction, (3) diabetes, (4) chronic renal failure, and (5) prior stroke.

[b] Initial combined therapy should be used cautiously in those at risk for orthostatic hypotension.

Data from Chobanian AV, Bakris GL, Black HR, et al. National Heart, Lung, and Blood Institute Joint National Committee on Prevention, Detection, Evaluation, and Treatment of High Blood Pressure; National High Blood Pressure Education Program Coordinating Committee. The seventh report of the Joint National Committee on Prevention, Detection, Evaluation, and Treatment of High Blood Pressure: the JNC 7 report. JAMA 2003;289:2560–72.

A meta-analysis of 18 long-term randomized trials found that both diuretics (hazard ratio, 0.49; 95% CI, 0.39–0.62) and β-blockers (hazard ratio, 0.71; 95% CI, 0.59–0.86) were effective in preventing stroke [12].

The Captopril Prevention Project (CAPPP) among 10,985 patients did not show a difference in efficacy in preventing cardiovascular morbidity and mortality between an ACEI-based therapeutic regimen captopril in comparison to the conventional therapy group (diuretics, β-blockers) in hypertension [14]. Interestingly, fatal and nonfatal stroke was more common with captopril (189 vs. 148; hazard ratio, 1.25; 95% CI, 1.01–1.55; $P = .044$).

The Systolic Hypertension in Europe (Syst-Eur) Trial showed a 42% stroke risk reduction in patients treated with a calcium channel blocker (nitrendipine) compared with placebo in patients with isolated systolic hypertension [15]. Data from the Controlled Onset Verapamil Investigation of Cardiovascular Endpoints (Convince) trial, however, did not demonstrate benefit in cardiovascular risk reduction of a calcium channel blocker (verapamil) compared with a diuretic or β-blocker treatment [16].

In the Anglo-Scandinavian Cardiac Output Trial—Blood Pressure–Lowering Arm (ASCOT-BPLA) with a primary cardiovascular outcome, a combination of atenolol (β-blocker) with a thiazide prevented more major cardiovascular events and induced less diabetes than amlodipine (a calcium channel blocker) with perindopril (ACEI) [17].

The Heart Outcomes Prevention Evaluation (HOPE) study conclusively demonstrated that ramipril (ACEI) reduces the risk of cardiovascular events in patients at risk for cardiovascular events but without heart failure [18]. The cardiovascular risk for patients treated with ACEI ramipril was reduced by approximately 20% compared with placebo. The Study to Evaluate Carotid Ultrasound Changes in Patients Treated With Ramipril and Vitamin E (Secure)substudy demonstrated that ramipril also reduced atherosclerosis [19].

The angiotensin II type 1 receptor antagonist (ARB) losartan has been shown in the Losartan Intervention for Endpoint Reduction in Hypertension (Life) study to decrease stroke risk in hypertensive patients to a substantially greater extent than conventional therapy with atenolol (β-blocker) for a similar reduction in blood pressure [10]. The Life study was a double-masked, randomized, parallel-group trial in 9193 participants aged 55 to 80 years with essential hypertension, and stroke occurred in 232 losartan and 309 atenolol patients (hazard ratio, 0.75; 95% CI, 0.63–0.89).

Achieving maximum benefit may require treatment with both an ACEI and ARB. The Ongoing Telmisartan Alone and in Combination With Ramipril Global Endpoint Trial (Ontarget) compared the benefits of ACEI treatment, ARB treatment, and treatment with an ACEI and ARB together. Meanwhile, a parallel study, Telmisartan Randomized Assessment Study in ACEI Intolerant Patients with Cardiovascular Disease (Transcend), randomized patients unable to tolerate an ACEI to receive telmisartan or placebo [20]. The results of these landmark trials have demonstrated that telmisartan, a second-generation ARB, is equally effective as the current standard, ramipril (ACEI), in reducing the risk of stroke, myocardial infarction, cardiovascular death, and hospitalization for congestive heart failure in a broad cross-section of high-risk cardiovascular patients with normal blood pressure or controlled high blood pressure, and resulted in fewer discontinuations (hazard ratio, 1.01; 95% CI, 0.94–1.09) [20]. Telmisartan is now the only ARB to have demonstrated cardiological and vascular risk reduction benefits beyond lowering blood pressure in this high-risk population. However, a combination of an ACEI ramapril and an ARB telmisartan did not show that dual renin-angiotensin system blockade provided additional risk-reduction benefit compared with single blockade. In addition, a higher discontinuation rate was observed if telmisartan and ramipril were combined [20].

The treatment of patients with hypertension is beneficial in younger but also in older patients. In the Hypertension in the Very Elderly Trial (Hyvet) among 3845 individuals 80 years of age or older with a sustained systolic blood pressure of 160 mm Hg or more, a 30% reduction in the rate of fatal or nonfatal stroke and a 39% reduction in the rate of death from stroke was achieved on active treatment (the diuretic indapamide with addition of ACEI perindopril if needed to achieve the target blood pressure of 150/80 mm Hg) in comparison to placebo [21]. In addition, fewer serious adverse events were reported in the active-treatment group. In the recent meta-analysis of 31 trials, with 190,606 participants, reduction of blood pressure produced benefits in younger (<65 years) and older (≥65 years) adults, with no strong evidence that protection against stroke and other vascular events varies substantially with age [22].

The recent Avoiding Cardiovascular Events Through Combination Therapy in Patients Living with Systolic Hypertension (Accomplish) Trial was the first trial designed to compare the effects on major fatal and nonfatal cardiovascular events of two forms of antihypertensive combination therapy: benazepril plus hydrochlorothiazide and amlodipine plus benazepril in 11,454 hypertensive patients at high cardiovascular risk [23]. The study was stopped early because combination ACEI plus the calcium channel blocker amlodipine was more effective than combination treatment with benazepril plus the thiazide diuretic hydrochlorothiazide (hazard ratio, 0.80; 95% CI, 0.71–0.90).

Direct comparisons among the various types of antihypertensive agents however are still limited. In several studies comparing ACEIs and calcium-antagonists with β-blockers, diuretic drugs, or both, primary outcome did not differ between treatment groups [7,24,25]. The optimal blood pressure lowering for primary stroke prevention and blood pressure targets are yet to be determined.

For secondary stroke prevention, the Perindopril Protection Against Recurrent Stroke Study (Progress) trial has confirmed that a perindopril (ACEI)–based regimen reduces the incidence of secondary stroke and primary myocardial infarction [26]. In addition, combination therapy with perindopril and indapamide (non–thiazide sulphonamide diuretic) produced larger blood pressure reductions and larger stroke reductions than monotherapy with perindopril alone. Treatment with these two agents should be considered routinely for all patients with a history of previous stroke or transient ischemic attack, whether hypertensive or normotensive.

Summary

It is well established that blood pressure lowering is effective for the primary prevention of stroke and other cardiovascular disorders. It has taken longer to prove that blood pressure lowering is equally effective for the prevention of recurrent stroke. Antihypertensive therapy has had a major impact on public health. Blood pressure control can be achieved in most patients, although most patients require combination therapy, often with more than two antihypertensive medications [27]. Despite this knowledge, blood pressure levels are controlled in less than 25% of the hypertensive population worldwide [28]. There is a real need to identify hypertensive subjects and treat them with blood pressure–lowering drugs for primary prevention. Lack of diagnosis and inadequate treatment are particularly evident in minority populations and in the elderly [6,29]. The real challenge now is to implement effective strategies for the control of blood pressure. Strategies should include lifestyle measures, such as exercising, losing weight, and stopping smoking [30]. Choice of a specific regimen must be individualized, but reduction in blood pressure is generally more important than the specific agent used to achieve this goal. However, it remains unclear whether specific classes of antihypertensive drugs offer, in addition to the blood pressure–lowering effects, special protection against stroke.

Diabetes

Individuals with type 2 diabetes are considered at high risk for vascular events and diabetes is a coronary heart disease (CHD) risk-equivalent with greater than 20% likelihood of a major coronary event or stroke in 10 years, according to the Adult Treatment Panel III (ATP III) of the National Cholesterol Education Program [31]. Individuals with type 2 diabetes also have an increased vulnerability to atherosclerosis and an increased prevalence of hypertension, obesity, and abnormal blood lipids. Since 1990, the prevalence of those diagnosed with diabetes rose 61%, with an increase of 8.2% from 2000 to 2001 [1].

Cardiovascular disease develops earlier in the presence of diabetes and, to reduce this increased risk, a multifactorial approach to the management of type 2 diabetes has been advocated [32]. The American Diabetes Association recommends not only good glycemic control, but also identification and aggressive treatment of associated cardiovascular risk factors, with more stringent target levels for lipids and blood pressure than those recommended for the general population [33]. Yet, data have been lacking on the effects of such a multifactorial approach to reduce risk of stroke among individuals with type 2 diabetes. In a small trial of multifactorial-intensive interventions with 160 patients with type 2 diabetes and microalbuminuria randomized to receive conventional care or intensive treatment, the risk of cardiovascular events was reduced almost by 50% (hazard ratio, 0.47; 95% CI, 0.22–0.74; $P = .01$) in those on intensive treatment [32]. Patients in the intensive-therapy group were treated with a stepwise introduction of lifestyle and pharmacologic interventions intended to maintain glycosylated hemoglobin values below 6.5%, blood pressure below 130/80 mm Hg, cholesterol levels below 175 mg/dL, and triglyceride levels below 150 mg/dL. Recommended lifestyle interventions included reduced intake of dietary fat, regular participation in light or moderate exercise, and cessation of smoking. All participants in the intensive-therapy group were advised to take aspirin and a dietary supplement, including vitamins E and C, folic acid, and chrome picolinate. In addition, individuals in the intensive-therapy group were given an ACEI (or, if contraindicated, an ARB), regardless of the level of blood pressure. The design of this study, however, did not allow identification of which intervention or combination of interventions was responsible for the benefits, or to what extent. The evidence that a multifactorial approach substantially reduces stroke and cardiovascular risk in type 2 diabetes is also supported by subgroup analyses of diabetic participants in large clinical trials. A reduction in major cardiovascular events, including stroke, was about 50% with blood pressure reduction, 25% with statin therapy, and 15% with aspirin therapy [34].

Certainly there is good justification for aggressive treatment of elevated blood pressure and lipid levels in diabetic patients with these risk factors. Several trials have compared the effect on stroke and other cardiovascular outcomes of tight control of blood glucose and blood pressure in type 2 diabetic patients versus less stringent management. In the UK Prospective Diabetes Study (UKPDS) Group, tight blood pressure control (mean blood pressure achieved, 144/82 mm Hg) resulted in a 44% reduction of fatal and nonfatal stroke as compared with more liberal control (mean blood pressure achieved, 154/87 mm Hg) [35]. Also, over 20% risk reduction was achieved with antihypertensive treatment in diabetic subjects in SHEP [36]. In a substudy of HOPE among diabetic patients, a 25% reduction of the primary combined outcome of myocardial infarction, stroke, and cardiovascular disease and a 33% risk reduction of stroke was achieved by the addition of ACEI to the current medical regimen of high-risk patients [37]. Whether these benefits were a specific effect of the ACEI or were an effect of blood pressure lowering is still the subject of debate. In a substudy of the Life study in diabetic patients, a 24% reduction in major vascular events and a nonsignificant 21% reduction in stroke were achieved among those treated with the ARB as compared with a β-blocker [11].

The evidence for lipid reduction in diabetes mellitus in relation to vascular disease has, until recently, come predominantly from subgroup analyses of clinical trials, which included people with diabetes. For people with established vascular disease, several trials of statins, and one trial of the fibrate drug gemfibrozil, have all shown significant reductions in coronary and cardiovascular events in people with diabetes comparable to that seen in those without diabetes [38–41]. The Medical Research Council/British Heart Foundation Heart Protection Study found that the addition of a statin to existing treatments in high-risk patients resulted in a 24% reduction in the rate of major vascular events and a 24% reduction in strokes [42]. This treatment effect was independent of baseline cholesterol. In a subgroup analysis of the Anglo-Scandinavian Cardiac Output Trial—Lipid-Lowering Arm (ASCOT-LLA) among diabetic individuals, there was a nonsignificant 16% reduction in the primary end point of vascular events. The trial, which was stopped early, had reduced statistical power and a lower number of primary end points [43]. The Collaborative Atorvastatin Diabetes Study (CARDS) is the only trial to date to evaluate statin therapy exclusively in diabetes in the primary prevention of vascular events. A total of 2838 people with type 2 diabetes and one risk factor (retinopathy, albuminuria, current smoking, or hypertension) were randomized to a statin or placebo [44]. Like the ASCOT-LLA trial, the CARDS trial was also stopped prematurely because the prespecified stopping rule for efficacy was met. In people with diabetes treated with a statin, the primary combined end point of acute coronary events, coronary revascularization, or stroke was reduced by 37% (hazard ratio, 0.63; 95% CI, 0.48–0.83). In particular, stroke was significantly reduced by 48%. Together, these trials provide convincing evidence that statin treatment is quite effective for prevention of stroke in individuals with diabetes mellitus.

Glycemic control is important for individuals with diabetes and ideally the glucose target is normoglycemia with the avoidance of hypoglycemia. Glycemic control is also effective way to reduce stroke risk. The UKPDS has shown that good glycemic control reduces the risk of stroke [45]. In type 1 diabetes, glucose control requires appropriate insulin therapy and concomitant professional dietary and lifestyle therapy. In type 2 diabetes, professional dietary advice, reduction of weight, and increased physical activity should be the first approach to achieve good glucose control. If these measures do not lead to a sufficient reduction of hyperglycemia, oral hypoglycemic drugs (biguanide, sulfonylurea, thiazolidinediones, or a combination) or insulin has to be added to the treatment regimen. In overweight and obese people, metformin is the drug of first choice [33]. Metformin in obese people with diabetes had a better cardiovascular outcome in an analysis of the UKPDS trial than those on treatment with insulin or a sulfonylurea [46]. There is also evidence of cardiovascular benefit with metformin for obese people as compared with conventional treatments. Second-line agents could include sulfonylureas, postprandial glucose regulators, and thiazolidinediones. A randomized controlled trial of a thiazolidinedione in 5238 people with type 2 diabetes did not achieve the composite primary end point (hazard ratio, 0.90; 95% CI, 0.80–1.02), but there was a reduction in the composite of all-cause mortality, nonfatal myocardial infarction, and stroke (hazard ratio, 0.84; 95% CI, 0.72–0.48). So there is now prospective trial evidence for another oral antidiabetic drug (in addition to metformin) in relation to cardiovascular events [47]. Insulin treatment should be considered as soon as treatment with oral agents fails to achieve the audit target hemoglobin A1c of 7.5% or less.

Summary

A comprehensive program that includes tight control of hypertension with ACEI or ARB treatment reduces the risk of stroke in individuals with diabetes. For adults with diabetes, especially those with additional risk factors, recommendations call for treatment with a statin to lower the risk of a first stroke [31]. The role of tight glycemic control in reducing the risk of stroke is still uncertain [48]. Glycemic control reduces microvascular complications, but evidence showing a reduction in stroke risk with tight glycemic control is lacking. Surely the most effective way to reduce cardiovascular risk associated with diabetes is to prevent diabetes itself. But for patients who already have diabetes or in whom it will develop, the advantages of a multifactorial approach to the reduction of cardiovascular risk are clear. The challenge is to ensure that this approach is widely adopted.

Dyslipidemia

Most epidemiologic studies find no consistent relationship between cholesterol levels and overall stroke risk. Some studies, however, have found a positive relationship between total and low-density lipoprotein (LDL) cholesterol levels and the risk of ischemic stroke [4,49–52]. Increased high-density lipoprotein (HDL) cholesterol levels are associated with reduced risk of ischemic stroke in men and women, in the elderly, and among different racial and ethnic groups [53–56]. These data add to the evidence relating lipids to stroke and support HDL cholesterol as an important modifiable stroke-risk factor. Triglyceride levels vary considerably, making elevated levels difficult to evaluate as a risk factor for stroke. Trends toward higher triglyceride levels in patients who subsequently experience ischemic stroke have been reported [4,50]. Elevated levels of triglycerides are one of the important components of the metabolic syndrome, a modifiable risk factor for stroke. The etiologic fraction estimates suggest that elimination of the metabolic syndrome would result in a 19% reduction in overall stroke, a 30% reduction of stroke in women, and a 35% reduction of stroke among Hispanics [57].

A compelling body of evidence documents that lipid-lowering agents reduce major cardiovascular events in both secondary and primary prevention of stroke and cardiovascular disease. Current evidence suggests that high-dose lipid-lowering agents can halt and, in some cases, reverse atherosclerotic progression. Furthermore, lipid-lowering agents are in general safe and well tolerated.

Statins (hydroxymethylglutaryl coenzyme A reductase inhibitors) are agents approved by the Food and Drug Administration for the prevention of ischemic stroke in patients with coronary artery disease. The rates were reduced 27% to 32% among subjects assigned to the statin as compared with placebo in ASCOT-LLA, which enrolled high-risk hypertensive subjects, and the Heart Protection Study, which enrolled high-risk subjects mostly with previous coronary events [43,58]. In a meta-analysis of nine trials including 70,070 patients, statin treatment provided 21% relative risk reductions of stroke and 0.9% absolute risk reduction [59]. It was estimated that statins prevent nine strokes per 1000 CHD or high-risk patients treated for 5 years. Although statins prevent recurrent stroke in patients with prior stroke or transient ischemic attack (the Stroke Prevention by Aggressive Reduction in Cholesterol Levels [SPARCL] trial) [60], they have not shown a definite benefit in the risk reduction of first stroke in the typical general population without known CHD.

However, in the population at high CHD risk but without documented CHD, statins were beneficial for first-stroke risk reduction [61]. Two (ASCOT-LLA and CARDS) out of five primary cardiovascular disease prevention statin trials showed a considerable reduction in stroke rates among individuals on 10 mg atorvastatin as compared with placebo [43,44]. In ASCOT-LLA, a relative risk reduction of stroke was 23%, and in CARDS (primary diabetic population), relative risk reduction of stroke was 48%. In two (Myocardial Ischemia Reduction With Aggressive Cholesterol Lowering [MIRACL] and Prevastatin or Atorvastatin Evaluation and Infection Therapy—Thrombolysis in Myocardial Infarction 22 [Prove-It]) out of five acute coronary syndrome trials, the prevention of first stroke was significant among individuals receiving a high-dose atorvastatin (80 mg) versus placebo (MIRACL) or versus pravastatin (Prove-It) [62]. Of secondary CHD prevention trials (Scandinavian Simvastatin Survival Study [4S], Cholesterol And Recurrent Events [CARE], Long-Term Intervention With Pravastatin in Ischaemic Disease [Lipid], the Heart Protection Study, Greek Atorvastatin and Coronoary Heart Disease Evaluation [Greace], and Treating to New Targets [TNT]), which together involved more than 50,000 patients with CHD, most showed a beneficial effect of statins in stroke prevention with the relative risk reduction of fatal or nonfatal stroke by 19% to 50% [4]. In the TNT trial, which randomized 10,001 individuals with stable CHD and an LDL cholesterol level of less than 130 mg/dL, the achieved LDL cholesterol levels were 101 mg/dL among those on low-dose atorvastatin and 77 mg/dL among those on high-dose treatment [63]. Those in the high-dose group had fewer major vascular events overall and fewer strokes (3.1% vs. 2.3%; hazard ratio, 0.75; 95% CI, 0.59–0.96). In addition to the stroke risk reduction by 25% ($P = .02$) on high-dose atorvastatin in the TNT trial, stroke was reduced by 47% ($P = .03$) relative to "usual" care in the Greace study [64].

In a recent review and meta-analysis of 42 randomized trials evaluating statin therapy for stroke prevention (N = 121,285), a pooled relative risk of statin therapy for all strokes was 0.84 (95% CI, 0.79–0.91) [65]. Eleven trials reported hemorrhagic stroke incidence (total N = 54,334; relative risk 0.94; 95% CI, 0.68–1.30) and 21 trials reported on fatal strokes (total N = 82,278; relative risk, 0.99; 95% CI, 0.80–1.21). This overview reinforces the need to consider prolonged statin treatment in patients at high risk of stroke and major vascular events, but caution remains for patients at risk of bleeds.

Nonstatin lipid-modifying therapies also may offer stroke protection, although the supporting data are less certain. Other lipid-modifying strategies include niacin, ezetimibe, bile acid sequestrants, cholesterol ester transfer protein inhibitors, and omega-3 fatty acids. Ezetimibe-statin combinations in particular provide superior lipid-modifying benefits compared with statin monotherapy in patients with atherogenic dyslipidemia [66]. Atherogenic dyslipidemia is associated with increased levels of chylomicrons and their remnants containing three main components: apolipoprotein B-48, triglycerides, and cholesterol ester of intestinal origin. Reduction in accessibility for one of them (specifically cholesteryl ester lessening due to ezetimibe administration) could lead to a decrease of the entire production of chylomicrons and result in a decrease of the hepatic body triglyceride pool as confirmed in a number of clinical studies. However, the Enhance study (Effect of Combination Ezetimibe and High-Dose Simvastatin Versus Simvastatin Alone on the Atherosclerotic Process in Patients with Heterozygous Familial Hypercholesterolemia) showed no difference in the progression of carotid atherosclerosis between ezetimibe and simvastatin versus simvastatin alone over a 2-year period [67]. Conclusions regarding ezetimibe and statin combinations, however, should not be made until the large clinical outcome trials are completed [68].

Niacin (nicotinic acid or vitamin B^3) treatment was associated with a 24% reduction in known or suspected stroke and transient ischemic attack [69]. The Veterans Administration HDL Intervention Trial (VA-HIT) reported a trend toward a reduction of stroke in the gemfibrozil (fibrate)–treated group (6.0% vs. 4.6%; hazard ratio, 0.75; 95% CI, 0.53–1.06; $P = .10$) of men with CHD and low levels of HDL cholesterol ($\leq$40 mg/dL) [70]. In addition, HDL cholesterol can be increased by 25% to 40% when multiple modalities are used, in particularly when niacin is added [71,72]. Because fibrates, niacin, ezetimibe, omega-3 fatty acids, and statins each regulate serum lipids by different mechanisms, combination therapy, selected on the basis of safety and effectiveness, could be more helpful in achieving comprehensive lipid control as compared with statin monotherapy.

In primary stroke prevention by lipid-lowering agents, surrogate markers of atherosclerosis, such as carotid intima-media thickness (IMT) and small nonstenotic carotid plaque measured by B-mode ultrasound, may be useful markers to monitor the effect of lipid-lowering therapies. Carotid IMT and plaque are preclinical surrogate markers of stroke and other atherosclerotic vascular diseases [73]. Lipoprotein levels and metabolic syndrome have been correlated with carotid IMT and plaque [74–77]. In clinical trials, colestipol-niacin combination therapy, statin monotherapy, and statin-niacin combination therapy each retarded the progression of carotid IMT [78–82]. In recent clinical trials that evaluated the effect of LDL reduction and HDL elevation, however, a beneficial effect resulting in halting carotid IMT progression or IMT regression was not observed. Paradoxically some individuals experienced the growth of atherosclerotic plaque and increased carotid IMT on a combination of a statin and cholesterol ester transfer protein inhibitor. More importantly, increased cardiovascular morbidity and mortality, despite achieving an aggressive reduction in LDL cholesterol and increased HDL cholesterol, was reported [67,83,84]. This evidence confirms the complex nature of an association between dyslipidemia, atherosclerosis, stroke, and cardiovascular diseases.

Summary

Lipid-modifying medications can substantially reduce the risk of stroke in patients with CHD. Treatment with statins is associated with the reduction in the risk of a first stroke in various populations of patients at increased risk of cardiovascular events. National Cholesterol Education Program III guidelines for the management of patients who have not had a stroke and who have elevated total cholesterol or elevated non–HDL cholesterol in the presence of hypertriglyceridemia are endorsed (Table 2) [31,85]. It is recommended that, in patients with known coronary artery disease and in high-risk hypertensive patients even with normal LDL cholesterol, therapy should be initiated with lifestyle measures and a statin. Suggested treatments for patients with known coronary artery disease and low-HDL cholesterol include weight loss, increased physical activity, smoking cessation, and possibly niacin or gemfibrozil administration.

Whether lipid lowering is effective in the primary prevention of stroke in the general population without CHD is still not clear. Whether the benefit of statins in reducing the risk of stroke is due to their potent lipid-lowering effects, pleiotropic effects, or a combination of the two cannot be determined based on current clinical trial data. From a benefit/risk perspective, the benefits of statin therapy outweigh the low risk of serious side effects. However, there are still populations, especially older persons (> 70 years of age) [86] and women, for whom more data on safety of lipid-lowering therapies are needed to clarify the risk associated with the effect of treatment.

Atrial fibrillation

Atrial fibrillation is an important well-documented risk factor for stroke. Atrial fibrillation is associated with a three- to fourfold increased risk of stroke [87]. Among those with atrial fibrillation but without prior stroke or transient ischemic attack, risk of first stroke is 2% to 4% per year [88]. Incidence of atrial fibrillation increases with age; approximately 6% to 10% of people older than 75 years have atrial fibrillation [89]. About one quarter of strokes in the very elderly (over 80 years) are due to atrial fibrillation [87].

Anticoagulation and antithrombotic therapies remain the main agents for stroke prevention in patients with atrial fibrillation. Several randomized controlled studies have shown that adjusted-dose warfarin reduces the overall risk of stroke by 68% with a 1% increase in the risk of major bleeds [89,90]. Risk of stroke is reduced by 20% with aspirin [91]. Warfarin reduces stroke by 45% as compared with aspirin [92]. However, reanalysis of pooled data suggests that the margin between expected benefit and harm may be less than originally believed. The reduction in annual incidence of major stroke was less than 1% and the increase in major bleeding was nearly

Table 2
Management recommendations for dyslipidemia according to National Cholesterol Education Program Adult Treatment Panel III

Factor	LDL cholesterol goal	Recommendations
0–1 CHD risk factor[a]	<160 mg/dL	Diet, weight loss, physical activity; drug therapy if LDL cholesterol remains ≥190 mg/dL; if LDL cholesterol 160–189 mg/dL, drug therapy optional
≥2 CHD risk factors and 10-y CHD risk <20%	<130 mg/dL	Diet, weight loss, physical activity; drug therapy if LDL cholesterol ≥160 mg/dL
≥2 CHD risk factors and 10-y CHD risk 10%–20%	<130 mg/dL, or <100 mg/dL	Diet, weight loss, physical activity; drug therapy if LDL cholesterol remains ≥130 mg/dL (or ≥100 mg/dL)
CHD or CHD risk equivalent[b] (10-y risk >20%)	<100 mg/dL, or <70 mg/dL	Diet, weight loss, physical activity; drug therapy if LDL cholesterol is ≥130 mg/dL and optional for LDL cholesterol 70–129 mg/dL
CHD or CHD risk equivalent[b] (10-y risk >20%)	<100 mg/dL, or <70 mg/dL	Diet, weight loss, physical activity; drug therapy if LDL cholesterol is ≥130 mg/dL and optional for LDL cholesterol 70–129 mg/dL
Non–HDL cholesterol in persons with triglycerides 200 mg/dL	Goals 30 mg/dL higher than LDL cholesterol	Same as LDL cholesterol with goal 30 mg/dL higher
Low HDL cholesterol	No consensus goal	Weight loss, physical activity; consider niacin or a fibrate in high-risk individuals with HDL cholesterol <40 mg/dL

[a] To screen for dyslipidemia, a fasting lipoprotein profile (cholesterol, triglycerides, HDL cholesterol, and LDL cholesterol) should be obtained every 5 years in adults. It should be obtained more often if two or more CHD risk factors are present (risk factors include cigarette smoking, hypertension, HDL cholesterol <40 mg/dL, CHD in a male first-degree relative <55 years old or in a female first-degree relative <65 years old, or age ≥45 years for men or ≥65 years for women) or if LDL cholesterol levels are borderline or high.

[b] CHD risk equivalents include diabetes or other forms of atherosclerotic disease (peripheral arterial disease, abdominal aortic aneurysm, and symptomatic carotid artery disease).

Data from Expert Panel on Detection, Evaluation, and Treatment of High Blood Cholesterol in Adults. Executive summary of the third report of the National Cholesterol Education Program (NCEP) Expert Panel on Detection, Evaluation, and Treatment of High Blood Cholesterol in Adults (Adult Treatment Panel III), JAMA. 2001;285:2486–97.

2% [93]. Although clinical trials have shown that an orally administered direct thrombin inhibitor ximelagatran is as effective as warfarin in atrial fibrillation, the Food and Drug Administration has not approved its use because of safety concerns (hepatotoxicity, a possible increased rate of myocardial infarction and coronary artery disease) [94,95].

Anticoagulation is underused in patients with atrial fibrillation in the community, and there is little information on treatment with anticoagulation in patients at low risk of stroke [96]. Several stroke risk–stratification schemes have been developed and validated [97,98]. The American College of Cardiology (ACC), the American Heart Association, and the European Society of Cardiology 2001 guideline recommends anticoagulation for patients with atrial fibrillation who are older than 60 years and have a history of hypertension, diabetes, coronary artery disease, impaired left ventricular systolic function, heart failure, or prior thromboembolism, and for all those with atrial fibrillation who are over 75 years of age [99]. However, this stratification model has not been validated. A new stratification model to assist clinicians in choosing patients for antithrombotic therapy, $CHADS_2$, has been recently proposed and validated [97,100]. $CHADS_2$ takes its name from C for congestive heart failure, H for hypertension, A for age (greater than 75 years), D for diabetes mellitis, and S_2 for prior stroke or transient ischemic attack. The $CHADS_2$ score was derived from independent predictors of stroke in patients with nonvalvular atrial fibrillation [100]. The score gives 1 point each for congestive heart failure, hypertension, age 75 years or over, and diabetes mellitus, and 2 points for prior stroke or transient ischemic attack. Before prescribing anticoagulation, several factors should be considered: the absolute risk of stroke, the estimated risk of bleeding, patient preferences, and access to an anticoagulation monitoring clinic. Risk stratification in these patients is the first step in the decision-making process (Table 3).

Most patients with atrial fibrillation who are less than 75 years of age and have no history of prior stroke or transient ischemic attack have a relatively low risk of stroke (1% to 2% per year) if given aspirin, and they do not benefit sufficiently from anticoagulation to warrant its use for primary stroke prevention [92,101]. It is generally agreed that atrial fibrillation patients whose estimated stroke risk exceeds 4% per year should be anticoagulated in the absence of contraindications [99].

However, warfarin therapy is underused in patients with atrial fibrillation. Only about half of patients with atrial fibrillation who are candidates for anticoagulation receive warfarin [102]. Anticoagulation is particularly underused in elderly patients [103]. In addition to age, poorly controlled hypertension and concomitant aspirin or nonsteroidal anti-inflammatory drug use confer higher bleeding risk during anticoagulation [4,98].

The optimal target international normalized ratio for primary prevention of stroke in patients with nonvalvular atrial fibrillation is in the 2 to 3 range for most atrial fibrillation patients [4,100,103,104]. Some recommend a lower

Table 3
Nonvalvular atrial fibrillation risk stratification by $CHADS_2$ scheme[a] and treatment recommendations

$CHADS_2$ score	Risk level	Stroke rate per year	Treatment recommendations based on risk stratification
0	Low	1.0%	Aspirin (75–325 mg/d)
1	Low–moderate	1.5%	Warfarin INR 2–3 or aspirin (75–325 mg/d)[b]
2[a]	Moderate	2.5%	Warfarin INR 2–3[b]
3	High	5.0%	Warfarin INR 2–3[c]
≥4	Very high	>7%	Warfarin INR 2–3[c]

One point for congestive heart failure, hypertension, age over 75 years, or diabetes; Two points for stroke or transient ischemic attack[b].

Abbreviation: INR, international normalized ratio.

[a] All nonvalvular atrial fibrillation patients with prior stroke or transient ischemic attack should be considered high risk and treated with anticoagulants; the $CHADS_2$ scheme should be applied for primary prevention.

[b] Consider patient preferences, bleeding risk, and access to INR monitoring.

[c] If patient is more than 75 years old, an INR target of 1.6 to 2.5 is recommended by some.

Data from Gage BF, Waterman AD, Shannon W, et al. Validation of clinical classification schemes for predicting stroke: results from the National Registry of Atrial Fibrillation. JAMA 2001;285:2864–70.

target international normalized ratio of 2 in the very elderly [105]. Control of hypertension in atrial fibrillation patients is also critically important, reducing both the risk of ischemic stroke and the risk of intracerebral hemorrhage [106].

All patients with mechanical heart valves, regardless of the presence of atrial fibrillation, require anticoagulation [107]. The rate of thromboembolism in patients with mechanical heart valves is 4.4 per 100 patient-years without antithrombotic therapy, 2.2 per 100 patient-years with antiplatelet drugs, and 1 per 100 patient-years with warfarin [108].

Summary

Atrial fibrillation is an important stroke risk factor and it can be treated successfully. Validated stroke risk-stratification models may help identify individuals with low risk (<2% per year) of first stroke who can be treated with aspirin. Anticoagulation reduces risk of stroke in those at high risk and without contraindications to this treatment. The development of safer, easier-to-use oral anticoagulants might improve the risk/benefit ratio.

Other cardiac conditions

Other types of cardiac disease that can contribute to the risk of thromboembolic stroke include myocardial infarction, dilated cardiomyopathy, valvular heart disease (eg, mitral valve prolapse, endocarditis, prosthetic cardiac valves), and intracardiac congenital defects (eg, patent foramen ovale, atrial septal defect, and aneurysm) [109]. Incidence of stroke is also increased in patients with reduced cardiac ejection fraction [110]. The use of warfarin for cardioembolic prophylaxis in patients with reduced left ventricular ejection fraction in the setting of idiopathic cardiomyopathy remains controversial, and clinical trials are in progress comparing warfarin with antiplatelet treatment [111]. Patients undergoing cardiac surgical procedures have a perioperative stroke risk of 1% to 7% [112]. Presence of aortic arch atheroma is also associated with increased risk of ischemic stroke [113].

Summary

Various guidelines recommend strategies to reduce the risk of stroke in patients with cardiac conditions. These include the management of patients with acute myocardial infarction [114], unstable and stable angina [115,116], and valvular heart disease [108]. Studies proving the benefits of specific prophylactic procedures for patients with a variety of cardiac conditions are lacking.

Asymptomatic carotid stenosis

Carotid stenosis of 50% or greater can be detected in about 5% to 10% of men and women older than 65 years of age, and stenosis of greater than 80% in 1% of the population [117–120]. An annual stroke risk between 1% and 3% occurs among individuals with asymptomatic CAS of 50% to 99% in the natural history studies [121] and is higher in those with CAS of greater than 75%, progression of CAS, and heart disease, and in men [122]. However, about 45% of ipsilateral strokes in patients with carotid stenosis could be attributable to lacunes or cardioembolism, emphasizing the need to fully evaluate patients with asymptomatic carotid stenosis for other treatable causes of stroke [120]. In summary, data from observational studies and clinical trials indicate an annual rate of stroke ipsilateral to a significant extracranial CAS of about 1% to 2%.

There have been two large published randomized controlled trials designed to assess the benefit of cardioembyonic antigen (CEA) in patients with asymptomatic CAS. In the Asymptomatic Carotid Atherosclerosis Study (ACAS) designed to test the efficacy of CEA in subjects with asymptomatic CAS 60% to 99%, 1662 subjects were randomized to CEA and best medical therapy (n = 828) or to medical therapy alone (n = 834) [123]. The overall risk of perioperative stroke or death was 2.7% (1.2% angiography-related complications and a 1.5% risk of stroke or death among those having CEA at 30 days). The study was stopped prematurely after a median follow-up of 2.7 years because there was a significant benefit of surgery over medical treatment alone. The aggregate rate of ipsilateral stroke, any perioperative stroke, or death was estimated at

5% over 5 years in surgically treated patients, and at 11% in medically treated patients (53% risk reduction, approximate 2% per year event rate was reduced to 1% per year; $P = .004$). The benefit began to accrue after 1 to 2 years. The study was not statistically powered to detect differences among patient subgroups. No surgical benefit was observed in relationship to the degree of CAS, but women appeared to benefit less than men (17% nonsignificant risk reduction in women; 95% CI, 4%–65%, vs. a 66% risk reduction in men, 95% CI, 36%–82%). This difference was partly due to a higher rate of perioperative complications in women (3.6% vs. 1.7%).

In the Medical Research Council Asymptomatic Surgery Trial (ACST), the largest randomized trial comparing a strategy of immediate versus deferred CEA, 3120 asymptomatic patients with CAS greater than 60% on carotid ultrasound were enrolled. There was a 3.1% (95% CI, 2.3%–4.1%) risk of stroke or death within 30 days of surgery [124]. Although the overall periprocedural complication rate was similar to that in ACAS, the surgical complication rate of the ACST was actually twice that of ACAS in which the complication rate of 1.5% was due to surgery only. The overall 5-year risk of any stroke or perioperative death was 11.8% with deferred surgery versus 6.4% with immediate endarterectomy ($P<.0001$; 2.4% per year reduced to 1.3% per year). The benefit began to accrue after about 2 years. Although subgroup analyses need to be interpreted with caution, as in ACAS, there did not appear to be any difference in benefit based on the degree of CAS. Women also appeared to benefit less than men after CEA (4.1% [95% CI, 0.7–7.4%] in women vs. 8.2% [95% CI, 5.6%–10.8%] in men) and had a somewhat higher but nonsignificant rate of perioperative complications (3.8% vs. 2.7%).

In the pooled analyses from ACAS and ACST, surgical benefit is greater in men than in women (men: pooled interaction $P = .01$, odds ratio 0.49 [95% CI, 0.36–0.60]; women: odds ratio 0.96 [95% CI, 0.63–1.45]) [125]. Data presented in the ACST publication also permit calculation of the comparative rates of any stroke or death. Similar to ACAS, the overall rate of any stroke or death was 31.2% for deferred endarterectomy versus 28.9% for immediate endarterectomy (relative risk reduction of 7%; 95% CI, 3%–17%; $P = .172$) and for any major stroke or death 25.5% versus 25.3% (relative risk reduction of 7%; 95% CI, –5%–18%; $P = .242$). These data must be taken into account when the procedure is considered.

The benefit of endarterectomy in asymptomatic CAS is very much dependent on surgical risk, with the benefit observed only if the periprocedural complication rates are less than 2.7% as observed in ACAS or less than 3.1% as in ACST. Community-wide scrutiny of CEA in asymptomatic CAS in 10 United States states shows an overall risk for stroke or death of 3.8% (including 1% mortality) [126]. Most physicians, however, are not aware of the CEA complication rates in their respective hospitals.

Since ACAS, "standard" medical therapy has been enhanced with widespread use of antiplatelet agents and of drugs that lower blood pressure and lipids. Therefore, the risk of stroke in asymptomatic CAS may be further reduced without CEA. Although screening of general populations for CAS may not be cost-effective [127], screening for "high-risk" individuals with asymptomatic CAS, such as screening for those with impaired cerebral vasoreactivity [128] or presence of microemboli on transcranial Doppler [129], may help select those who may benefit from CEA.

Carotid angioplasty with stenting has been available for over 10 years, but data from clinical studies proving its equivalence or superiority to CEA in asymptomatic CAS are still limited. The Stenting and Angioplasty with Protection in Patients at High Risk for Endarterectomy (Sapphire) trial showed that stenting was not inferior (within 3%, $P = .004$) to CEA among CAS subjects at high risk for the surgery [130]. About 70% of the enrolled subjects had asymptomatic CAS, with 5.4% rates of stroke, myocardial infarction, or death with stenting versus 10.2% in CEA group at 30 days ($P = .20$), and 9.9% versus 21.5% at 1 year, respectively ($P = .02$). Because, the outcome in Sapphire included myocardial infarction, the results are not directly comparable to those from ACAS or ACST. But even in the stenting arm of Sapphire with lower rates of combined major cardiovascular outcomes of 9.9% at 1 year, it is considerably higher than the stroke risk associated with asymptomatic CAS (1% to 2% per year) in ACAS or ACST. The study did not include medically treated controls, so a comparison to the best medical treatment could not be performed.

Although pivotal stenting trials, including Sapphire, were initially limited by a lack of equipment dedicated to carotid artery stenting, including embolic protection filters, their results have compared favorably to both direct and historical surgical controls [131]. While this has led to Food and Drug Administration approval of several carotid stent systems in the United States, recent European randomized carotid stenting trials (Space [Stent-Supported Percutaneous Angioplasty of the Carotid Artery Versus Endarterectomy] and EVA-3S [Endarterectomy Versus Angioplasty in Patients With Severe Symptomatic Carotid Stenosis]) had mixed results because they failed to prove noninferiority of stenting compared with CEA and confused the perception of the place of this technology in the care of asymptomatic CAS patients [132]. The carotid stent registries with a wide range of operator experience, and patient enrollment based on surgical risk criteria (Capture II [Carotid Acculink/Accunet Post Approval Trial to Uncover Rare Events], Exact [Emboshield and Xact Post Approval Carotid Stent Trial], Cabernet [Carotid Artery Revascularization Using the Boston Scientific FilterWire and the EndoTex NexStent]) were able to meet the guidelines of 3% procedural events in the asymptomatic CAS [133]. Ongoing carotid stenting trials in the United States will further contribute to our understanding of the benefit of stent therapy in CAS patients.

Summary

In individuals with asymptomatic CAS who are at low risk for surgery, CEA in a combination with "usual medical care" is superior to "usual medical care" alone for reduction of ischemic stroke if the perioperative complication rate is lower than 3% (Table 4) [134]. The total 5-year risk of stroke or procedural morbidity after CEA is 11.5% for deferred endarterectomy versus 6.0% for immediate endarterectomy (5.5% absolute difference, which means that to prevent one event 18 subjects need to be treated over 5 years) [124]. Perioperative risk is not balanced by benefit for 2 years. Patient selection, comorbidities, life expectancy, and patient preferences should be discussed, and the risks and benefits of the procedure should be carefully considered. The benefit of CEA in patients with asymptomatic CAS seems to be more pronounced in men, and it still

Table 4
Guideline management recommendations

Factor	Goal	Recommendation
Asymptomatic CAS	No CAS	Endarterectomy may be considered in selected patients with ≥60% stenosis without occlusion, performed by a surgeon with surgical morbidity and mortality <3%; careful patient selection should be guided by individual factors, including comorbid conditions, life expectancy, and patient preference
Cigarette smoking	Cessation	Counseling, nicotine replacement, varenicline, and formal programs are recommended
Diet/nutrition	Well-balanced diet	A diet containing ≥5 servings of fruits and vegetables per day may reduce the risk of stroke
Physical activity	≥30 min of moderate activity/d	Moderate exercise (eg, brisk walking, jogging, cycling, or other aerobic activity)
Alcohol	Moderation	No more than 2 drinks per day for men, and no more than 1 drink per day for women
Drug abuse	Cessation	A history of substance abuse should be part of health evaluation
Sleep apnea	Treatment for OSA	Overnight sleep study in patients with snoring, excessive daytime sleepiness, body mass index over 30, and drug-resistant hypertension; continuous positive airway pressure treatment

remains uncertain whether there is benefit of CEA in women. One must keep in mind that women have been underrepresented in CEA trials, and some observational data have suggested benefit of CEA for women. Carotid angioplasty with stenting may be a reasonable alternative to CEA in asymptomatic CAS at high risk for the surgical procedure.

Cigarette smoke

Cigarette smoking is a well-recognized and modifiable risk factor for ischemic and hemorrhagic stroke [87,135–137]. A meta-analysis of 32 studies estimated a twofold increased risk of ischemic stroke for smokers versus nonsmokers and a threefold increased risk for subarachnoid hemorrhage [138]. Passive cigarette smoke is a risk factor for stroke [139]. The stroke risk for passive smoking is close to the risk for active smoking, suggesting that tobacco exposure may have "threshold" rather than a dose–response relationship [140].

The most effective preventive measures are to never smoke and to minimize exposure to environmental smoke. The risk of stroke is also reduced with smoking cessation. Smoking cessation is associated with a rapid reduction in the risk of stroke to a level that approaches, although never reaches, the risk of those who never smoked within 2 to 5 years of cessation [141]. Sustained smoking cessation is difficult to achieve. A combination of nicotine replacement therapy, social support, and behavioral treatments offers an effective management for smoking cessation (Table 4) [142]. Varenicline is a novel smoking-cessation agent that acts at a number of nicotinic acetylcholine receptors and recently has been shown to be superior to the current standard patch in achieving abstinence and in reducing withdrawal phenomena, such as urges to smoke and withdrawal symptoms [143]. Varenicline may be an additional treatment option and is likely to become popular with patients and clinicians.

Summary

Cigarette smoking is clearly associated with the risk of stroke. Comprehensive smoking cessation programs are effective. Data, however, on the effects of these programs on reduction of the risk of stroke are lacking.

Diet and nutrition

Diet is associated with the risk of stroke. Increased fruit and vegetable consumption is associated with a reduced risk of stroke in a dose-response manner [144]. For each 1-serving-per-day increment in fruit and vegetable intake, the risk of stroke was reduced by 6% in the Nurses' Health Study and the Health Professionals' Follow-Up Study [145]. A higher level of sodium and lower level of potassium intake is associated with an increased risk of stroke, possibly mediated through mechanisms dependent on blood pressure [146]. Diets rich in fruits and vegetables lower blood pressure and therefore may decrease risk of stroke [147]. Other dietary factors may affect the risk of stroke, but specific evidence is lacking. The Dietary Approaches to Stop Hypertension diet includes high consumption of fruits, vegetables, and low-fat dairy products, and reduced intake of total and saturated fat (Table 4) [147].

Summary

Diets rich in fruits and vegetables and with increased potassium but reduced sodium and fat may reduce the risk of stroke. Dietary trials specifically focused to reducing the risk of stroke are lacking.

Physical inactivity

Physical inactivity is a well-established and modifiable risk factor for stroke [148]. The protective effects of physical activity have been reported for different ages, sexes, and race/ethnicities in large studies, including the National Health and Nutrition Examination Survey Study and the Northern Manhattan Stroke Study [149,150]. In the Northern Manhattan Stroke Study, a dose–response relationship was reported as more intensive physical activity provided additional benefits compared with light to moderate physical activity. The protective effect of physical activity may be mediated through reduced blood pressure and weight and control of diabetes [151].

The benefits of physical activity are outlined in the Centers for Disease Control and Prevention and the National Institutes of Health guidelines (Table 4) [152,153], which recommend moderate exercise for at least 30 minutes per day. The benefits for stroke are evident for light to moderate activities, such as walking.

Summary

Although clinical trials examining how physical activity affects risk of stroke do not exist, it is clear that a sedentary lifestyle increases the risk of stroke. Physical activity is beneficial in reduction of risk factors, and therefore is recommended to reduce risk of first stroke.

Management of less well documented modifiable risk factors to prevent first stroke

Obesity and metabolic syndrome

Obesity is a risk factor for stroke (relative risks, 1.5–2.0) and is associated with increased risk of hypertension, dyslipidemia, hyperinsulinemia, and glucose intolerance [154]. In addition, higher weight during young adulthood and weight gain after young adulthood are associated with an increased risk of stroke [155]. Recent studies have also reported the association between measures of the distribution of body fat, such as the waist-to-hip ratio, as a measure of abdominal obesity [156] and increased risk of stroke. About one in three adults in the United States is overweight, and the prevalence of obesity has been steadily increasing [157].

Obesity is an important component of the metabolic syndrome, a potentially modifiable risk factor for stroke. Metabolic syndrome is defined as the presence of more than three of the following: (1) abdominal obesity as determined by waist circumference greater than 102 cm or greater than 40 in for men and greater than 88 cm or greater than 35 in for women; (2) triglycerides 150 mg/dL or more; (3) HDL cholesterol less than 40 mg/dL for men and less than 50 mg/dL for women; (4) blood pressure 130/85 mm Hg or higher; and (5) fasting glucose of 110 mg/dL or more [31]. Insulin resistance is an important marker of the metabolic syndrome and may be a prevalent risk factor for stroke [57]. Insulin resistance has been incorporated into the World Health Organization definition of metabolic syndrome. Drugs that can reduce insulin resistance may also be effective in preventing stroke [158]. The metabolic syndrome is highly prevalent in the United States. Age-adjusted prevalence of metabolic syndrome is 23.7%. The highest prevalence is in Mexican Americans (31.9%) and in African American women (57%) [159].

Weight reduction is beneficial in reducing risk factors, reducing metabolic syndrome, and, therefore, in possibly reducing the risk of stroke. Clinical trials to test the effects of weight reduction on reducing the risk of stroke do not exist. Numerous studies, however, report the beneficial effects of weight reduction on blood pressure. In a meta-analysis of 25 clinical trials, blood pressure was reduced by 3.6 to 4.4 mm Hg with an average weight loss of 5.1 kg [160].

Summary

Obesity and metabolic syndrome are associated with an increased risk of stroke. Individual components of the metabolic syndrome have been associated with an increased risk of ischemic stroke, and therefore should be treated by lifestyle measures and pharmacotherapy as recommended by JNC 7 and ATP III guidelines [6,31]. Despite a lack of clinical trials on the effects of weight reduction and stroke risk, weight reduction is important for lowering blood pressure and metabolic syndrome risk, which may lead to reduction of stroke risk. In addition to exercise and diet, glycemic and lipid control are important factors in reducing the risk of first stroke.

Alcohol and drug abuse

The J-shaped relation of alcohol consumption to the risk of stroke has been reported [161]. The relative risk of ischemic stroke associated with moderate alcohol consumption (one to two drinks per day), as compared with nondrinking, is between 0.3 and 0.5 in some populations and increases to two for persons consuming three or more drinks per day. For hemorrhagic stroke, the relative risk varies from 2 to 4, with some increased risk at all levels of intake [162]. Alcoholism is a major public health problem in the United States. Over 10 million adults have alcoholism and alcohol-related diseases, such as hypertension and cirrhosis [163]. Despite the potential benefit of moderate alcohol consumption, alcohol should not be considered as a preventive agent for stroke, given the health risks associated with excessive intake.

Compared to no alcohol consumption, light-to-moderate alcohol consumption (one or fewer drinks per day for women and two or fewer drinks per day for men) can increase HDL cholesterol, reduce platelet aggregation, and lower plasma fibrinogen concentration [164]. Heavy alcohol consumption can lead to hypertension, hypercoagulability, reduced cerebral blood flow, and a greater likelihood of atrial fibrillation [165]. In a meta-analysis of 35 observational studies, consumption of less than one drink per day (one drink defined as 12 g of alcohol), but not abstention, was associated with a 20% reduced risk of stroke (95% CI, 0.67–0.96) and consumption of one to two drinks per day with 28% risk reduction (95% CI, 0.57–0.91) [166]. As compared with abstainers, those who consumed more than five drinks per day had a 69% increased stroke risk (risk ratio, 1.69; 95% CI, 1.34–2.15).

Abuse of drugs, such as heroin, cocaine, and amphetamines, is associated with an increased risk of ischemic and hemorrhagic stroke [167,168]. These drugs may cause metabolic and hematologic changes, including increased platelet aggregation and changes in blood pressure, and can lead to vasculopathy or cerebral embolization from various sources [169].

Summary

Compared to no alcohol consumption, light to moderate alcohol consumption is associated with a reduced risk of stroke while heavier consumption is associated with an increased risk of stroke. Alcoholism is a major public health problem as alcohol consumption can induce dependence. Reduction of alcohol consumption in heavy drinkers is recommended [170]. A suggested consumption of alcohol in those who consume alcohol is no more than two drinks per day for men and no more than one drink per day for nonpregnant women (Table 4).

Identification and management of drug abuse is challenging. Long-term treatment strategies based on medication, psychologic support, and outreach programs play an important part in treatment of drug dependency (Table 4). When a patient is identified as having a drug addiction problem, referral for appropriate counseling is recommended.

Sleep apnea

Sleep-related breathing disorders are highly prevalent in patients with established cardiovascular disease. Obstructive sleep apnea (OSA) is being increasingly recognized as an important risk factor for stroke. It is a less well documented but modifiable risk factor. The evidence of the association of OSA with first ischemic stroke is primarily derived from the association with heart disease. OSA affects an estimated 15 million adult Americans and is present in a large proportion of patients with hypertension, obesity, and cardiovascular disease [171]. Prevalence of OSA in these populations ranges between 3% and 7%. Factors that increase vulnerability for OSA include age, male sex, obesity, family history, menopause, craniofacial abnormalities, and certain health behaviors, such as cigarette smoking and alcohol use.

OSA is characterized by repetitive interruption of ventilation during sleep caused by collapse of the pharyngeal airway or central nervous system dysfunction. The overnight polysomnogram is the standard diagnostic test for OSA. A diagnosis of OSA syndrome is made when a person has an apnea-hypopnea index (number of apneas and hypopneas per hour of sleep) greater than five and symptoms of excessive daytime sleepiness [172]. A recent analysis from more than 6000 adults participating in the Sleep Heart Health Study showed that hypopneas accompanied by oxyhemoglobin desaturation of more than 4% were associated with prevalent cardiovascular disease and stroke independent of confounders [173].

Habitual snoring and daytime sleepiness are risk factors for ischemic stroke [174]. Snoring may be a marker for sleep apnea, which can secondarily increase the risk of stroke by worsening hypertension and heart disease; reducing cerebral blood flow and autoregulation; impairing endothelial function; accelerating atherosclerosis, hypercoagulability, and inflammation; and causing paradoxical embolism in patients with patent foramen ovale [172].

Treatment of OSA is individualized and includes noninvasive continuous positive airway pressure ventilation, bilevel positive airway pressure, and automatic control of airway pressure delivery with continuous positive airway pressure devices. A variety of surgical interventions and prosthetic oral devices are available.

Summary

OSA is associated with vascular risk factors and an increased risk of cardiovascular disease. Individuals with abdominal obesity and hypertension, snoring, and daytime sleepiness are more likely to have OSA and should be referred to a sleep specialist for further evaluation (Table 4). Prospective randomized studies regarding the effect of treatment of sleep apnea on stroke risk reduction do not exist. However, successful treatment of OSA can lead to a reduction in blood pressure, which may lead to a reduced risk of first stroke.

Hyperhomocysteinemia

Elevated plasma levels of homocysteine (hyperhomocysteinemia) are increasingly recognized as a potential risk for atherothrombotic vascular diseases, including stroke [175,176]. In the Northern Manhattan Stroke Study, the adjusted hazard ratio of 2.0 (95% CI, 1.0–4.1) was reported for ischemic stroke among those with a homocysteine level greater than 15 μmol/L compared with less than 10 μmol/L (95% CI, 1.00–4.05) [176]. The vascular effects of homocysteine were greatest among whites and Hispanics, but least among blacks.

A key event in the vascular pathobiology of hyperhomocysteinemia seems to involve the induction of endothelial dysfunction due to a reduction of the endogenous antiatherothrombotic molecular nitric oxide [177]. Elevated homocysteine levels can be efficiently and safely reduced in most hyperhomocysteinemic patients by supplementation with folic acid and cobalamin. This reduction is associated with an improvement in endothelial function and other surrogate markers of atherothrombosis, such as carotid plaque area [178]. Whether or not this translates into clinical benefits, is still under investigation. On the basis of the results of several recent clinical trials (eg, Vitamin Intervention for Stroke Prevention [VISP] trial or from ongoing Vitamins to Prevent Stroke [Vitatops] trial, which did not show a reduction of inflammatory markers by reducing homocysteine), many researchers doubt that vitamin therapy designed to lower total homocysteine concentrations is effective in reducing the risk of stroke and cardiovascular events [179,180]. However, these trials were not designed for secondary and not primary stroke prevention but rather for preventing secondary strokes, when hyperhomocysteinemia may have been less important than other factors.

In a detailed assessment of the results of the recent HOPE-2 trial and a reanalysis of the VISP trial restricted to patients capable of responding to vitamin therapy, it has been suggested that higher doses of vitamin B_{12} and perhaps new approaches to lowering total homocysteine, besides routine vitamin therapy with folate, vitamin B_6, and vitamin B_{12}, could reduce the risk of stroke [181]. Thus, therapy to lower homocysteine could still help to prevent stroke. Unfortunately, many major trials of homocysteine lowering in the general cardiovascular literature have not shown benefit of vitamin therapy for reduction of major vascular endpoints.

A single-nucleotide polymorphism in the methylenetetrahydrofolate reductase gene reduces activity of the enzyme that metabolizes homocysteine, producing an increase in serum homocysteine [182]. This single-nucleotide polymorphism can be found in 10% to 12% of the population and is associated with a 25% higher homocysteine level than in those with a wild-type genotype. In a recent meta-analysis of 72 studies, a 5-μmol/L increase in homocysteine was associated with a 1.6-fold increased risk of stroke (95% CI, 1.2–2.0) [182]. In addition, a 3-μmol/L decrement of homocysteine level was associated with a 24% risk reduction of stroke [183].

The current American Heart Association guidelines [4] recommend daily intake of folate (400 μg/d), B_6 (1.7 mg/d), and B_{12} (2.4 μg/d) by consumption of vegetables, fruits, legumes, meats, fish, and fortified grains and cereals. This diet may be useful in reducing the risk of stroke.

Summary

No randomized trials have shown that lowering elevated homocysteine levels reduces the risk of a first stroke. Until the results of more clinical trials are available, the question of whether homocysteine is a risk predictor or a modifiable risk factor for stroke remains unanswered. However, there is consistent evidence regarding overall relationship between homocysteine levels and vascular risk, and a benefit of treatment of elevated homocysteine levels cannot be excluded. There are insufficient data to recommend specific treatments to reduce the risk of first stroke in patients with elevated homocysteine. Use of folic acid and B vitamins in persons with known elevated homocysteine levels is safe and may be useful in primary stroke prevention.

Aspirin for primary stroke prevention

Despite conclusive evidence of the benefits of aspirin in the secondary prevention of stroke, only a few clinical trials have addressed aspirin use in primary prevention. In the United States, the Physicians' Health Study [184] showed that the relative risk of ischemic stroke was 1.11 (95% CI, 0.82–1.50) among men using 325 mg of aspirin every other day for an average of 60.2 months versus placebo; and the relative risk of stroke of all types was 1.22 (95% CI, 0.93–1.60) on aspirin versus placebo. The risk of hemorrhagic stroke was increased (relative risk 2.14; 95% CI, 0.96–4.77). In the British Doctors' Trial with a daily dose of 500 mg of aspirin for 6 years, no significant difference in the incidence of stroke between the treatment and control groups was found, but a higher incidence of disabling stroke among those taking aspirin was reported (relative risk, 2.58; $P < .05$) [185]. In a recent meta-analysis of six randomized trials (the Physicians' Health Study, the British Doctors' Trial, the Thrombosis Prevention Trial, the Hypertension Optimal Treatment study, the Primary Prevention Project, and the Women's Health Study) that evaluated the benefits of aspirin for primary prevention in a combined sample of 47,293 subjects on aspirin and 45,580 on placebo (or nonaspirin), superiority of aspirin was suggested for total cardiovascular events but there was no significant difference in the incidence of stroke [186]. Many of the patients in these studies, however, were at relatively low risk, and a study of persons at moderate risk might show a benefit of aspirin therapy.

The effects and the risk/benefit ratio of aspirin in primary prevention may be different in women and men. In the Women's Health Study [187] among 39,876 asymptomatic women 45 years old or older who were followed for 10 years for a first major vascular event, a 17% reduction in the risk of stroke (95% CI, 0.69–0.99) was found among those who received 100 mg of aspirin compared with placebo, but a nonsignificant 9% reduction (95% CI, 0.80–1.03) in the risk of the combined primary end point. The risk of hemorrhagic stroke was nonsignificant (relative risk, 1.24; 95% CI, 0.82–1.87). The overall average stroke rates were 0.11% per year in aspirin-treated patients and 0.13% per year in placebo-treated patients (absolute risk reduction 0.02% per year, and a number needed to treat of 5000). The average gastrointestinal hemorrhage rates were 0.06% per year for aspirin and 0.05% per year for placebo (absolute risk increase 0.01% per year, number needed to harm of 10,000). The most consistent benefit for aspirin was among women 65 years old or older, a history of hypertension, hyperlipidemia, diabetes, or a 10-year cardiovascular risk of at least 10%.

Summary

Aspirin is not recommended for the prevention of a first stroke in men [4]. The use of aspirin 75 mg/d is recommended for cardiovascular (including but not specific to stroke) prophylaxis for persons whose risk is sufficiently high for the benefits to outweigh the risks associated with treatment (a 10-year risk of cardiovascular events of >6%–10%) [188]. There is no evidence that this class of drugs reduces the risk of stroke in the general population of persons at low risk [188]. Aspirin can be useful for prevention of a first stroke among women whose risk is sufficiently high for the benefits to outweigh the risks associated with treatment. The reasons for the differences between men and women remain uncertain.

Assessing the risk of a first stroke

Many therapeutic options exist for risk factor management to prevent a first stroke. The choice of an appropriate risk modification program depends on individual stroke risk. Each individual should have an assessment of risk of first stroke. Many factors can contribute to stroke risk. Many individuals have more than one risk factor, some of which are well documented and some less well documented. Several stroke risk assessment tools are available to use for primary stroke prevention screening programs [189]. These stroke risk estimation tools generally focus on several major vascular risk factors and do not include the full range of contributing factors, and especially do not consider different characteristics of various race/ethnic populations. The Framingham Stroke Profile is gender specific and provides a gender-specific 1-, 5-, or 10-year cumulative stroke risk [190]. Independent stroke predictors included in the Framingham Stroke Profile are age, systolic blood pressure, hypertension, diabetes mellitus, current smoking, established cardiovascular disease (any one of myocardial infarction, angina or coronary insufficiency, congestive heart failure, or intermittent claudication), atrial fibrillation, and left ventricular hypertrophy on EKG. It has been updated to include the use of antihypertensive therapy and the risk of stroke or death among individuals with atrial fibrillation (Table 5) [191]. Although very useful in some populations, the Framingham Stroke Profile has not been sufficiently studied in different race/ethnic groups.

Table 5
Modified Framingham Stroke Profile

Risk factor	Points
Age	
54–56 y	0
57–59 y	1
60–62 y	2
63–65 y	3
66–68 y	4
69–71 y	5
72–74 y	6
75–77 y	7
78–80 y	8
81–83 y	9
84–86 y	10
Systolic blood pressure	
95–105 mm Hg	0
106–116 mm Hg	1
117–126 mm Hg	2
127–137 mm Hg	3
138–148 mm Hg	4
149–159 mm Hg	5
160–170 mm Hg	6
171–181 mm Hg	7
182–191 mm Hg	8
192–202 mm Hg	9
203–213 mm Hg	10
Treated systolic pressure	2
Diabetes mellitus	2
Cigarette smoking	3
CHD	3
Atrial fibrillation	4
Left ventricular hypertrophy on EKG	6

Data from Wang TJ, Massaro JM, Levy D, et al. A risk score for predicting stroke or death in individuals with new-onset atrial fibrillation in the community: the Framingham Heart Study. JAMA 2003;290:1049–56.

Alternative prediction models using Framingham risk factors and adding continuous levels of risk factors have been developed in other cohorts but their validity has not been well tested. [3,192,193]

Summary

A goal is to develop a generally applicable and simple tool for assessing stroke risk. Such tools that exist each have limitations and none is widely accepted. New risk factors associated with the risk of stroke are emerging and they would need to be considered in newer stroke risk assessment tools. Validation of the current stroke risk assessment tools is needed in different age, gender, and race/ethnic groups. The complexity of risk factors predicting stroke in an individual makes development of new stroke risk assessment tools a challenging task.

References

[1] Sacco RL, Benjamin EJ, Broderick JP, et al. American Heart Association Prevention Conference. IV. Prevention and rehabilitation of stroke risk factors. Stroke 1997;28:1507–17.

[2] American Heart Association. Heart disease and stroke statistics—2004 update. Dallas (TX): American heart association; 2003.

[3] Sacco RL. The 2006 William Feinberg Lecture: shifting the paradigm from stroke to global vascular risk estimation. Stroke 2007;38(6):1980–7.

[4] Larry B, Goldstein LB, Adams R, et al. A guideline from the American Heart Association/American Stroke Association Stroke Council: cosponsored by the Atherosclerotic Peripheral Vascular Disease Interdisciplinary Working Group; Cardiovascular Nursing Council; Clinical Cardiology Council; Nutrition, Physical Activity, and Metabolism Council; and the Quality of Care and Outcomes Research Interdisciplinary Working Group: the American Academy of Neurology affirms the value of this guideline. Stroke 2006;37:1583–633.

[5] Vasan RS, Beiser A, Seshadri S, et al. Residual lifetime risk for developing hypertension in middle-aged women and men: the Framingham Heart Study. JAMA 2002;287:1003–10.

[6] Chobanian AV, Bakris GL, Black HR, et al. National Heart, Lung, and Blood Institute Joint National Committee on Prevention, Detection, Evaluation, and Treatment of High Blood Pressure; National High Blood Pressure Education Program Coordinating Committee. The seventh report of the Joint National Committee on Prevention, Detection, Evaluation, and Treatment of High Blood Pressure: the JNC 7 report. JAMA 2003;289:2560–72.

[7] Neal B, MacMahon S, Chapman N. Blood Pressure Lowering Treatment Trialists' Collaboration. Effects of ACE inhibitors, calcium antagonists, and other blood-pressure–lowering drugs: results of prospectively designed overviews of randomised trials. Blood Pressure Lowering Treatment Trialists' Collaboration. Lancet 2000;356:1955–64.

[8] ALLHAT Officers and Coordinators for the ALLHAT Collaborative Research Group. Major outcomes in high-risk hypertensive patients randomized to angiotensin-converting enzyme inhibitor or calcium channel blocker vs diuretic: the Antihypertensive and Lipid-Lowering Treatment to Prevent Heart Attack Trial (ALLHAT) [published corrections appear in JAMA. 2003;289:178 and JAMA. 2004;18:2196]. JAMA 2002;288:2981–97.

[9] Black HR, Elliott WJ, Grandits G, et al. Convince Research Group. Principal results of the Controlled Onset Verapamil Investigation of Cardiovascular End Points (CONVINCE) trial. JAMA 2003;289:2073–82.

[10] Dahlof B, Devereux RB, Kjeldsen SE, et al. Life Study Group. Cardiovascular morbidity and mortality in the Losartan Intervention For Endpoint reduction in hypertension study (LIFE): a randomised trial against atenolol. Lancet 2002;359:995–1003.

[11] Turnbull F. Blood Pressure Lowering Treatment Trialists' Collaboration. Effects of different blood-pressure–lowering regimens on major cardiovascular events: results of prospectively-designed overviews of randomised trials. Lancet 2003;362:1527–35.

[12] Psaty BM, Smith NL, Siscovick DS, et al. Health outcomes associated with antihypertensive therapies used as first-line agents. A systematic review and meta-analysis. JAMA 1997;277:739–45.

[13] SHEP Cooperative Research Group. Prevention of stroke by antihypertensive drug treatment in older persons with isolated systolic hypertension: final results of the Systolic Hypertension in the Elderly Program (SHEP). JAMA 1991;265:3255–64.

[14] Hansson L, Lindholm LH, Niskanen L, et al. Effect of angiotensin-converting-enzyme inhibition compared with conventional therapy on cardiovascular morbidity and mortality

in hypertension: the Captopril Prevention Project (CAPPP) randomised trial. Lancet 1999; 353(9153):611–6.

[15] Staessen JA, Fagard R, Thijs L, et al. Randomised double-blind comparison of placebo and active treatment for older patients with isolated systolic hypertension: the Systolic Hypertension in Europe (Syst-Eur) Trial Investigators. Lancet 1997;350:757–64.

[16] Principal results of the Controlled Onset Verapamil Investigation of Cardiovascular End Points (CONVINCE) trial. 2003; 289(16):2073–82.

[17] Dahlöf B, Sever PS, Poulter NR, et al. ASCOT Investigators. Prevention of cardiovascular events with an antihypertensive regimen of amlodipine adding perindopril as required versus atenolol adding bendroflumethiazide as required, in the Anglo-Scandinavian Cardiac Outcomes Trial—Blood Pressure Lowering Arm (ASCOT-BPLA): a multicentre randomised controlled trial. Lancet 2005;366(9489):895–906.

[18] The Heart Outcomes Prevention Evaluation Study Investigators. Effects of an angiotensin-converting-enzyme inhibitor, ramipril, on cardiovascular events in high-risk patients. N Engl J Med 2000;342:145–53.

[19] Lonn E, Yusuf S, Dzavik V, et al. SECURE Investigators. Effects of ramipril and vitamin E on atherosclerosis: the Study to Evaluate Carotid Ultrasound Changes in Patients Treated with Ramipril and Vitamin E (SECURE). Circulation 2001;103(7):919–25.

[20] The ONTARGET Investigators. Telmisartan, ramipril, or both in patients at high risk for vascular events. N Engl J Med 2008;358:1547–59.

[21] Beckett NS, Peters R, Fletcher AE, et al. Hyvet Study Group. Treatment of hypertension in patients 80 years of age or older. N Engl J Med 2008;358(18):1887–98.

[22] Turnbull F, Neal B, Ninomiya T, et al. Blood Pressure Lowering Treatment Trialists' Collaboration. Effects of different regimens to lower blood pressure on major cardiovascular events in older and younger adults: meta-analysis of randomised trials. BMJ 2008; 336(7653):1121–3.

[23] Weber MA, Bakris GL, Dahlöf B, et al. Baseline characteristics in the avoiding cardiovascular events through combination therapy in patients living with Systolic Hypertension (ACCOMPLISH) trial: a hypertensive population at high cardiovascular risk. Blood Press 2007;16(1):13–9.

[24] Yusuf S. From the HOPE to the ONTARGET and the TRANSCEND studies: challenges in improving prognosis. Am J Cardiol 2002;89(2A):18A–25A.

[25] Chalmers J, Chapman N. Challenges for the prevention of primary and secondary stroke: the importance of lowering blood pressure and total cardiovascular risk. Blood Press 2001; 10(5–6):344–51.

[26] PROGRESS Collaborative Group. Randomised trial of a perindopril-based blood-pressure-lowering regimen among 6,105 individuals with previous stroke or transient ischaemic attack. Lancet 2001;358(9287):1033–41.

[27] Cushman WC, Ford CE, Cutler JA, et al. ALLHAT Collaborative Research Group. Success and predictors of blood pressure control in diverse North American settings: the Antihypertensive and Lipid-Lowering Treatment to Prevent Heart Attack Trial (ALLHAT). J Clin Hypertens 2002;4:393–404.

[28] Cutler DM, Long G, Berndt E, et al. The value of antihypertensive drugs: a perspective on medical innovation. Health Aff 2007;26:97–110.

[29] Douglas JG, Bakris GL, Epstein M, et al. Management of high blood pressure in African Americans: consensus statement of the Hypertension in African Americans Working Group of the International Society on Hypertension in Blacks. Arch Intern Med 2003; 163:525–41.

[30] Whelton PK, He J, Appel LJ, et al. Primary prevention of hypertension: clinical and public health advisory from the National High Blood Pressure Education Program. JAMA 2002; 288:1882–8.

[31] Expert panel on detection, evaluation, and treatment of high blood cholesterol in adults, executive summary of the third report of the National Cholesterol Education Program

(NCEP) expert panel on detection, evaluation, and treatment of high blood cholesterol in adults (Adult Treatment Panel III). JAMA 2001;285:2486–97.
[32] Gaede P, Vedel P, Larsen N, et al. Multifactorial intervention and cardiovascular disease in patients with type 2 diabetes. N Engl J Med 2003;348:383–93.
[33] American Diabetes Association. Standards of medical care for patients with diabetes mellitus. Diabetes Care 2003;26(Suppl 1):S33–50.
[34] Solomon CG. Reducing cardiovascular risk in type 2 diabetes. N Engl J Med 2003;348(5): 457–9.
[35] Effect of intensive blood-glucose control with metformin on complications in overweight patients with type 2 diabetes (UKPDS 34). UK Prospective Diabetes Study (UKPDS) Group. Lancet 1998;352:854–65, [published correction appears in Lancet. 1998;352:1558].
[36] Curb JD, Pressel SL, Cutler JA, et al. Effect of diuretic-based antihypertensive treatment on cardiovascular disease risk in older diabetic patients with isolated systolic hypertension. Systolic Hypertension in the Elderly Program Cooperative Research Group [published correction appears in JAMA. 1997;277:1356]. JAMA 1996;276:1886–92.
[37] Effects of ramipril on cardiovascular and microvascular outcomes in people with diabetes mellitus: results of the HOPE study and MICRO-HOPE substudy. Heart Outcomes Prevention Evaluation Study Investigators [published correction appears in Lancet. 2000;356:860]. Lancet 2000;355:253–9.
[38] Pyorala K, Pedersen TR, Kjekshus J, et al. Cholesterol lowering with simvastatin improves prognosis of diabetic people with coronary heart disease. A subgroup analysis of the Scandinavian Simvastatin Survival Study (4S). Diabetes Care 1997;20:614–20.
[39] Lewis SJ, Moye LA, Sacks FM, et al. Effect of pravastatin on cardiovascular events in older people with myocardial infarction and cholesterol levels in the average range. Results of the Cholesterol And Recurrent Events (CARE) trial. Ann Intern Med 1998;129:681–9.
[40] LIPID Study Group. Prevention of cardiovascular events and death with pravastatin in people with coronary heart disease and a broad range of initial cholesterol levels. The Long-term Intervention with Pravastatin in Ischaemic Disease (LIPID) study group. N Engl J Med 1998;339:1349–57.
[41] Frick MH, Elo O, Haapa K, et al. Helsinki Heart Study: primary-prevention trial with gemfibrozil in middle-aged men with dyslipidemia. Safety of treatment, changes in risk factors, and incidence of coronary heart disease. N Engl J Med 1987;317:1237–45.
[42] Medical Research Council, British Heart Foundation. MRC/BHF heart protection study of cholesterol lowering with simvastatin in 20,536 high-risk individuals: a randomised placebo-controlled trial. Lancet 2002;360:7–22.
[43] Sever PS, Dahlof B, Poulter NR, et al. Prevention of coronary and stroke events with atorvastatin (ASCOT-LLA). Lancet 2003;361:1149–58.
[44] Colhoun H, Betteridge D, Durrington P, on behalf of the CARDS Investigators. Primary prevention of cardiovascular disease with atorvastatin in type 2 diabetes in the Collaborative Atorvastatin Diabetes Study (CARDS): multicentre randomised placebo-controlled trial. Lancet 2004;364:685–96.
[45] Turner RC, Cull CA, Frighi V, et al. Glycemic control with diet, sulfonylurea, metformin, or insulin in people with type 2 diabetes mellitus: progressive requirement for multiple therapies (UKPDS 49). UK Prospective Diabetes Study (UKPDS) group. JAMA 1999;281: 2005–12.
[46] UK Prospective Diabetes Study (UKPDS) Group. Effect of intensive blood-glucose control with metformin on complications in overweight people with type 2 diabetes (UKPDS 34). Lancet 1998;352:854–65.
[47] Dormandy JA, Charbonnel B, Eckland DJA, et al. Secondary prevention of macrovascular events in patients with type 2 diabetes in the PROactive study (prospective pioglitazone clinical trial in macrovascular events): a randomised controlled trial. Lancet 2005;366:1279–89.
[48] Lukovits TG, Mazzone TM, Gorelick TM. Diabetes mellitus and cerebrovascular disease. Neuroepidemiology 1999;18(1):1–14.

[49] Leppala JM, Virtamo J, Fogelholm R, et al. Different risk factors for different stroke subtypes: association of blood pressure, cholesterol, and antioxidants. Stroke 1999;30: 2535–40.
[50] Gordon T, Kannel WB, Castelli WP, et al. Lipoproteins, cardiovascular disease, and death. The Framingham Study. Arch Intern Med 1981;141:1128–31.
[51] Shahar E, Chambless LE, Rosamond WD, et al. Plasma lipid profile and incident ischemic stroke: the Atherosclerosis Risk in Communities (ARIC) Study. Stroke 2003;34:623–31.
[52] Koren-Morag N, Tanne D, Graff E, et al. Low- and high-density lipoprotein cholesterol and ischemic cerebrovascular disease: the bezafibrate infarction prevention registry. Arch Intern Med 2002;162:993–9.
[53] Wannamethee SG, Shaper AG, Ebrahim S. HDL-cholesterol, total cholesterol, and the risk of stroke in middle-aged British men. Stroke 2000;31:1882–8.
[54] Soyama Y, Miura K, Morikawa Y, et al. Oyabe Study. High-density lipoprotein cholesterol and risk of stroke in Japanese men and women: the Oyabe Study. Stroke 2003;34:863–8.
[55] Sacco RL, Benson RT, Kargman DE, et al. High-density lipoprotein cholesterol and ischemic stroke in the elderly: the Northern Manhattan Stroke Study. JAMA 2001;285(21): 2729–35.
[56] Lindenstrom E, Boysen G, Nyboe J. Influence of total cholesterol, high density lipoprotein cholesterol, and triglycerides on risk of cerebrovascular disease: the Copenhagen City Heart Study [published correction appears in BMJ1994;309:1619]. BMJ 1994;309:11–5.
[57] Boden-Albala B, Sacco RL, Lee HS, et al. Metabolic syndrome and ischemic stroke risk: Northern Manhattan Study. Stroke 2008;39(1):30–5.
[58] Collins R, Armitage J, Parish S, et al. Heart Protection Study Collaborative Group. Effects of cholesterol-lowering with simvastatin on stroke and other major vascular events in 20536 people with cerebrovascular disease or other high-risk conditions. Lancet 2004;363:757–67.
[59] Amarenco P, Tonkin AM. Statins for stroke prevention: disappointment and hope. Circulation 2004;109(23 Suppl 1):III44–9.
[60] Amarenco P, Bogousslavsky J, Callahan A 3rd, et al. Stroke Prevention by Aggressive Reduction in Cholesterol Levels (SPARCL) Investigators. High-dose atorvastatin after stroke or transient ischemic attack. N Engl J Med 2006;355(6):549–59.
[61] Nassief A, Marsh JD. Statin therapy for stroke prevention. Stroke 2008 Mar;39(3):1042–8.
[62] Gotto AM Jr, Farmer JA. Reducing the risk for stroke in patients with myocardial infarction: a Myocardial Ischemia Reduction with Aggressive Cholesterol Lowering (MIRACL) substudy. Circulation 2002;106(13):1595–8.
[63] LaRosa JC, Grundy SM, Waters DD, et al. Treating to New Targets (TNT) Investigators. Intensive lipid lowering with atorvastatin in patients with stable coronary disease. N Engl J Med 2005;352:1425–35.
[64] Spencer FA, Allegrone J, Goldberg RJ, et al. GRACE Investigators. Association of statin therapy with outcomes of acute coronary syndromes: the GRACE study. Ann Intern Med 2004;140(11):857–66.
[65] O'Regan C, Wu P, Arora P, et al. Statin therapy in stroke prevention: a meta-analysis involving 121,000 patients. Am J Med 2008;121(1):24–33.
[66] Tenenbaum A, Fisman EZ, Motro M, et al. Optimal management of combined dyslipidemia: what have we behind statins monotherapy? Adv Cardiol 2008;45:127–53.
[67] Kastelein J, Akdim F, Stroes E, et al. Simvastatin with or without ezetimibe in familial hypercholesterolemia. N Engl J Med 2008;358:1431–43.
[68] Philip Greenland P, Lloyd-Jones D. Critical lessons from the ENHANCE Trial. JAMA 2008;299(8):953–5.
[69] Clofibrate and niacin in coronary heart disease. JAMA 1975;231:360–81.
[70] Bloomfield Rubins H, Davenport J, Babikian V, et al. Study Group. Reduction in stroke with gemfibrozil in men with coronary heart disease and low HDL cholesterol: the Veterans Affairs HDL Intervention Trial (VA-HIT). Circulation 2001;103:2828–33.

[71] Guyton JR, Blazing MA, Hagar J, et al. Extended-release niacin vs gemfibrozil for the treatment of low levels of high-density lipoprotein cholesterol. Niaspan-Gemfibrozil Study Group. Arch Intern Med 2000;160:1177–84.
[72] Kashyap ML, McGovern ME, Berra K, et al. Long-term safety and efficacy of a once-daily niacin/lovastatin formulation for patients with dyslipidemia. Am J Cardiol 2002;89:672–8.
[73] Rundek T, Arif H, Boden-Albala B, et al. Carotid plaque, a subclinical precursor of vascular events: the Northern Manhattan Study. Neurology 2008;70(14):1200–7.
[74] Heiss G, Sharrett AR, Barnes R, et al. Carotid atherosclerosis measured by B-mode ultrasound in populations: associations with cardiovascular risk factors in the ARIC study. Am J Epidemiol 1991;134:250–6.
[75] Sacco RL, Roberts JK, Boden-Albala B, et al. Race-ethnicity and determinants of carotid atherosclerosis in a multiethnic population. The Northern Manhattan Stroke Study. Stroke 1997;28(5):929–35.
[76] Jeng JS, Sacco RL, Kargman DE, et al. Apolipoproteins and carotid artery atherosclerosis in an elderly multiethnic population: the Northern Manhattan Stroke Study. Atherosclerosis 2002;165(2):317–25.
[77] Rundek T, White H, Boden-Albala B, et al. Sacco RL. The metabolic syndrome and subclinical carotid atherosclerosis: the Northern Manhattan Study. J Cardiometab Syndr. Winter 2007;2(1):24–9.
[78] Blankenhorn DH, Selzer RH, Crawford DW, et al. Beneficial effects of colestipol-niacin therapy on the common carotid artery. Two- and four-year reduction of intima-media thickness measured by ultrasound. Circulation 1993;88:20–8.
[79] Crouse JR III, Byington RP, Bond MG, Espeland MA, et al. Pravastatin, Lipids, and Atherosclerosis in the Carotid Arteries (PLAC-II). Am J Cardiol 1995;75:455–9.
[80] Furberg CD, Adams HP Jr, Applegate WB, et al. Effect of lovastatin on early carotid atherosclerosis and cardiovascular events. Asymptomatic Carotid Artery Progression Study (ACAPS) Research Group. Circulation 1994;90:1679–87.
[81] Hodis HN, Mack WJ, LaBree L, et al. Reduction in carotid arterial wall thickness using lovastatin and dietary therapy: a randomized controlled clinical trial. Ann Intern Med 1996;124:548–56.
[82] Taylor AJ, Sullenberger LE, Lee HJ, et al. Arterial Biology for the Investigation of the Treatment Effects of Reducing Cholesterol (ARBITER) 2: a double-blind, placebo-controlled study of extended-release niacin on atherosclerosis progression in secondary prevention patients treated with statins [published correction appears in Circulation. 2004;110:3615]. Circulation 2004;110:3512–7.
[83] Nissen SE, Tardif J-C, Nichlis SJ, et al. Effect of torcetrapid on the progression of coronary arthrosclerosis. N Engl J Med 2007;356:1304–16.
[84] Barter PJ, Caulfield M, Eriksson M, et al. Effects of torcetrapib in patients at high risk for coronary events. N Engl J Med 2007;357(21):2109–22.
[85] Grundy SM, Cleeman JI, Merz CN, et al. Coordinating Committee of the National Cholesterol Education Program. Implications of recent clinical trials for the national cholesterol education program adult treatment panel III guidelines. Arterioscler Thromb Vasc Biol 2004;24:e149–61.
[86] Walker DB, Jacobson TA. Initiating statins in the elderly: the evolving challenge. Curr Opin Endocrinol Diabetes Obes 2008;15(2):182–7.
[87] Wolf PA, Abbott RD, Kannel WB. Atrial fibrillation as an independent risk factor for stroke: the Framingham Study. Stroke 1991;22:983–8.
[88] Go AS, Hylek EM, Chang Y, et al. Anticoagulation therapy for stroke prevention in atrial fibrillation: How well do randomized trials translate into clinical practice? JAMA 2003;290: 2685–92.
[89] Sudlow M, Thomson R, Thwaites B, et al. Prevalence of atrial fibrillation and eligibility for anticoagulants in the community. Lancet 1998;352:1167–71.

[90] Feinberg WM. Anticoagulation for prevention of stroke. Neurology 1998;51(suppl 3): S20–2.
[91] Hart RG, Benavente O, McBride R, et al. Antithrombotic therapy to prevent stroke in patients with atrial fibrillation: a meta-analysis. Ann Intern Med 1999;131:492–501.
[92] van Walraven C, Hart RG, Singer DE, et al. Oral anticoagulants vs aspirin in nonvalvular atrial fibrillation: an individual patient meta-analysis. JAMA 2002;288:2441–8.
[93] Green CJ, Hadorn DC, Bassett K, et al. Anticoagulation in chronic non-valvular atrial fibrillation: a critical appraisal and meta-analysis. Can J Cardiol 1997;13:811–5.
[94] Albers GW, SPORTIF Investigators. Stroke prevention in atrial fibrillation: pooled analysis of SPORTIF III and V trials. Am J Manag Care 2004;10(Suppl 14):S462–9 [discussion S469–S73].
[95] Gurewich V. Ximelagatran—promises and concerns. JAMA 2005;293:736–9.
[96] Brass LM, Krumholz HM, Scinto JM, et al. Warfarin use among patients with atrial fibrillation. Stroke 1997;28:2382–9.
[97] Gage BF, van Walraven C, Pearce L, et al. Selecting patients with atrial fibrillation for anticoagulation: stroke risk stratification in patients taking aspirin. Circulation 2004;110: 2287–92.
[98] Hart RG, Halperin JL, Pearce LA, et al. Stroke Prevention in Atrial Fibrillation Investigators. Lessons from the Stroke Prevention in Atrial Fibrillation trials. Ann Intern Med 2003; 138:831–8.
[99] Fuster V, Ryden LE, Asinger RW, et al. American College of Cardiology/American Heart Association Task Force on Practice Guidelines; European Society of Cardiology Committee for Practice Guidelines and Policy Conferences (Committee to Develop Guidelines for the Management of Patients With Atrial Fibrillation); North American Society of Pacing and Electrophysiology. ACC/AHA/ESC Guidelines for the Management of Patients With Atrial Fibrillation: Executive Summary. A report of the American College of Cardiology/American Heart Association Task Force on Practice Guidelines and the European Society of Cardiology Committee for Practice Guidelines and Policy Conferences (Committee to Develop Guidelines for the Management of Patients With Atrial Fibrillation) developed in collaboration with the North American Society of Pacing and Electrophysiology. Circulation 2001;104:2118–50.
[100] Gage BF, Waterman AD, Shannon W, et al. Validation of clinical classification schemes for predicting stroke: results from the National Registry of Atrial Fibrillation. JAMA 2001; 285:2864–70.
[101] Patients with nonvalvular atrial fibrillation at low risk of stroke during treatment with aspirin: Stroke Prevention in Atrial Fibrillation III Study. The SPAF III Writing Committee for the Stroke Prevention in Atrial Fibrillation Investigators. JAMA 1998;279:1273–7.
[102] Gage BF, Boechler M, Doggette AL, et al. Adverse outcomes and predictors of underuse of antithrombotic therapy in Medicare beneficiaries with chronic atrial fibrillation. Stroke 2000;31:822–7.
[103] Hart RG. Warfarin in atrial fibrillation: underused in the elderly, often inappropriately used in the young. Heart 1999;82:539–40.
[104] Hylek EM, Go AS, Chang Y, et al. Effect of intensity of oral anticoagulation on stroke severity and mortality in atrial fibrillation. N Engl J Med 2003;349:1019–26.
[105] Hart RG. Intensity of anticoagulation to prevent stroke in patients with atrial fibrillation. Ann Intern Med 1998;128:408.
[106] Arima H, Hart RG, Colman S, et al. Perindopril-based blood pressure lowering reduces major vascular events in patients with atrial fibrillation and prior stroke or transient ischemic attack. Stroke 2005;36:2164–9.
[107] Bonow RO, Carabello B, de Leon AC Jr, et al. ACC/AHA guidelines for the management of patients with valvular heart disease: a report of the American College of Cardiology/American Heart Association Task Force on Practice Guidelines (Committee

on Management of Patients With Valvular Heart Disease). J Am Coll Cardiol 1998; 32(5):1486–588.

[108] Cannegieter SC, Rosendaal FR, Briet E. Thromboembolic and bleeding complications in patients with mechanical heart valve prostheses. Circulation 1994;89:635–41.

[109] Di Pasquale G, Urbinati S, Pinelli G. Cardiac investigation in patients with cerebrovascular disease. In: Ginsberg M, Bogousslavsky J, editors. Cerebrovascular disease: pathophysiology, diagnosis, and management. Malden (MA):: Blackwell Science; 1998.

[110] Loh E, Sutton MS, Wun CC, et al. Ventricular dysfunction and the risk of stroke after myocardial infarction. N Engl J Med 1997;336:251–7.

[111] Pullicino P, Thompson JL, Barton B, et al. Warfarin versus aspirin in patients with reduced cardiac ejection fraction (WARCEF): rationale, objectives, and design. J Card Fail 2006; 12(1):39–46.

[112] Wolman RL, Nussmeier NA, Aggarwal A, et al. Cerebral injury after cardiac surgery: identification of a group at extraordinary risk. Multicenter Study of Perioperative Ischemia Research Group (McSPI) and the Ischemia Research Education Foundation (IREF) Investigators. Stroke 1999;30:514–22.

[113] Di Tullio MR, Sacco RL, Gersony D, et al. Aortic atheromas and acute ischemic stroke: a transesophageal echocardiographic study in an ethnically mixed population. Neurology 1996;46:1560–6.

[114] Antman EM, Anbe DT, Armstrong PW, et al. ACC/AHA guidelines for the management of patients with ST-elevation myocardial infarction: a report of the American College of Cardiology/American Heart Association Task Force on Practice Guidelines (Committee to Revise the 1999 Guidelines for the Management of Patients with Acute Myocardial Infarction). J Am Coll Cardiol 2004;44:E1–211.

[115] Braunwald E, Antman EM, Beasley JW, et al. American College of Cardiology/American Heart Association Task Force on Practice Guidelines (Committee on the Management of Patients With Unstable Angina). ACC/AHA 2002 guideline update for the management of patients with unstable angina and non–ST-segment elevation myocardial infarction: a report of the American College of Cardiology/American Heart Association Task Force on Practice Guidelines (Committee on the Management of Patients With Unstable Angina). Circulation 2002;106:1893–900.

[116] Gibbons RJ, Abrams J, Chatterjee K, et al. American College of Cardiology; American Heart Association Task Force on Practice Guidelines. Committee on the Management of Patients With Chronic Stable Angina. ACC/AHA 2002 guideline update for the management of patients with chronic stable angina: a report of the American College of Cardiology/American Heart Association Task Force on Practice Guidelines (Committee to Update the 1999 Guidelines for the Management of Patients with Chronic Stable Angina). Circulation 2003;107:149–58.

[117] O'Leary DH, Polak JF, Kronmal RA, et al. Distribution and correlates of sonographically detected carotid artery disease in the Cardiovascular Health Study. The CHS Collaborative Research Group. Stroke 1992;23:1752–60.

[118] Fine-Edelstein JS, Wolf PA, O'Leary DH, et al. Precursors of extracranial carotid atherosclerosis in the Framingham Study. Neurology 1994;44:1046–50.

[119] Inzitari D, Eliasziw M, Gates P, et al. The causes and risk of stroke in patients with asymptomatic internal-carotid-artery stenosis. North American Symptomatic Carotid Endarterectomy Trial Collaborators. N Engl J Med 2000;342:1693–700.

[120] Barnett HJ, Gunton RW, Eliasziw M, et al. Causes and severity of ischemic stroke in patients with internal carotid artery stenosis. JAMA 2000;283:1429–36.

[121] Autret A, Pourcelot L, Saudeau D, et al. Stroke risk in patients with carotid stenosis. Lancet 1987;1:888–90.

[122] Chambers BR, Norris JW. Outcome in patients with asymptomatic neck bruits. N Engl J Med 1986;315:860–5.

[123] Endarterectomy for asymptomatic carotid artery stenosis. Executive Committee for the Asymptomatic Carotid Atherosclerosis Study. JAMA 1995;273:1421–8.
[124] Halliday A, Mansfield A, Marro J, et al. Asymptomatic Carotid Surgery Trial (ACST) Collaborative Group. Prevention of disabling and fatal strokes by successful carotid endarterectomy in patients without recent neurological symptoms: randomised controlled trial. Lancet 2004;363:1491–502.
[125] Rothwell PM, Goldstein LB. Carotid endarterectomy for asymptomatic carotid stenosis: asymptomatic carotid surgery trial. Stroke 2004;35:2425–7.
[126] Goldstein LB, Bonito AJ, Matchar DB, et al. US national survey of physician practices for the secondary and tertiary prevention of ischemic stroke. Design, service availability, and common practices. Stroke 1995;26:1607–15.
[127] Perry JR, Szalai JP, Norris JW. Consensus against both endarterectomy and routine screening for asymptomatic carotid artery stenosis. Canadian stroke consortium. Arch Neurol 1997;54:25–8.
[128] Marshall RS, Rundek T, Sproule DM, et al. Monitoring of cerebral vasodilatory capacity with transcranial Doppler carbon dioxide inhalation in patients with severe carotid artery disease. Stroke 2003;34(4):945–9.
[129] Spence JD, Tamayo A, Lownie SP, et al. Absence of microemboli on transcranial Doppler identifies low-risk patients with asymptomatic carotid stenosis. Stroke 2005;36(11):2373–8.
[130] Yadav JS, Wholey MH, Kuntz RE, et al. Stenting and Angioplasty with Protection in Patients at High Risk for Endarterectomy Investigators. Protected carotid-artery stenting versus endarterectomy in high-risk patients. N Engl J Med 2004;351:1493–501.
[131] Gray WA. Clinical trials: past, present, and future. Semin Vasc Surg 2008;21(2):80–7.
[132] Mansour MA. Carotid artery stenting in the SPACE and EVA-3S trials: analysis and update. Perspect Vasc Surg Endovasc Ther 2008;20(1):11–4.
[133] Holey MH, Barbato JE, Al-Khoury GE. Treatment of asymptomatic carotid disease with stenting: pro. Semin Vasc Surg 2008;21(2):95–9.
[134] Gray WA, Moussa ID. Carotid artery stenting in patients with asymptomatic carotid artery stenosis. In: Mooussa ID, Rundek T, Mohr JP, editors. Asymptomatic carotid artery stenosis. Risk stratification and management. Informa; 2007. p. 175–96.
[135] Manolio TA, Kronmal RA, Burke GL, et al. Short-term predictors of incident stroke in older adults: the cardiovascular health study. Stroke 1996;27:1479–86.
[136] Broderick JP, Viscoli CM, Brott T, et al. Hemorrhagic Stroke Project Investigators. Major risk factors for aneurysmal subarachnoid hemorrhage in the young are modifiable. Stroke 2003;34:1375–81.
[137] The Centers for Disease Control. The Surgeon General's 1989 Report on Reducing the Health Consequences of Smoking: 25 Years of Progress. MMWR Morb Mortal Wkly Rep 1989;38(suppl 2):1–32.
[138] Shinton R, Beevers G. Meta-analysis of relation between cigarette smoking and stroke. BMJ 1989;298:789–94.
[139] Bonita R, Duncan J, Truelsen T, et al. Passive smoking as well as active smoking increases the risk of acute stroke. Tob Control 1999;8:156–60.
[140] Howard G, Thun MJ. Why is environmental tobacco smoke more strongly associated with coronary heart disease than expected? A review of potential biases and experimental data. Environ Health Perspect 1999;107(suppl 6):853–8.
[141] Fagerstrom K. The epidemiology of smoking: health consequences and benefits of cessation. Drugs 2002;62(suppl 2):1–9.
[142] Fiore MC. US Public Health Service clinical practice guideline: treating tobacco use and dependence. Respir Care 2000;45:1200–62.
[143] Aubin J-H, Bobak A, Britton JR, et al. Varenicline versus transdermal nicotine patch for smoking cessation: results from a randomised, open-label trial. Thorax 2008;63: 717–24.

[144] Steffen LM, Jacobs DR Jr, Stevens J, et al. Associations of whole-grain, refined-grain, and fruit and vegetable consumption with risks of all-cause mortality and incident coronary artery disease and ischemic stroke: the Atherosclerosis Risk in Communities (ARIC) Study. Am J Clin Nutr 2003;78:383–90.
[145] Joshipura KJ, Ascherio A, Manson JE, et al. Fruit and vegetable intake in relation to risk of ischemic stroke. JAMA 1999;282:1233–9.
[146] Khaw KT, Barrett-Connor E. Dietary potassium and stroke-associated mortality. A 12-year prospective population study. N Engl J Med 1987;316:235–40.
[147] Appel LJ, Moore TJ, Obarzanek E, et al. A clinical trial of the effects of dietary patterns on blood pressure. DASH collaborative research group. N Engl J Med 1997;336:1117–24.
[148] Fletcher GF. Exercise in the prevention of stroke. Health Rep 1994;6:106–10.
[149] Gillum RF, Mussolino ME, Ingram DD. Physical activity and stroke incidence in women and men. The NHANES I epidemiologic follow-up study. Am J Epidemiol 1996;143:860–9.
[150] Sacco RL, Gan R, Boden-Albala B, et al. Leisure-time physical activity and ischemic stroke risk: the Northern Manhattan Stroke Study. Stroke 1998;29:380–7.
[151] Shinton R, Sagar G. Lifelong exercise and stroke [published correction appears in BMJ. 1993;307:706]. BMJ 1993;307:231–4.
[152] NIH develops consensus statement on the role of physical activity for cardiovascular health. Am Fam Physician 1996;54:763–4, 767.
[153] Pate RR, Pratt M, Blair SN, et al. Physical activity and public health: a recommendation from the Centers for Disease Control and Prevention and the American College of Sports Medicine. JAMA 1995;273:402–7.
[154] Wolf PA, Cobb JL, D'Agostino RB. Epidemiology of stroke. In: Barnett HJM, Mohr JP, Stein BM, editors. Stroke: pathophysiology, diagnosis, and management. 2nd edition. New York: Churchill Livingstone; 1992. p. 3–27.
[155] Heyden S, Hames CG, Bartel A, et al. Weight and weight history in relation to cerebrovascular and ischemic heart disease. Arch Intern Med 1971;128:956–60.
[156] Suk SH, Sacco RL, Boden-Albala B, et al. Northern Manhattan Stroke Study. Abdominal obesity and risk of ischemic stroke: the Northern Manhattan Stroke Study. Stroke 2003; 34(7):1586–92.
[157] Kuczmarski RJ, Flegal KM, Campbell SM, et al. Increasing prevalence of overweight among US adults: the national health and nutrition examination surveys, 1960 to 1991. JAMA 1994;272:205–11.
[158] Kernan WN, Inzucchi SE, Viscoli CM, et al. Insulin resistance and risk for stroke. Neurology 2002;59:809–15.
[159] Ford ES, Giles WH, Dietz WH. Prevalence of the metabolic syndrome among US adults: findings from the third National Health and Nutrition Examination Survey. JAMA 2002; 287:356–9.
[160] Neter JE, Stam BE, Kok FJ, et al. Influence of weight reduction on blood pressure: a meta-analysis of randomized controlled trials. Hypertension 2003;42:878–84.
[161] Sacco RL, Elkind M, Boden-Albala B, et al. The protective effect of moderate alcohol consumption on ischemic stroke. JAMA 1999;281:53–60.
[162] Berger K, Ajani UA, Kase CS, et al. Light-to-moderate alcohol consumption and risk of stroke among US male physicians. N Engl J Med 1999;341:1557–64.
[163] National Institute on Alcohol Abuse and Alcoholism. Sixth special report to the U.S. Congress on alcohol and health from the Secretary of Health and Human Services. Washington (DC): Government Printing Office; 1987 [DHHS publication no. (ADM) 87-1519].
[164] US Department of Health and Human Services. US Department of Agriculture. Available at: http://www.healthierus.gov/dietaryguidelines. Accessed April 21, 2006.
[165] Djousse L, Levy D, Benjamin EJ, et al. Long-term alcohol consumption and the risk of atrial fibrillation in the Framingham Study. Am J Cardiol 2004;93:710–3.

[166] Reynolds K, Lewis B, Nolen JD, et al. Alcohol consumption and risk of stroke: a meta-analysis [published correction appears in JAMA. 2003;289:2798]. JAMA 2003;289:579–88.

[167] Brust JCM. Neurological aspects of substance abuse. 2nd edition. Philadelphia: Butterworth-Heinemann; 2004.

[168] Levine SR, Brust JC, Futrell N, et al. Cerebrovascular complications of the use of the "crack" form of alkaloidal cocaine. N Engl J Med 1990;323:699–704.

[169] Neiman J, Haapaniemi HM, Hillbom M. Neurological complications of drug abuse: pathophysiological mechanisms. Eur J Neurol 2000;7:595–606.

[170] US Preventive Services Task Force. Screening and behavioral counseling interventions in primary care to reduce alcohol misuse: recommendation statement. Available at: http://www.preventiveservices.ahrq.gov. Accessed April 21, 2006.

[171] Somers VK, White DP, Amin R, et al. An American Heart Association/American College of Cardiology Foundation Scientific Statement From the American Heart Association Council for High Blood Pressure Research Professional Education Committee, Council on Clinical Cardiology, Stroke Council, and Council on Cardiovascular Nursing Council. Circulation 2008;118.

[172] Sleep-related breathing disorders in adults: recommendations for syndrome definition and measurement techniques in clinical research. The report of an American Academy of Sleep Medicine Task Force. Sleep 1999;22:667–89.

[173] Punjabi NM, Newman AB, Young TB, et al. Sleep-disordered breathing and cardiovascular disease: an outcome-based definition of hypopneas. Am J Respir Crit Care Med 2008; 177(10):1150–5.

[174] Partinen M, Palomaki H. Snoring and cerebral infarction. Lancet 1985;2:1325–6.

[175] Homocysteine Studies Collaboration. Homocysteine and risk of ischemic heart disease and stroke: a meta-analysis. JAMA 2002;288:2015–22.

[176] Sacco RL, Anand K, Lee HS, et al. Homocysteine and the risk of ischemic stroke in a triethnic cohort: the NOrthern MAnhattan Study. Stroke 2004;35(10):2263–9.

[177] Spence JD. Homocysteine-lowering therapy: a role in stroke prevention? Lancet Neurol 2007;6(9):830–8.

[178] Spence JD, Blake C, Landry A, et al. Measurement of carotid plaque and effect of vitamin therapy for total homocysteine. Clin Chem Lab Med 2003;41(11):1498–504.

[179] Toole JF, Malinow MR, Chambless LE, et al. Lowering homocysteine in patients with ischemic stroke to prevent recurrent stroke, myocardial infarction, and death: the Vitamin Intervention for Stroke Prevention (VISP) randomized controlled trial. JAMA 2004;291: 565–75.

[180] Dusitanond P, Eikelboom JW, Hankey GJ, et al. Homocysteine-lowering treatment with folic acid, cobalamin, and pyridoxine does not reduce blood markers of inflammation, endothelial dysfunction, or hypercoagulability in patients with previous transient ischemic attack or stroke: a randomized substudy of the VITATOPS trial. Stroke 2005;36(1):144–6.

[181] Lonn E, Yusuf S, Arnold MJ, et al. Heart Outcomes Prevention Evaluation (HOPE) 2 Investigators. Homocysteine lowering with folic acid and B vitamins in vascular disease. N Engl J Med 2006;354(15):1567–77.

[182] Brattstrom L, Wilcken DE, Ohrvik J, et al. Common methylenetetrahydrofolate reductase gene mutation leads to hyperhomocysteinemia but not to vascular disease: the result of a meta-analysis. Circulation 1998;98:2520–6.

[183] Wald DS, Law M, Morris JK. Homocysteine and cardiovascular disease: evidence on causality from a meta-analysis. BMJ 2002;325:1202.

[184] Steering Committee of the Physicians' Health Study Research Group. Final report on the aspirin component of the ongoing Physicians' Health Study. N Engl J Med 1989;321: 129–35.

[185] Peto R, Gray R, Collins R, et al. Randomised trial of prophylactic daily aspirin in British male doctors. BMJ 1988;296:313–6.

[186] Bartolucci AA, Howard G. Meta-analysis of data from the six primary prevention trials of cardiovascular events using aspirin. Am J Cardiol 2006;98(6):746–50.
[187] Ridker PM, Cook NR, Lee IM, et al. A randomized trial of low-dose aspirin in the primary prevention of cardiovascular disease in women. N Engl J Med 2005;352:1293–304.
[188] Hayden M, Pignone M, Phillips C, et al. Aspirin for the primary prevention of cardiovascular events: a summary of the evidence for the US Preventive Services Task Force. Ann Intern Med 2002;136:161–72.
[189] Grundy SM, Pasternak R, Greenland P, et al. AHA/ACC scientific statement: assessment of cardiovascular risk by use of multiple-risk-factor assessment equations: a statement for healthcare professionals from the American Heart Association and the American College of Cardiology. J Am Coll Cardiol 1999;34:1348–59.
[190] Wolf PA, D'Agostino RB, Belanger AJ, et al. Probability of stroke: a risk profile from the Framingham Study. Stroke 1991;22:312–8.
[191] Wang TJ, Massaro JM, Levy D, et al. A risk score for predicting stroke or death in individuals with new-onset atrial fibrillation in the community: the Framingham Heart Study. JAMA 2003;290:1049–56.
[192] Lumley T, Kronmal RA, Cushman M, et al. A stroke prediction score in the elderly: validation and Web-based application. J Clin Epidemiol 2002;55:129–36.
[193] Stroke Risk in Atrial Fibrillation Working Group. Comparison of 12 risk stratification schemes to predict stroke in patients with nonvalvular atrial fibrillation. Stroke 2008; 39(6):1901–10.

ELSEVIER
SAUNDERS

Neurol Clin 26 (2008) 1047–1077

NEUROLOGIC
CLINICS

Use of Antiplatelet Agents for Prevention of Ischemic Stroke

R. Charles Callison, MD, Harold P. Adams, Jr, MD*

Division of Cerebrovascular Diseases Department of Neurology, Carver College of Medicine University of Iowa, 200 Hawkins Drive, Iowa City, IA 52242, USA

Effective prevention may be the most cost-effective strategy for managing patients who have ischemic cerebrovascular disease, because it helps eliminate the costs of acute care and rehabilitation and the economic impact of lost productivity from premature death or disability. In addition, prevention avoids human suffering associated with ischemic stroke. Although no intervention may entirely eliminate the risk for ischemic stroke, therapies are available that have been proven to lower the likelihood of a cerebrovascular event.

Interventions are prescribed to a broad range of persons who have not experienced ischemic neurologic symptoms (primary prevention) and to those who have already experienced a stroke or the warning symptoms (secondary prevention) (Box 1) [1]. The division between primary and secondary prevention is rather arbitrary, because patients who have symptomatic coronary artery disease may undergo therapies to prevent myocardial infarction (secondary prevention) and ischemic stroke (primary prevention). On the other hand, besides secondary prevention of recurrent ischemic stroke, management is also aimed at lessening the likelihood of myocardial infarction, symptomatic ischemia in other vascular territories, or vascular death [2]. Most medical interventions to lower the risk for stroke are prescribed similarly in either the setting of primary or secondary prevention.

Overall management to lower risk for ischemic stroke is multifaceted. Management includes measures to treat risk factors for accelerated atherosclerosis and stroke, antithrombotic therapies to lower the risk for

Dr. Adams was a co-investigator in trials sponsored by Boerhinger-Ingelheim and Sanofi-Aventis/Bristol-Myers Squibb.

* Corresponding author.

E-mail address: harold-adams@uiowa.edu (H.P. Adams).

0733-8619/08/$ - see front matter
doi:10.1016/j.ncl.2008.06.005 ***neurologic.theclinics.com***

Box 1. Stroke risk factors

Nonmodifiable
Age
Male gender
Race
Low birth weight
Family history of stroke or other ischemic disease
Prior stroke, transient ischemic attack (TIA), ischemic heart disease, peripheral (leg) artery disease

Modifiable
Cardiovascular disease
Hypertension
Diabetes mellitus
Hyperlipidemia
Cigarette smoking
Atrial fibrillation
Physical inactivity
Sickle cell disease
Postmenopausal use of estrogen-progesterone medications

thromboembolism, and surgery to treat a defined arterial or cardiac lesion (Box 2). Treatment decisions are made on a case-by-case basis, with most patients receiving some combination of medication and recommendations for lifestyle modification. Some patients will also undergo surgical or endovascular interventions. This article discusses antithrombotic treatment for ischemic stroke prevention, placing major emphasis on the indications for and administration of antiplatelet therapy.

Antithrombotic therapy: general considerations

Antithrombotic medications are the keystone of management to lower risk for ischemic stroke, myocardial infarction, and vascular death among patients who have ischemic cerebrovascular disease. Virtually all patients who experience a stroke or the warning symptoms should be treated with these medications (see Box 2). Choices include anticoagulants and antiplatelet agents. These medications should be used in combination with treatments aimed at modifying cardiovascular and stroke risk factors, and surgical procedures. These medications may be prescribed as a single agent or in combinations.

Atithrombotic medication is selected based on several factors that must be considered for each patient (Box 3). The presumed underlying cause of the patient's neurologic symptoms is especially important. Long-term

Box 2. Stroke prevention

Risk factor modification
Lifestyle changes (weight loss, diet, exercise)
Smoking cessation
Antihypertensives
Oral and injectable hypoglycemics
Lipid-lowering agents

Antithrombotic agents
Aspirin
Clopidogrel or ticlopidine
Dipyridamole
Oral anticoagulants (most commonly warfarin)

Surgical procedures
Carotid endarterectomy
Endovascular surgery
Other cardiac procedures

administration of oral anticoagulants is recommended for most patients who have cerebral ischemia secondary to high-risk cardiac disorders, including atrial fibrillation [2]. In general, the benefit of lowering the risk for stroke is considerably greater when using adjusted doses of oral anticoagulants compared with antiplatelet agents. However, antiplatelet agents may be prescribed for patients who have a contraindication to oral anticoagulants [2]. Depending on the nature of the underlying coagulation disorder, either oral anticoagulants or antiplatelet agents are prescribed. Data are limited on the usefulness of antithrombotic medications in patients who have hypercoagulable disorders. In general, antiplatelet agents are preferred for treating patients who have intracranial or extracranial arterial disease [2]. Antiplatelet agents are usually administered to individuals who have stroke of undetermined origin. The presumed vascular territory (carotid versus vertebrobasilar circulation) has less influence on the selection of antithrombotic medications.

Plans for surgical or endovascular interventions also affect management with antithrombotic agents. Antiplatelet agents are usually prescribed in the pre- and postoperative management of patients undergoing carotid endarterectomy or other vascular operations. Combinations of antiplatelet agents (eg, aspirin plus clopidogrel) usually are given to patients undergoing angioplasty and stenting.

Use of antithrombotic medications at the time of a new stroke also affects decisions about subsequent treatment. A new stroke may be considered a failure of previous antithrombotic treatment, and a different medication is often

Box 3. Side effects and other concerns of commonly used antithrombotic agents

Aspirin
Bleeding and bruising
Epigastric distress
Gastrointestinal ulcer and hemorrhage
Intracranial hemorrhage
Allergic nasal polyposis and anaphylaxis
Teratogenicity in the first trimester of pregnancy

Dipyridamole
Headache
Epigastric distress
Bleeding and bruising[a]
Intracranial hemorrhage[a]

Ticlopidine
Bleeding and bruising
Allergic urticaria
Intracranial hemorrhage
Thrombotic thrombocytopenia purpura
Agranulocytosis
Cholestatic hepatitis
Diarrhea

Clopidogrel
Bleeding and bruising
Allergic urticaria
Intracranial hemorrhage
Thrombotic thrombocytopenic purpura[b]
Agranulocytosis[b]

Warfarin
Bleeding and bruising
Intracranial hemorrhage
Gastrointestinal or urinary hemorrhage
Warfarin-associated skin necrosis
Hemorrhagic fatty necrosis
Frequent laboratory monitoring and dose adjustments
Interactions with medications and food
Teratogenicity

[a] Bleeding is a complication of dipyridamole when used in combination with aspirin. This may be from the action of aspirin alone or the combination of the two agents.

[b] The frequency of thrombotic thrombocytopenic purpura and agranulocytosis with clopidogrel is substantially lower than with ticlopidine and does not require laboratory monitoring.

prescribed. In addition, patients may have contraindications to a specific medication. For example, patients may have a history of allergy or intolerance to aspirin. Cognitively impaired patients, those considered at high risk for falls, and those who have problems with a complex treatment regimen also may not be able to take some medications, such as oral anticoagulants. In addition, the presence of concomitant diseases, including coronary or peripheral artery disease, may affect treatment decisions.

Although oral anticoagulants remain an important treatment option for patients at high risk for stroke, use is restricted largely to those who have cardioembolic events and some whose neurologic symptoms are caused by an inherited or acquired coagulation disorder [2]. Oral anticoagulants have not been effective in preventing stroke among patients in whom it occurs secondary to arterial diseases, such as extracranial or intracranial large artery atherosclerosis, or among those who have symptoms despite treatment with antiplatelet therapy [3–6]. Anticoagulants are currently not a treatment option for most patients who experience stroke secondary to arterial disease, and therefore this article focuses on the use of antiplatelet agents. In some instances, antiplatelet agents are combined with oral anticoagulants to treat persons at especially high risk for stroke.

Antiplatelet agents have been tested in a broad range of subjects who have symptomatic or ischemic vascular disease, including those who recently experienced TIA or ischemic stroke. These agents reduce the risk for nonfatal myocardial infarction, nonfatal ischemic stroke, and vascular death by approximately 25% [7]. They also lower the need for major vascular operations, including reconstructive surgery or endovascular procedures. However, these medications have established efficacy as adjuncts for preventing thromboembolic complications of these operations [8].

Responses to antiplatelet therapy are not influenced by the patient's gender or age. Patients who are hypertensive and nonhypertensive, and diabetic and nondiabetic respond equally well [7]. Unfortunately, despite their proven track record, antiplatelet agents are underused [8]. Given the low cost of aspirin, financial considerations should not be the reason antiplatelet agents are not prescribed in patients who have ischemic disease. The Joint Commission now includes the initiation of antithrombotic therapy (most commonly an antiplatelet agent) before discharge as a quality of care marker for patients hospitalized with a TIA or ischemic stroke [9].

Aspirin

Aspirin (acetylsalicylic acid) was first developed in the 19th century for treating inflammatory diseases and managing symptomatic pain. In the mid-1950s, Craven [10] described the potential usefulness of aspirin for preventing heart attack and stroke in a general practice setting. Aspirin was then found to have a profound effect on inhibiting the actions of cyclo-oxygenase-1 on platelet function, and could therefore be used as an antithrombotic agent [11,12].

Aspirin is the most extensively studied medication for the primary or secondary prevention of ischemic vascular events [7]. It has been tested in a broad spectrum of patients and has been found to be effective when given in a broad range of doses. For many years, aspirin has been the standard against which other medical or surgical interventions are compared. Aspirin has several advantages: it is an inexpensive over-the-counter medication, it is easy to administer, and no specific monitoring is required.

Pharmacology

Suppression of cyclo-oxygenase activity leads to decreased production of prostaglandins and thromboxane A2, which in turn limits platelet aggregation. The effects on platelets and megakaryocytes are irreversible, and therefore the antiplatelet aggregating actions of aspirin persist the 7 to 10 days of the platelet's life. These effects persist even if the blood levels of aspirin have declined. Aspirin is readily absorbed from the gastrointestinal tract, with a slower rate when using an enteric-coated preparation.

Platelet function inhibition may be detected within 1 hour of administration of a 325-mg non–enteric-coated aspirin tablet. Because starting treatment at a lower dose (eg, 81 mg) will not suppress platelet function for several days, a rationale exists for starting treatment with one 325-mg tablet of aspirin (loading dose) and maintaining therapy with an 81-mg dosage. If immediate antiplatelet effects are strongly desired, aspirin could be given in a rapid-release formulation, but the necessity of this approach is unclear [13].

Larger doses of aspirin exceeding 600 mg also have an inhibitory but reversible effect of the endothelial production of prostacyclin, which could have a theoretic prothrombotic effect [14]. Other nonsteroidal anti-inflammatory agents, including ibuprofen, may interfere with the antiplatelet effects of aspirin [15,16]. Using these medications may contribute to aspirin resistance or aspirin response variability. Although the clinical implications of these interactions are unclear, it seems that these medications should not be given within 8 hours of aspirin administration.

The anti-inflammatory actions of aspirin also may affect white blood cell function and thus may help stabilize atherosclerotic plaques [17,18]. Therefore, aspirin could lower the risk for ischemic events in ways other than preventing platelet aggregation. Aspirin also may have some neuroprotective effects, although this attribute has not been established with any certainty [19].

Aspirin resistance or variability of response

Considerable interest has been shown in the concept of aspirin resistance, which is now referred to by some experts as *aspirin variability of response* (AVR) [20–22]. The antiplatelet aggregating actions of aspirin may vary among individuals; some may be relatively insensitive to the effects of aspirin whereas others may develop resistance with prolonged use [23]. The prevalence and importance of AVR are unknown [24–26]. Chen and colleagues [27] concluded that AVR may be associated with an increased risk for ischemic events among persons who have coronary artery disease. In general, aspirin resistance is defined as the retention of normal platelet function despite aspirin use.

Presumably, a relative resistance to aspirin's pharmacologic actions could explain some recurrent strokes among persons taking the medication. A potential relationship may exist between the aspirin dose or use of an enteric-coated preparation and the finding of AVR [28]. Based on the findings that many other medications, including oral anticoagulants, have different therapeutic effects in different patients, a possible individual resistance to aspirin's actions or a dosage relationship makes sense.

Responses to aspirin may be affected by factors such as patient compliance, smoking, hyperglycemia, hyperlipidemia, or concomitant medications [25,29]. A potential genetic factor that directly or indirectly affects platelet cyclo-oxygenase also may be present [30]. However, a leading explanation may be lack of compliance with the treatment regimen rather than failure of the medication to inhibit platelet function [20,31].

The diagnosis of AVR is currently based primarily on the findings of a laboratory evaluation examining platelet function [20,32–34]. However, no agreement exists about the best test to screen for platelet function or when the tests should be performed [25]. Currently, no standard method to diagnose AVR is available [29]. Considerable confusion exists about the importance of AVR in the development of recurrent ischemic events among persons taking the medication [35]. Much additional research is needed to determine if the syndrome of AVR is clinically important and to establish the best response to this phenomenon. Therefore, according to current evidence-based guidelines, routine point-of-care or other platelet function tests to monitor therapy with aspirin or other antiplatelet agents are not recommended in general practice [36].

Safety

The safety profile of aspirin is very well-known. Although it has been available for more than a century and is an over-the-counter medication that many people have used, it is a potent medication and patients should be warned about possible adverse reactions. Some people may experience allergic reactions, including rash or anaphylaxis. Those who have a history of nasal polyps or asthma may be at higher risk. Epigastric pain, gastritis, and upper gastrointestinal hemorrhage are the most common side effects and may require discontinuance. Sze and colleagues [37] estimated that prolonged use of aspirin increases the risk for peptic ulcer disease by approximately 350%.

Because aspirin is a potent inhibitor of platelet function, bleeding is a potential complication. The estimated risk for major bleeding is 3.5 per 100 patient-years [38]. Bleeding, including intracranial hemorrhage, may occur with a broad range of daily doses. This relationship should not be unexpected, because aspirin has potent effects on platelet function, even at low doses. Clinical trials testing aspirin treatment initiated within a few hours after stroke onset show a modest association with the development of hemorrhagic transformation or other intracranial bleeding [39,40]. Trials of aspirin in the primary prevention of ischemic events have reported a slight increase in risk for hemorrhagic stroke [41]. The risk for intracranial hemorrhage has been estimated to be 12 in 10,000 [42].

Aspirin may also aggravate surgery-associated bleeding, and surgeons often request that patients stop taking the medication before an elective operation. No dosage relationship exists with bleeding other than for gastrointestinal hemorrhage, which is correlated with doses greater than 325 mg/d. Using enteric-coated preparations may lower the risk for upper gastrointestinal complications. In addition, patients may be prescribed antacids or gastroprotective medications to lower the gastric side effects of aspirin. Aspirin may have teratogenic effects, but it can be administered after the first trimester of pregnancy [43].

Potential indications and efficacy

Aspirin is used for the primary prevention of myocardial infarction in men and the primary prevention of ischemic stroke in women [41,44]. The differences in responses to aspirin between men and women probably reflect the natural history of atherosclerotic disease in the two genders. Because men have a higher rate of early myocardial infarction, aspirin's impact on preventing these events would be more apparent than among women. The best dosage for preventing myocardial infarction is 75 to 325 mg/d, and the same dosage is probably equally effective for preventing ischemic stroke [45–47].

Based on a meta-analysis of trials enrolling several thousand subjects, the Antiplatelet Trialists Group concluded that aspirin was equally effective in reducing vascular events in men and women [7]. Although national guidelines do not recommend aspirin for primary prevention of stroke in men, it remains an important therapy for preventing ischemia in high-risk asymptomatic individuals, especially among men older than 50 years [1,48–50]. Besides reducing the risk for ischemic stroke, aspirin may lower the likelihood of myocardial infarction or other causes of vascular death.

Additional research is underway to test the role of aspirin in primary prevention of vascular events [51]. The Aspirin to Reduce the Risk of Initial Vascular Events (ARRIVE) is a placebo-controlled primary prevention trial studying the benefits of 100 mg of aspirin over 10 years among men and women who have a 10% to 20% risk for cardiovascular events.

Many clinical trials have tested aspirin's ability to prevent ischemic stroke among persons who experienced a TIA or stroke, and most have tested the medication in patients who have symptomatic large artery atherosclerosis or lacunar disease. The first clinical trials tested a dosage of 1300 mg/d [52–54]. Lower daily dosages (30–325 mg/d) were then tested and shown to be equally effective [55–57]. In addition, the lower doses were associated with fewer gastrointestinal side effects. The Aspirin Carotid Endarterectomy Trial found that lower dosages of aspirin (81–325 mg/d) were superior to larger doses (650–1300 mg/d) in reducing cardiac and cerebrovascular events [58]. In the Second European Stroke Prevention Study, aspirin in a dosage of 50 mg/d was found to reduce the risk for stroke by approximately 16% compared with placebo [59].

The trials have consistently shown a benefit from aspirin in reducing the risk for ischemic stroke among high-risk patients. Based on a meta-analysis, Algra and van Gijn [60] estimated that aspirin reduces risk for major stroke by approximately 16%.

In addition to lowering the likelihood of stroke, aspirin also has been shown to reduce the chances of myocardial infarction or vascular death. In addition, evidence suggests that low-dose aspirin is equal or superior to larger doses in prophylaxis against stroke [2,61,62]. Based on these findings, the guidelines do not recommend increasing the dose of aspirin in patients who experience ischemic symptoms while taking low-dose aspirin.

Aspirin also has been shown to be superior in preventing non–cardioembolic stroke. The Warfarin-Aspirin Recurrent Stroke Study showed no difference between aspirin and the oral anticoagulant. Although a trend was seen toward a lower event rate and fewer bleeding complications in the aspirin group, these differences were not statically significant [3].

Another head-to-head trial studying the prevention of recurrent stroke among patients who had symptomatic intracranial atherosclerosis found no difference between aspirin and warfarin in terms of primary event rate, but a significantly higher rate of major hemorrhage was seen in the warfarin group [6,63,64]. In an international study, antiplatelet therapy was superior to warfarin in preventing stroke among patients who had arterial disease [4].

Recent use of aspirin is not a contraindication for emergency treatment of acute ischemic stroke with intravenous thrombolytic therapy. On the other hand, national guidelines recommend that aspirin therapy not be initiated within 24 hours of treatment with tissue plasminogen activator (tPA) [9]. One clinical trial found that concomitant administration of aspirin increased the risk for serious bleeding after treatment with streptokinase [65].

Several trials have administered aspirin within the first hours after onset of stroke; in this setting, aspirin often was used as the control to which an anticoagulant was compared [39,40,66–69]. In these studies, aspirin seemed to be equal to or more effective than the anticoagulant. A meta-analysis of two large trials of aspirin showed that initiation of aspirin within 48 hours of stroke was associated with a modest but statistically significant improvement in outcomes [39,40]. Much of aspirin's benefit may have been in preventing early recurrent stroke. One study evaluating the efficacy of aspirin in halting progression of neurologic worsening noted no impact on outcomes [70]. Current guidelines recommend that most patients receive aspirin within 48 hours after the onset of stroke [9].

Although no large-scale clinical trials have tested aspirin among patients who have moyamoya disease, arterial dissections, or other vasculopathies, it is often prescribed. The potential for intracranial bleeding from collateral vessels in patients who have moyamoya disease and the presumed lower risk for hemorrhage with aspirin may favor its use over anticoagulants. Although some physicians prescribe oral anticoagulants to patients who have arterial dissection, the relatively low risk for recurrent stroke among these patients may also favor the use of aspirin. No data from randomized trials are available to provide information about the possible use of either antiplatelet agents or anticoagulants in treating patients who have arterial dissection.

Aspirin is not effective for preventing intraventricular thrombus among patients who have experienced a recent myocardial infarction. It is also not effective in preventing embolic events among patients who have mechanical prosthetic cardiac valves, especially in the mitral position [71]. However, aspirin seems to be the appropriate antithrombotic therapy for patients who have aortic bioprosthetic valves [72], and although Brueck and colleagues [73] concluded that it was not necessary among these patients, most physicians prescribe it.

No difference has been shown between aspirin and oral anticoagulants in preventing recurrent stroke among persons who have patent foramen ovale (PFO) and neurologic symptoms [74]. A French trial administered aspirin to several groups of young adults who had PFO and ischemic stroke [75]. The rates of recurrent embolic events were similar among patients who had PFO and those who did not experience the cardiac change. These results suggest that aspirin may be useful in treating patients who have cardiac diseases that have a relatively low risk for embolization.

Several trials have tested the efficacy of aspirin among persons who have atrial fibrillation [76–79]. At a daily dosage of 325 mg, aspirin reduces the risk for ischemic stroke by approximately 20%. Still, aspirin is not as effective as oral anticoagulants [80,81], even among older persons who have atrial fibrillation [82]. Currently, aspirin should be reserved for treating patients who have atrial fibrillation and a high risk for complications from oral anticoagulants. The currently recommended dosage of aspirin, which is the only one tested in trials of atrial fibrillation, is 325 mg/d [2].

Dipyridamole

Dipyridamole was the second antiplatelet agent extensively tested for preventing stroke among high-risk patients. The medication was initially tested as a monotherapy, given as a relatively short-acting formulation. Early trials were generally negative and the enthusiasm for dipyridamole waned. However, ensuing trials tested either conventional or sustained-release formation of dipyridamole alone or in combination with aspirin, and results have provided the strongest evidence for the role of dipyridamole in secondary prevention of stroke.

Pharmacology

A potent vasodilator, dipyridamole also has antiplatelet effects through the inhibition of cyclic nucleotide phosphodiesterase. As a result, cyclic adenosine monophosphate builds up within the platelet, preventing aggregation [83]. It also blocks the uptake of adenosine within the platelet [11]. Dipyridamole also may prolong survival of platelets, affect the synthesis of prostaglandins, and have vasoprotective properties.

Because of variable absorption of dipyridamole, systemic bioavailability may be low. The use of a sustained-release preparation increases its bioavailability. Dipyridamole is metabolized in the liver. Its effects on platelet function are reversible and the aggregation drops after the medication is stopped. The half-life of dipyridamole is approximately 10 hours. Thus, the medication must be given in a twice-daily regimen to maintain therapeutic effects on platelet function. A currently marketed preparation is 25 mg of aspirin and 200 mg of sustained-released dipyridamole.

Safety

Bleeding is not a major complication of dipyridamole [84]; headache is the most frequent and troublesome side effect. In some instances, the headache can be sufficiently severe to indicate possible subarachnoid hemorrhage. Usually the headache develops within the first days of treatment. Patients who have a history of migraine may not be able to tolerate the medication. In some patients who have a history of headache, clinicians may initiate treatment with one tablet of the combination of aspirin and dipyridamole given daily [85] and later increase the dosage to the twice-daily regimen.

Dipyridamole may also cause epigastric distress in some patients. Because of its vasodilatory effects on coronary arteries, concern exists that dipyridamole may increase the likelihood of myocardial ischemia. However, studies have not shown an increased risk for myocardial infarction with the aspirin/dipyridamole combination [86,87].

Because the daily dosage of aspirin in the combination is 50 mg, some cardiologists have recommended supplementing it with an additional 81-mg tablet, either whole or half, to assure that the patient is receiving at least 75 mg of aspirin per day. Although it has vasodilatory actions, dipyridamole does not lower blood pressure with long-term administration [88]. No laboratory monitoring is required.

Potential indications and efficacy

The results of the first trials did not show dipyridamole to be efficacious [89,90]. Thereafter, a European trial found that the combination of aspirin and dipyridamole was superior to placebo, but whether the effect was related primarily to the aspirin was unclear [91]. In the Second European Stroke Prevention Study, sustained-release dipyridamole, 200 mg, taken twice daily resulted in an approximately 16% reduction in ischemic events compared with placebo; the effectiveness was approximately the same as with aspirin, 25 mg, administered twice daily [59].

The same trial found that the combination of aspirin and dipyridamole was superior to either medication when given alone. Furthermore, an approximate 23% relative risk reduction for stroke was seen, favoring aspirin plus sustained-release dipyridamole over aspirin alone. Subsequently, an investigator-initiated international trial also showed the combination of aspirin and dipyridamole to be superior to aspirin monotherapy [92].

Although the combination has not been shown to reduce the risk for myocardial infarction or vascular death, the studies were not statistically powered to prove these reductions.

Recently, the results of the Prevention Regimen for Effectively Avoiding Second Strokes (PRoFESS) trial [93] were presented at a large international meeting. The trial compared aspirin plus sustained-release dipyridamole to clopidogrel for preventing recurrent stroke events among patients who had non–cardioembolic ischemic stroke. Over a mean follow-up of approximately 2.5 years, the rates of recurrent stroke were 9.0% among individuals taking aspirin and dipyridamole and 8.8% for those prescribed clopidogrel. No differences were noted in the composite end points of recurrent stroke, myocardial infarction, or vascular death.

This trial showed a higher rate of major bleeding events, including intracranial hemorrhages, among patients taking aspirin and dipyridamole (4.1%) than those taking clopidogrel (3.6%). Approximately 6% of patients taking the aspirin/dipyridamole combination had to discontinue the medication prematurely because of headaches. How the results of PRoFESS will affect future plans for selecting antiplatelet agents for preventing recurrent stroke is unclear. Clopidogrel and the combination of aspirin and dipyridamole seem to be roughly equal in efficacy.

Ticlopidine

Ticlopidine was the first thienopyridine developed as an antiplatelet aggregating agent. It was tested in two large trials of secondary prevention of stroke among patients who experienced TIA or stroke [94,95]. Ticlopidine also was evaluated as an adjunctive antiplatelet agent for treating patients who had ischemic heart disease [96,97]. Subsequent concerns about the safety of ticlopidine, particularly its association with the development of thrombotic thrombocytopenia purpura (TTP), have reduced ticlopidine's role in clinical practice for preventing stroke.

Pharmacology

Ticlopidine blocks in vivo platelet responses to ADP-induced aggregation and signal transduction [98–100]. The medication affects binding of fibrinogen to the platelet glycoprotein IIb/IIIa receptor [99]. It irreversibly alters platelet function and prolongs the bleeding time. Almost 90% of a single 250-mg dose of ticlopidine is absorbed rapidly and reaches a peak plasma concentration within 1 to 3 hours [99]. The usual daily dose is 250 mg twice daily, and it has a half-life of approximately 24 to 36 hours.

The antiplatelet actions of ticlopidine gradually increase after starting treatment, and inhibition of platelet aggregation is delayed by 24 to 48 hours after starting treatment [100]. Maximal suppression of platelet function does not occur until 1 to 2 weeks after starting treatment. Therefore, ticlopidine is not an effective therapy for the acute treatment of patients who have ischemic vascular disease. The antiplatelet effects of ticlopidine disappear over approximately 1 week after stopping treatment.

Safety

Because ticlopidine is a potent antiplatelet agent, hemorrhage is a potential complication. Bleeding may occur in any site, including inside the cranial vault. Risk for gastrointestinal bleeding is less than with aspirin. Although abdominal pain can accompany ingestion of ticlopidine, it does not cause gastritis or peptic ulcer disease.

Unusual complications of ticlopidine include pulmonary disease, cholestatic hepatitis, and jaundice [101,102]. Skin eruptions, including urticaria, most commonly develop within the first 2 weeks of starting ticlopidine. Potentially life-threatening hematologic complications may also occur, most commonly within the first 3 to 4 months of treatment [103]. Neutropenia, including agranulocytosis, may develop in 0.5% of cases. Because of the risk for neutropenia and TTP, complete blood cell and platelet counts must be monitored every 2 weeks during the initial 3 months of treatment.

Although some persons, especially African Americans, may have a benign cyclical neutropenia, the development of neutropenia usually prompts stopping of the medication. Patients who have severe ticlopidine-associated neutropenia usually require hospitalization and often receive granulocyte colony-stimulating factor to reduce the risk for infectious complications [104]. The use of ticlopidine is complicated by TTP at a frequency of approximately 0.02% [105,106]. Seriously affected patients also may have hemolytic uremic syndrome [107]. Most patients who have TTP require hospitalization, and early intervention may be lifesaving. Treatment is centered on plasma exchange, although relapses of TTP may occur despite intervention.

Potential indications and efficacy

Clinical trials have shown the efficacy of ticlopidine in treating patients who have ischemic heart disease, peripheral artery disease, and diabetic retinopathy in addition to those who have ischemic cerebrovascular disease [96,97,108]. The medication has been tested as monotherapy (usually compared with aspirin) or in combination with aspirin.

In a trial that enrolled patients who experienced recent ischemic stroke, the Canadian-American Ticlopidine Study found that ticlopidine reduced the risk for recurrent stroke by approximately 30% compared with placebo [95]. In a trial comparing aspirin or ticlopidine in preventing stroke among patients experiencing warning symptoms, ticlopidine was found to reduce the risk for new ischemic events by approximately 14% [94]. Most benefit was found within the first few months of starting treatment.

More recently, a large trial tested the efficacy of aspirin or ticlopidine for preventing stroke among African Americans [109,110]. Recurrent stroke, myocardial infarction, or vascular death was diagnosed in 14.7% of subjects taking ticlopidine and 12.3% taking aspirin. Overall, the trial showed that ticlopidine was not better than aspirin among these high-risk patients.

Clopidogrel

Clopidogrel, another thienopyridine, is widely used for treating patients who have ischemic vascular disease, including those at risk for stroke. It was initially tested in a large trial that enrolled subjects who had symptomatic coronary artery, cerebrovascular, and peripheral vascular disease [111]. Since the approval of clopidogrel by regulatory bodies, it has been tested alone or in combination with aspirin in several clinical settings.

Pharmacology

Clopidogrel has a chemical structure and pharmacologic actions similar to ticlopidine. Clopidogrel is administered orally at a usual daily dose of 75 mg. The pharmacokinetic properties of clopidogrel differ slightly from ticlopidine [99]. It is rapidly absorbed and metabolized. The antiplatelet effects of clopidogrel can be detected within 2 hours of a loading dose of 300 to 400 mg [112,113].

An acutely ill or unstable patient may be treated with an initial dose of 300 to 600 mg of clopidogrel; thus, this therapy may be useful in emergency treatment of ischemia [114,115]. For instance, Kennedy and colleagues [116] administered a loading dose of clopidogrel in combination with aspirin for the emergency treatment of patients who experienced recent TIA. Thereafter, a daily dose of 75 mg maintains the antiplatelet effects.

The effects on platelet aggregation disappear approximately 1 week after clopidogrel is stopped. Using caffeine after administering a loading dose of clopidogrel may further enhance platelet inhibition, probably through synergistic actions on cyclic AMP [117].

Atorvastatin, lovastatin, and simvastatin, which have effects on the CYP3A4 pathway, may lessen the antiplatelet effects of clopidogrel. However, Saw and colleagues [118] did not find any impact on the frequency of either ischemic or bleeding events in patients receiving clopidogrel and one of the statin agents. Other studies found that statin medications do not affect the antiplatelet activity of loading or maintenance doses of clopidogrel [119,120].

The antiplatelet aggregating effects of clopidogrel are not affected by the angiotensin-converting enzyme inhibitors. Administering omeprazole as a gastroprotective agent was found to lessen the actions of clopidogrel on platelet function [121]. Conversely, cilostazol seems to increase the antiplatelet effects of clopidogrel given in conjunction with aspirin [122].

Clopidogrel resistance

Cases of potential clopidogrel resistance have been reported [28,30,123,124]. Similar to patients who have presumed aspirin resistance, this diagnosis is based on the results of platelet aggregation testing. In one study of 50 patients receiving clopidogrel as part of preprocedural treatment before stenting, 14 were found to be resistant to clopidogrel [125]. Among patients who had diabetes, a sizable percentage treated with the combination of aspirin and clopidogrel retained platelet function [126–128]. A Hungarian study could not find a specific genetic polymorphism that might explain the resistance of platelets to treatment with clopidogrel [129]. Barnes and colleagues [26] could not find any evidence of resistance to dual antiplatelet agents as a distinct clinical syndrome.

Safety

Bleeding, including intracranial hemorrhage, is a potential complication of treatment with clopidogrel, particularly when the medication is given with aspirin. A large trial found that clopidogrel was associated with a lower risk for gastrointestinal hemorrhage than aspirin [111]. Vilahur and colleagues [130] tested the ability of platelet concentrates to reverse the antithrombotic effects of clopidogrel. They found that 10 and 12.5 platelet concentrate units would respectively inhibit 300 or 600 mg loading doses of clopidogrel-induced platelet disaggregation.

Many complications associated with ticlopidine also can occur with clopidogrel, although the frequency seems less. A Japanese study found that clopidogrel was safer than ticlopidine [131]. Because the risk for neutropenia is low, patients receiving clopidogrel do not require hematologic monitoring.

Cases of TTP have been reported, including those with complicating hemolytic uremic syndrome [132–134]. Overall, the risk for TTP is considerably less than with ticlopidine. TTP usually develops within the first 2 weeks of starting treatment with clopidogrel. Plasma exchange is the usual management for patients who have clopidogrel-associated TTP, with repeated exchanges needed in some instances. Fatal aplastic anemia may also occur [135].

Potential indications and efficacy

An international trial showed that clopidogrel was more effective than aspirin in preventing ischemic events (5.32% versus 5.83%) [111]. The primary benefit was found among the subgroup of patients who had symptomatic peripheral vascular disease; no difference between the treatment groups was found among the subjects who had ischemic stroke as their qualifying event.

In a subgroup analysis, Ringleb and colleagues [136] found that clopidogrel was superior among patients who had ischemic symptoms. Several trials have compared clopidogrel with other antithrombotic agents in patients who had ischemic heart disease, with clopidogrel added to aspirin in some instances [127,137–140]. Overall, data suggest that clopidogrel is slightly more effective than aspirin in preventing recurrent ischemic events among high-risk persons, although the difference is modest.

Because its antiplatelet effects occur rapidly when the agent is administered with a loading dose of 300 to 600 mg, clopidogrel has become a standard intervention for treating patients who have acute myocardial ischemia. However, the efficacy of clopidogrel in the emergency management of acute ischemic stroke has not been tested on a large-scale basis [141]. Current guidelines do not recommend use of clopidogrel for emergency treatment of stroke, and advise that antiplatelet agents not be initiated within 24 hours after treatment with intravenous tPA [9].

Prasugrel

Prasugrel is a new thienopyridine that was recently tested in patients who had ischemic heart disease. This potent antiplatelet agent may be tested in a wide range of patients who have ischemic vascular disease. It seems to have advantages over clopidogrel [142].

Pharmacology

Like ticlopidine and clopidogrel, prasugrel is a prodrug that is inactive in vitro [143,144]. The medication rapidly and irreversibly binds the platelet P2Y12 receptor and blocks ADP-induced platelet activation and aggregation. Morel and colleagues [145] found that it inhibited ADP-induced platelet aggregation at a higher level than clopidogrel.

Prasugrel was estimated to be 10 to 100 times more potent than either clopidogrel or ticlopidine [143]. Wiviott and colleagues [146] found that

60 mg of prasugrel resulted in a greater inhibition of platelet aggregation than a 600-mg loading dose of clopidogrel. They also found that a daily dose 10 mg of prasugrel had more effect on platelet function than 150 mg of clopidogrel. Another study found that a 60/10 mg regimen of prasugrel has greater inhibition of platelet aggregation than a 600/75 mg regimen of clopidogrel [147]. A study comparing clopidogrel and prasugrel in normal volunteers found the platelet inhibitory actions of prasugrel to be similar, but that the range of responses was smaller with prasugrel [148].

Safety

Serious bleeding seems to be more frequent with prasugrel than the other thienopyridine medications [149]. No differences in the rates of intracranial bleeding were found with prasugrel or clopidogrel; however, older persons who experienced stroke may be at higher risk for bleeding with this agent. Stopping the combination of prasugrel and aspirin may be associated with rebound platelet activation [150].

Potential indications and efficacy

A clinical trial compared aspirin and prasugrel with aspirin and clopidogrel in the treatment of patients who had acute coronary artery syndromes and underwent endovascular treatment [149]. The group of patients receiving prasugrel experienced significant reductions in myocardial infarction, urgent revascularization operations, and stent thrombosis. No differences in the rate of nonfatal stroke were found between the treatment groups. No trials have tested prasugrel in the long-term prevention of ischemic events or in persons at high risk for ischemic stroke. Additional research on the short- or long-term administration of prasugrel is warranted.

Other antiplatelet agents

A Canadian trial tested sulfinpyrazone alone and in combination with aspirin [52]. The medication, which is a uricosuric agent that has antiplatelet effects, was not found to be as effective as aspirin and further study was abandoned.

Cannon and colleagues [151] tested AZD6140, a reversible oral adenosine diphosphate receptor antagonist, in patients who had non–ST segment elevation myocardial infarction. Compared with clopidogrel, AZD6140 was associated with a slight increase in minor bleeding and is now being tested in a large clinical trial.

Indobufen, an anti-inflammatory agent that also inhibits cyclo-oxygenase, was also evaluated but found to be less effective than ticlopidine [152,153].

Cilostazol increases the cyclic adenosine monophosphate induction of platelet aggregation [122,154]. It has been used in combination with aspirin and clopidogrel to treat patients who have coronary artery disease [155]. The combination was associated with a reduction in adverse cardiac events.

Cilostazol in combination with aspirin was compared with clopidogrel combined with aspirin in patients undergoing stenting of the coronary arteries [156]. The cilostazol therapy was superior to the combination of aspirin and clopidogrel for preventing restenosis of the arteries. Cilostazol has also been studied in secondary ischemic stroke prevention. In a placebo-controlled trial, Gotoh and colleagues [157] found it to be effective and safe.

A clinical trial comparing trifusal with aspirin found it to have no net benefit [158]. Several orally administered glycoprotein IIb/IIIa receptor blockers were tested in nonstroke populations, but high rates of bleeding and mortality were reported [159–161]. The glycoprotein IIb/IIIa receptor blockers also may induce thrombocytopenia. These agents have not been tested subsequently for long-term prevention. Valencia and colleagues [162] found that the combination of eptifibatide, aspirin, and clopidogrel could be given safely to patients who underwent recent coronary artery angioplasty and stenting.

Combinations of antiplatelet agents

Because the antiplatelet agents inhibit aggregation through different mechanisms, the facts that their actions could be synergistic and that a combination of medications would be more effective in preventing thromboembolic disease and ischemia than would each agent administered alone have a natural appeal. In addition, because the actions of the antiplatelet agents could be complementary to the inhibition of coagulation factors by oral anticoagulants, this antithrombotic combination could be given to especially high-risk patients.

Potential indications for combinations of antiplatelet agents or antiplatelet agents and anticoagulants could include emergency treatment for patients experiencing crescendo or recent TIA, recent stroke, acute myocardial ischemia, or unstable angina; adjunctive treatment of patients undergoing endovascular interventions; or management of patients who have very high-risk cardiac circumstances, such as those who have prosthetic valves. The combination of medications also may be used if a patient has ischemic symptoms despite treatment with an individual antiplatelet agent or anticoagulant.

Several recent clinical trials have focused on testing combinations of antiplatelet agents rather than performing head-to-head comparisons of the efficacy and safety of the medications. Although combinations of medications may be more effective in preventing ischemia, they probably will be associated with a higher risk for serious bleeding complications than among persons taking one medication. Thus, the potential benefit in preventing ischemia must be weighed against the risk of serious hemorrhage, including intracranial bleeding.

Oral anticoagulants and antiplatelet agents

The use of warfarin and an antiplatelet agent is relatively common among patients who have cardiovascular disease. Johnson and colleagues [163] found that approximately 40% of patients taking warfarin also were receiving an antiplatelet agent. Most of these patients have symptomatic coronary artery disease and risk factors for cardioembolic stroke, such as atrial fibrillation or a dilated cardiomyopathy. These patients also had symptomatic artery disease and recent endovascular interventions.

Data on the safety and efficacy of oral anticoagulants and antiplatelet agents are limited. Most experience involves the administration of aspirin, and most studies involved subjects who had symptomatic heart disease or were considered at high risk for cardioembolic stroke. Testa and colleagues [164] found the combination of warfarin and aspirin to be comparable to that of aspirin and clopidogrel in preventing death, bleeding adverse experiences, and recurrent myocardial infarction among persons who had symptomatic coronary artery disease.

The combination of warfarin and single or dual antiplatelet therapy (most commonly aspirin and/or clopidogrel) was evaluated among patients undergoing coronary artery stenting [165]. No major increase in bleeding complications or decline in ischemic events was noted. However, Khurram and colleagues [166] found that combining warfarin, clopidogrel, and aspirin was associated with more serious bleeding complications than treatment with just two antiplatelet agents. Delaney and colleagues found adding aspirin to warfarin to be associated with a marked increase in the risk for gastrointestinal bleeding.

O'Connor and colleagues [168] found that the combination of fixed-dose warfarin and 81 mg of aspirin was inferior to aspirin 160 mg/d in preventing stroke among patients who experienced recent myocardial infarction. Aspirin was also added to adjusted-dose warfarin to prevent thromboembolic events among patients who had prosthetic heart valves. A common scenario would be to add aspirin after a patient has an embolic stroke, despite treatment with warfarin at a therapeutic level of anticoagulation.

One study administering low-dose aspirin (100 mg/d) in conjunction with anticoagulants to reach an international normalized ratio of approximately 2.5 showed that the combination may be as effective as higher-intensity anticoagulation in preventing embolic events among persons who have mechanical cardiac valves [169]. A systemic review found that the combination of low-dose aspirin (75–81 mg) and warfarin is effective in lowering the risks for embolic events or stroke among persons who have prosthetic heart valves [170]. Dipyridamole was also used as an adjunct to oral anticoagulants to lower the risk for embolic events among high-risk patients who have mechanical heart valves [171].

Dipyridamole has been shown to have additive effects on inhibiting platelet aggregation among patients taking aspirin [172]. Because the data on the efficacy of dipyridamole as a monotherapy are limited, most trials of dipyridamole in stroke prevention (immediate or sustained-release formulation) have focused on its combination with aspirin [173,174]. Two European studies found that the combination of aspirin and dipyridamole was superior to placebo, with one showing that the combination was more effective than either medication given as a monotherapy [59,175].

Subsequently, an investigator-initiated trial of dipyridamole and aspirin found that the combination was more effective than aspirin monotherapy in preventing stroke among high-risk patients who had symptomatic cerebrovascular disease [92]. Bleeding complications were not a major problem.

These three trials provide solid evidence that the combination of aspirin and dipyridamole is an effective choice for stroke prophylaxis among high-risk persons. Indirect evidence suggests that the combination is more effective than clopidogrel in preventing stroke [176]. The large international PRoFESS trial compared the combination of sustained-release dipyridamole and aspirin with clopidogrel [177].

Studies tested the efficacy of the combination of ticlopidine and aspirin primarily in the treatment of patients who had acute heart disease [95,96]. These studies showed that the combination was more efficacious in preventing arterial occlusion and ischemic symptoms than aspirin monotherapy. Although interest in the use of ticlopidine has waned, primarily because of concerns about safety, research continues on the efficacy of combining aspirin and ticlopidine [178].

Serebrauany and colleagues [179] found that adding clopidogrel to an 81-mg dose of aspirin had more effects on platelet function than adding clopidogrel to a 325-mg dose. Clopidogrel provides further inhibition of platelet function among patients undergoing long-term treatment with aspirin [180], which is associated with an increased risk for bleeding complications. For example, Delaney and colleagues [167] found that combining clopidogrel and aspirin was associated with an approximately doubled risk for gastrointestinal bleeding compared with either medication alone. A trial comparing the safety and efficacy of combining aspirin and clopidogrel versus clopidogrel alone among patients who experienced recent TIA or stroke found that the combination was associated with an increased risk for major bleeding complications [181].

Another large trial compared the efficacy of adding clopidogrel to aspirin versus aspirin alone in a broad range of subjects who had symptomatic atherosclerotic disease or asymptomatic patients at high risk for ischemic events [182]. Overall the trial did not show a reduction in ischemic events associated with the combination therapy, although a trend among the subgroup of symptomatic persons may have favored the combination.

A second trial that enrolled only subjects who had a history of TIA or stroke was unable to show that adding aspirin to clopidogrel was superior to clopidogrel alone in preventing recurrent ischemic events [181]. The combination of aspirin and clopidogrel was tested against monotherapy with aspirin in a series of patients who had symptomatic carotid stenosis. The marker of success was a reduction in microembolic signals detected with transcranial Doppler ultrasonography [183]. The combination reduced the number of recurrent events compared with aspirin. Kennedy and colleagues [116] tested the efficacy of the combination of clopidogrel and aspirin for emergency treatment of patients who experienced recent TIA. Although a modest increase in bleeding complications was noted with the combination, the frequency of stroke within 90 days was 10.8% for patients treated with aspirin only and 7.1% among those treated with both medications. Another trial is testing the combination of clopidogrel and aspirin for treating patients who have recent TIA [114].

A German study that surveyed outcomes in 7559 patients found that the combination of clopidogrel and aspirin was superior to aspirin alone in preventing death, nonfatal recurrent myocardial infarction, and nonfatal stroke among patients who had acute ST-elevation myocardial infarction [115]. These changes were found regardless of reperfusion strategy (thrombolysis or endovascular treatment). The combination of medications was associated with a higher risk for bleeding than aspirin alone (7.1% versus 3.4%). Bhatt and colleagues [184] concluded that the combination of clopidogrel and aspirin was superior to aspirin alone among patients in the CHARISMA trial who had symptomatic atherosclerotic disease.

The combination of clopidogrel and aspirin is often prescribed for patients undergoing endovascular interventions [185,186]. Fares and colleagues [187] concluded that the combination of clopidogrel and aspirin is justified in high-risk patients, but the exact dose regimen and duration of treatment has not been established. Another analysis concluded that adding clopidogrel to aspirin results in a small reduction in all-cause mortality in patients who had ST-elevation myocardial infarction and a modest reduction in stroke or recurrent myocardial infarction in patients who had symptomatic cardiovascular disease [188,189]. The combination was not associated with an excess rate of intracranial or fatal hemorrhages.

The combination of clopidogrel and aspirin has been compared with adjusted dose warfarin in the treatment of patients who have atrial fibrillation [190,191]. Not only was the combination found to be less effective than adjusted-dose oral anticoagulant treatment, the frequency of bleeding events was higher among patients taking the combination of aspirin and clopidogrel.

Summary

Antithrombotic therapy is a major component of ischemic stroke prevention. Oral anticoagulants are typically reserved for patients who have a known cardioembolic source. Antiplatelet agents are the most widely prescribed medications for preventing first or recurrent stroke among patients who have arterial diseases. They also are prescribed to patients who have cardiac sources of embolization, either as an adjunct to oral anticoagulants or as an alternative for patients who have contraindications to oral anticoagulants.

Because of its well-studied side-effect profile, widespread availability, and low cost, many regard aspirin as the first-line agent for preventing ischemic cardiovascular disease, including stroke. In general, the desired dose of aspirin is 50 to 325 mg/d. No evidence shows that higher doses of aspirin are more effective, but larger doses may be associated with an increased risk for upper gastrointestinal side effects.

The 2008 American Heart Association/American Stroke Association evidence-based guideline update [192] indicates that aspirin, aspirin plus sustained-release dipyridamole, or clopidogrel may be used as initial long-term therapy for recurrent ischemic stroke prevention if anticoagulants are not indicated. However, some reserve antiplatelet agents other than aspirin for patients who experience aspirin failure, those at high risk for recurrent events, or those unable to tolerate aspirin.

The other commonly prescribed antiplatelet agents are clopidogrel and the combination of aspirin and sustained-release dipyridamole. The combination of aspirin and clopidogrel has not been shown to be superior to either agent alone and has a higher risk for causing major bleeding, including intracerebral hemorrhage. A recent large trial showed that the efficacy of clopidogrel was approximately the same as that of sustained-release dipyridamole plus aspirin. Therefore, evidence shows that either clopidogrel monotherapy or the combination of aspirin and sustained-release dipyridamole is a reasonable choice for patients who are not treated with aspirin alone.

References

[1] Goldstein LB, Adams R, Alberts MJ, et al. Primary prevention of ischemic stroke: a guideline from the American heart association/American stroke association stroke council: cosponsored by the atherosclerotic peripheral vascular disease interdisciplinary working group; cardiovascular nursing council; clinical cardiology council; nutrition, physical activity, and metabolism council; and the quality of care and outcomes research interdisciplinary working group: the American academy of neurology affirms the value of this guideline. Stroke 2006;37:1583–633.

[2] Sacco RL, Adams R, Albers G, et al. Guidelines for prevention of stroke in patients with ischemic stroke or transient ischemic attack: a statement for healthcare professionals from the American heart association/American stroke association council on stroke: co-sponsored by the council on cardiovascular radiology and intervention: the American academy of neurology affirms the value of this guideline. Stroke 2006;37:577–617.

[3] Mohr JP, Thompson JL, Lazar RM, et al. A comparison of warfarin and aspirin for the prevention of recurrent ischemic stroke. N Engl J Med 2001;345:1444–51.

[4] Algra A. Medium intensity oral anticoagulants versus aspirin after cerebral ischaemia of arterial origin (ESPRIT): a randomised controlled trial. Lancet Neurol 2007;6:115–24.

[5] Algra A, De Schryver EL, van Gijn J, et al. Oral anticoagulants versus antiplatelet therapy for preventing further vascular events after transient ischemic attack or minor stroke of presumed arterial origin. Stroke 2003;34:234–5.
[6] Chimowitz MI, Lynn MJ, Howlett-Smith H, et al. Comparison of warfarin and aspirin for symptomatic intracranial arterial stenosis. N Engl J Med 2006;353:1305–16.
[7] Antiplatelet trialists' collaboration collaborative overview of randomised trials of antiplatelet therapy–i: prevention of death, myocardial infarction, and stroke by prolonged antiplatelet therapy in various categories of patients. BMJ 1994;308:81–106.
[8] Assadian A, Eidher U, Senekowitsch C, et al. Antiplatelet therapy prior to carotid endarterectomy–still room for improvement. Vasa 2006;35:96–100.
[9] Adams HP Jr, del Zoppo G, Alberts MJ, et al. Guidelines for the early management of adults with ischemic stroke: a guideline from the American heart association/American stroke association stroke council, clinical cardiology council, cardiovascular radiology and intervention council, and the atherosclerotic peripheral vascular disease and quality of care outcomes in research interdisciplinary working groups: the American academy of neurology affirms the value of this guideline as an educational tool for neurologists. Stroke 2007;38:1655–711.
[10] Craven LL. Prevention of coronary thrombosis and cerebral thrombosis. Mississippi Valley Medical Journal 1956;78:213–5.
[11] Patrono C, Coller B, Dalen JE, et al. Platelet-active drugs. Chest 2001;119:39S–63S.
[12] Awtry EH, Loscalzo J. Aspirin. Circulation 2000;101:1206–18.
[13] Brandon RA, Eadie MJ. The basis for aspirin dosage in stroke prevention. Clin Exp Neurol 1987;23:47–54.
[14] Heavey DJ, Barrow SE, Hickling NE, et al. Aspirin causes short-lived inhibition of bradykinin-stimulated prostacyclin production in man. Nature 1985;318:186–8.
[15] Capone ML, Sciulli MG, Tacconelli S, et al. Pharmacodynamic interaction of naproxen with low-dose aspirin in healthy subjects. J Am Coll Cardiol 2005;45:1295–301.
[16] Cryer B, Verlin RG, Cooper SA, et al. Double-blind, randomized, parallel, placebo-controlled study of ibuprofen effects on thromboxane B2 concentrations in aspirin-treated healthy adult volunteers. Clin Ther 2005;27:185–91.
[17] Zhao J, Qi R, Wu W, et al. Protective effects of aspirin against oxidized LDL-induced inflammatory protein expression in human endothelial cells. J Cardiovasc Pharmacol 2008;51:32–7.
[18] Cyrus T, Sung S, Zhao L, et al. Effect of low-dose aspirin on vascular inflammation, plaque stability, and atherogenesis in low-density lipoprotein receptor-deficient mice. Circulation 2002;106:1282–7.
[19] Gomes I. Aspirin: a neuroprotective agent at high doses? Natl Med J India 1998;11:14–7.
[20] Hohlfeld T, Weber AA, Junghans U, et al. Variable platelet response to aspirin in patients with ischemic stroke. Cerebrovasc Dis 2007;24:43–50.
[21] Patrono C, Rocca B. Aspirin: promise and resistance in the new millennium. Arteroscler Thromb Vasc Biol 2008;28:525–32.
[22] Pamukcu B, Oflaz H, Onur I, et al. Clinical relevance of aspirin resistance in patients with stable coronary artery disease: a prospective follow-up study (PROSPECTAR). Blood Coagul Fibrinolysis 2007;18:187–92.
[23] Assadian A, Lax J, Meixner-Loicht U, et al. Aspirin resistance among long-term aspirin users after carotid endarterectomy and controls: flow cytometric measurement of aspirin-induced platelet inhibition. J Vasc Surg 2007;45:1142–7.
[24] Sanderson S, Emery J, Balin T, et al. Narrative review: aspirin resistance and its clinical implications. Ann Intern Med 2005;142:370–80.
[25] Coma-Canella I, Velasc A. Variability in individual responsiveness to aspirin: clinical implications and treatment. Cardiovasc Hematol Disord Drug Targets 2007;7:274–87.
[26] Barnes GD, Li J, Kline-Rogers E, et al. Dual antiplatelet agent failure: a new syndrome or clinical nonentity. Am Heart J 2007;154:732–5.

[27] Chen WH, Cheng X, Lee PY, et al. Aspirin resistance and adverse clinical events in patients with coronary artery disease. Am J Med 2007;120:631–5.
[28] Gurbel PA, Bliden KP, DiChiara J, et al. Evaluation of dose-related effects of aspirin on platelet function: results from the aspirin-induced platelet effect (ASPECT) study. Circulation 2007;115:3156–64.
[29] Patel D, Moonis M. Clinical implications of aspirin resistance. Expert Rev Cardiovasc Ther 2007;5:969–75.
[30] Fitzgerald DJ, Maree A. Aspirin and clopidogrel resistance. Hematology Am Soc Hematol Educ Program 2007;2007:114–20.
[31] Cattaneo M. Resistance to antiplatelet drugs: molecular mechanisms and laboratory detection. J Thromb Haemost 2007;5:230–7.
[32] Alberts MJ, Bergman DL, Molner E, et al. Antiplatelet effect of aspirin in patients with cerebrovascular disease. Stroke 2004;35:175–8.
[33] Helgason CM, Bolin KM, Hoff JA, et al. Development of aspirin resistance in persons with previous ischemic stroke. Stroke 1994;25:2331–6.
[34] Helgason CM, Tortorice KL, Winkler SR, et al. Aspirin response and failure in cerebral infarction. Stroke 1993;24:345–50.
[35] Rao GH, Michiels JJ. Aspirin resistance: does it exist? Semin Thromb Hemost 2007;33: 210–4.
[36] Patrono C, Bachmann F, Baigent C, et al. Expert consensus document on the use of antiplatelet agents: the task force on the use of antiplatelet agents in patients with atherosclerotic cardiovascular disease of the European society of cardiology. Eur Heart J 2004;25: 166–81.
[37] Sze PC, Reitman D, Pincus MM, et al. Antiplatelet agents in the secondary prevention of stroke: meta-analysis of the randomized control trials. Stroke 1988;19:436–42.
[38] Petty GW, Brown RD Jr, Whisnant JP, et al. Frequency of major complications of aspirin, warfarin, and intravenous heparin for secondary stroke prevention. Ann Intern Med 1999; 130:14–22.
[39] CAST (Chinese Acute Stroke Trial) collaborative group CAST: randomised placebo-controlled trial of early aspirin use in 20,000 patients with acute ischaemic stroke. Lancet 1997;349:1641–9.
[40] International stroke trial collaborative group the international stroke trial (IST): a randomised trial of aspirin, subcutaneous heparin, both, or neither among 19435 patients with acute ischaemic stroke. Lancet 1997;349:1569–81.
[41] Steering committee of the physicians' health study research group final report on the aspirin component of the ongoing physicians' health study. N Engl J Med 1989;321:129–35.
[42] He J, Whelton PK, Vu B. Aspirin and risk of hemorrhagic stroke. J Am Med Assoc 1998; 280:1930–5.
[43] CLASP collaborative group low dose aspirin in pregnancy and early childhood development: follow up of the collaborative low dose aspirin study in pregnancy. Br J Obstet Gynaecol 1995;102:861–8.
[44] Ridker PM, Cook NR, Lee IM, et al. A randomized trial of low-dose aspirin in the primary prevention of cardiovascular disease in women. N Engl J Med 2005;352:1293–304.
[45] Patrono C. Prevention of myocardial infarction and stroke by aspirin: different mechanisms? Different dosage? Thromb Res 1998;92:S7–12.
[46] Hart R, Halperin J, McBride R. Aspirin for the primary prevention of stroke and other major vascular events. Arch Neurol 2000;57:326–32.
[47] Hennekens CH, Schneider WR. The need for wider and appropriate utilization of aspirin and statins in the treatment and prevention of cardiovascular disease. Expert Rev Cardiovasc Ther 2008;6:95–107.
[48] Goldstein LB, Rothwell PM. Primary prevention and health services delivery. Stroke 2007; 38:222–4.

[49] Ambrosi P, Villani P, Bouvenot G, et al. Antiplatelet therapy for primary prevention in diabetes. Diabete Metab 2006;32:2S52–6.
[50] De Berardis G, Sacco M, Evangelista V, et al. Aspirin and Simvastatin Combination for Cardiovascular Events Prevention Trial in Diabetes (ACCEPT-D): design of a randomized study of the efficacy of low-dose aspirin in the prevention of cardiovascular events in subjects with diabetes mellitus treated with statins. Trials 2007;8:21–30.
[51] Morimoto T, Nakayama M, Saito Y, et al. Aspirin for primary prevention of atherosclerotic disease in Japan. J Atheroscler Thromb 2007;14:159–66.
[52] The Canadian cooperative study group a randomized trial of aspirin and sulfinpyrazone in threatened stroke. N Engl J Med 1978;299:53–9.
[53] Fields WS, Lemak NA, Frankowski RF, et al. Controlled trial of aspirin in cerebral ischemia. Part II: surgical group. Stroke 1978;9:309–19.
[54] Fields WS, Lemak NA, Frankowski RF, et al. Controlled trial of aspirin in cerebral ischemia. Circulation 1980;62:V90–6.
[55] The SALT collaborative group Swedish aspirin low-dose trial (SALT) of 75 mg aspirin as secondary prophylaxis after cerebrovascular ischaemic events. Lancet 1991;338: 1345–9.
[56] The Dutch TIA study group. The Dutch TIA trial: protective effects of low-dose aspirin and atenolol in patients with transient ischemic attacks or nondisabling stroke. Stroke 1988;19: 512–7.
[57] United Kingdom Transient Ischaemic Attack (UK-TIA) aspirin trial: interim results. UK-TIA Study Group. Br Med J 1988;296:316–20.
[58] Taylor DW, Barnett HJM, Haynes RB, et al. Low-dose and high-dose acetylsalicylic acid for patients undergoing carotid endarterectomy: a randomised controlled trial. Lancet 1999;353:2179–84.
[59] Diener HC, Cunha L, Forbes C, et al. Dipyridamole and acetylsalicylic acid in the secondary prevention of stroke. J Neurol Sci 1996;143:1–13.
[60] Algra A, van Gijn J. Aspirin at any dose above 30 mg offers only modest protection after cerebral ischaemia. J Neurol Neurosurg Psychiatr 1996;60:197–9.
[61] Adams HP Jr, Bendixen BH. Low- versus high-dose aspirin in prevention of ischemic stroke. Clin Neuropharmacol 1993;16:485–500.
[62] Johnson ES, Lanes SF, Wentworth CE, et al. A metaregression analysis of the dose-response effect of aspirin on stroke. Arch Intern Med 1999;159:1248–53.
[63] Kasner SE, Lynn MJ, Chimowitz MI, et al. Warfarin vs aspirin for symptomatic intracranial stenosis: subgroup analyses from WASID. Neurology 2006;67:1275–8.
[64] Chimowitz MI, Lynn MJ, Howlett-Smith H, et al. Comparison of warfarin and aspirin for symptomatic intracranial arterial stenosis. N Engl J Med 2005;352:1305–16.
[65] Multicentre Acute Stroke Trial–Italy (MAST-I) group randomised controlled trial of streptokinase, aspirin, and combination of both in treatment of acute ischaemic stroke. Lancet 1995;346:1509–14.
[66] Berge E, Abdelnoor M, Nakstad PH, et al. Low molecular-weight heparin versus aspirin in patients with acute ischaemic stroke and atrial fibrillation: a double-blind randomised study. Lancet 2000;355:1205–10.
[67] Berge E, Sandercock P. Anticoagulants versus antiplatelet agents for acute ischaemic stroke. Cochrane Database Syst Rev 2002;(4):CD003242.
[68] Bath PM, Lindenstrom E, Boysen G, et al. Tinzaparin in Acute Ischaemic Stroke (TAIST): a randomised aspirin-controlled trial. Lancet 2001;358:683–4.
[69] Wong KS, Chen C, Ng PW, et al. Low-molecular-weight heparin compared with aspirin for the treatment of acute ischaemic stroke in Asian patients with large artery occlusive disease: a randomised study. Lancet 2007;6:407–13.
[70] Roden-Jullig A, Britton M, Malmkvist K, et al. Aspirin in the prevention of progressing stroke: a randomized controlled study. J Intern Med 2003;254:584–90.

[71] Stein PD, Alpert JS, Dalen JE, et al. Antithrombotic therapy in patients with mechanical and biological prosthetic heart valves. Chest 1998;114:602S–10S.
[72] di Marco F, Grendene S, Feltrin G, et al. Antiplatelet therapy in patients receiving aortic bioprostheses: a report of clinical and instrumental safety. J Thorac Cardiovasc Surg 2007;133:1597–603.
[73] Brueck M, Kramer W, Vogt P, et al. Antiplatelet therapy early after bioprosthetic aortic valve replacement is unnecessary in patients without thromboembolic risk factors. Eur J Cardiothorac Surg 2007;32:108–12.
[74] Homma S, Sacco R, Di Tuillo M, et al. Effect of medical treatment in stroke patients with patent foramen ovale. Patent foramen ovale in cryptogenic stroke study. Circulation 2002; 105:2625–31.
[75] Mas J-L, Cabanes L, Coste J, et al. Patent foramen ovale, atrial septal aneurysm, and recurrent stroke. N Engl J Med 2002;346:1331–2.
[76] The atrial fibrillation investigators. The efficacy of aspirin in patients with atrial fibrillation. Analysis of pooled data from 3 randomized trials. Arch Intern Med 1997;157:1237–40.
[77] The SPAF III Writing Committee for Stroke Prevention in Atrial Fibrillation Investigators. Patients with nonvalvular atrial fibrillation at low risk of stroke during treatment with aspirin. Stroke Prevention in Atrial Fibrillation III Study. JAMA 1998;279:1273–7.
[78] Petersen P, Boysen G, Godtfredsen J, et al. Placebo-controlled, randomised trial of warfarin and aspirin for prevention of thromboembolic complications in chronic atrial fibrillation. The Copenhagen AFASAK study. Lancet 1989;1:175–9.
[79] Petersen P. Thromboembolic complications in atrial fibrillation. Stroke 1990;21:4–13.
[80] Mant J, Hobbs FR, Fletcher K, et al. Warfarin versus aspirin for stroke prevention in an elderly community population with atrial fibrillation (the Birmingham atrial fibrillation treatment of the aged study, BAFTA): a randomised controlled trial. Lancet 2007;370: 493–503.
[81] Rash A, Downes T, Portner R, et al. A randomised controlled trial of warfarin versus aspirin for stroke prevention in octogenarians with atrial fibrillation (WASPO). Age Ageing 2007;36:117–9.
[82] Mant J, Hobbs FD, Fletcher K, et al. Warfarin versus aspirin for stroke prevention in an elderly community population with atrial fibrillation (the Birmingham atrial fibrillation treatment of the aged study, BAFTA): a randomised controlled trial. Lancet 2007;370: 493–503.
[83] Rivey MP, Alexander MR, Taylor JW. Dipyridamole: a critical evaluation. Drug Intell Clin Pharm 1984;18:869–80.
[84] Fleck JD, Biller J. Choices in medical management for prevention of acute ischemic stroke. Curr Neurol Neurosci Rep 2001;1:33–8.
[85] Theis JG, Deichsel G, Marshall S. Rapid development of tolerance to dipyridamole associated headaches. Br J Clin Pharmacol 1999;48:750–5.
[86] Humphreys DM, Street J, Schumacher H, et al. Dipyridamole may be used safely in patients with ischaemic heart disease. Int J Clin Pract 2002;56:121–7.
[87] Diener HC, Darius H, Bertrand-Hardy JM, et al. Does early high dosage dipyridamole in prevention of secondary stroke induce cardiac events? Z Kardiol 2001;90:348–51.
[88] De Schryver EL, ESPRIT Study Group. Dipyridamole in stroke prevention: effect of dipyridamole on blood pressure. Stroke 2003;34:2339–42.
[89] The Persantine-Aspirin Reinfarction Study (PARIS) research group. The Persantine-Aspirin Reinfarction Study. Circulation 1980;62:V85–8.
[90] The American-Canadian co-operative study group persantine aspirin trial in cerebral ischemia. Part II: endpoint results. Stroke 1985;16:406–15.
[91] The ESPS group. The European stroke prevention study. Lancet 1987;2:1351–4.
[92] ESPRIT Study Group. Aspirin plus dipyridamole versus aspirin alone after cerebral ischaemia of arterial origin (ESPRIT): randomised controlled trial. Lancet 2006;367:1665.
[93] Sacco R. European Stroke Conference, Nice France, May 14, 2008.

[94] Hass WK, Easton JD, Adams HP Jr, et al. A randomized trial comparing ticlopidine hydrochloride with aspirin for the prevention of stroke in high-risk patients. Ticlopidine aspirin stroke study group. N Engl J Med 1989;321:501–7.
[95] Gent M, Blakely JA, Easton JD, et al. The Canadian American ticlopidine study (CATS) in thromboembolic stroke. Lancet 1989;1:1215–20.
[96] van de Loo A, Nauck M, Noory E, et al. Enhancement of platelet inhibition of ticlopidine plus aspirin vs aspirin alone given prior to elective PTCA. Eur Heart J 1998;19:96–102.
[97] Goods CM, al-Shaibi KF, Liu MW, et al. Comparison of aspirin alone versus aspirin plus ticlopidine after coronary artery stenting. Am J Cardiol 1996;78:1042–4.
[98] Harker LA. Therapeutic inhibition of platelet function in stroke. Cerebrovasc Dis 1998; 8(Suppl 5):8–18.
[99] Patrono C, Coller B, Dalen JE, et al. Platelet-active drugs: the relationships among dose, effectiveness, and side effects. Chest 1998;114:470S–88S.
[100] Quinn MJ, Fitzgerald DJ. Ticlopidine and clopidogrel. Circulation 1999;100:1667–72.
[101] Iqbal M, Goenka P, Young MF, et al. Ticlopidine-induced cholestatic hepatitis: report of three cases and review of the literature. Dig Dis Sci 1998;43:2223–6.
[102] Persoz CF, Cornella F, Kaeser P, et al. Ticlopidine-induced interstitial pulmonary disease: a case report. Chest 2001;119:1963–5.
[103] Love BB, Biller J, Gent M. Adverse haematological effects of ticlopidine. Prevention, recognition and management. Drug Saf 1998;19:89–98.
[104] Hung MJ, Wang CH, Cherng WJ. Granulocyte colony stimulating factor treatment for delayed recovery of ticlopidine-related neutropenia. Int J Clin Pract 2002;56:70–1.
[105] Bennett CL, Weinberg PD, Rozenberg-Bendror K, et al. Thrombotic thrombocytopenia purpura associated with ticlopidine. Ann Intern Med 1998;128:541–4.
[106] Steinhubl SR, Tan WA, Foody JM, et al. Incidence and clinical course of thrombotic thrombocytopenic purpura due to ticlopidine following coronary stenting. EPISTENT Investigators. Evaluation of platelet IIb/IIIa inhibitor for stenting. J Am Med Assoc 1999;281:806–10.
[107] Medina PJ, Sipols JM, George JN. Drug-associated thrombotic thrombocytopenic purpura-hemolytic uremic syndrome. Curr Opin Hematol 2001;8:286–93.
[108] Janzon L. The STIMS trial: the ticlopidine experience and its clinical applications. Swedish ticlopidine multicenter study. Vasc Med 1996;1:141–3.
[109] Gorelick PB, Richardson D, Kelly M, et al. Aspirin and ticlopidine for prevention of recurrent stroke in black patients: a randomized trial. JAMA 2003;289:2947–57.
[110] Gorelick PB, Richardson D, Kelly M, et al. Aspirin and ticlopidine for prevention of recurrent stroke in black patients. JAMA 2006;289:2947–57.
[111] CAPRIE steering committee a randomised, blinded, trial of clopidogrel versus aspirin in patients at risk of ischaemic events (CAPRIE). Lancet 1996;348:1329–39.
[112] Helft G, Osende JI, Worthley SG, et al. Acute antithrombotic effect of a front-loaded regimen of clopidogrel in patients with atherosclerosis on aspirin. Arterioscler Thromb Vasc Biol 2000;20:2316–21.
[113] Pache J, Kastrati A, Mehilli J, et al. Clopidogrel therapy in patients undergoing coronary stenting: value of a high-loading-dose regimen. Catheter Cardiovasc Interv 2002;55:436–41.
[114] Meyer DM, Albright KC, Allison TA, et al. LOAD: a pilot study of the safety of loading of aspirin and clopidogrel in acute ischemic stroke and transient ischemic attack. J Stroke Cerebrovasc Dis 2008;17:26–9.
[115] Zeymer U, Arntz H, Darius H, et al. Efficacy and safety of clopidogrel 600 mg administered pre-hospitally to improve primary percutaneous coronary intervention in patients with acute myocardial infarction (CIPAMI): study rationale and design. Cardiology 2007;108: 265–72.
[116] Kennedy J, Hill MD, Ryckborst KJ, et al. Fast Assessment of Stroke and Transient Ischaemic Attack to Prevent Early Recurrence (FASTER): a randomised controlled pilot trial. Lancet Neurol 2007;6:961–9.

[117] Lev EI, Arikan ME, Vaduganathan M, et al. Effect of caffeine on platelet inhibition by clopidogrel in healthy subjects and patients with coronary artery disease. Am Heart J 2007;154:694.e1–694.e7.

[118] Saw J, Brennan DM, Steinhubl SR, et al. Lack of evidence of a clopidogrel-statin interaction in the CHARISMA trial. J Am Coll Cardiol 2007;50:291–5.

[119] Trenk D, Hochholzer W, Frundi D, et al. Impact of cytochrome P450 3A4-metabolized statins on the antiplatelet effect of a 600-mg loading dose clopidogrel and on clinical outcome in patients undergoing elective coronary stent placement. Thromb Haemost 2008;99:174–81.

[120] Wenaweser P, Windecker S, Billinger M, et al. Effect of atorvastatin and pravastatin on platelet inhibition by aspirin and clopidogrel treatment in patients with coronary stent thrombosis. Am J Cardio 2007;99:353–6.

[121] Gilard M, Arnaud B, Cornily JC, et al. Influence of omeprazole on the antiplatelet action of clopidogrel associated with aspirin: the randomized, double-blind OCLA (Omeprazole Clopidogrel Aspirin) study. J Am Coll Cardiol 2008;51:256–60.

[122] Kim JY, Lee K, Shin M, et al. Cilostazol could ameliorate platelet responsiveness to clopidogrel in patients undergoing primary percutaneous coronary intervention. Circ J 2007;71: 1867–72.

[123] Shenkman B, Matetzky S, Fefer P, et al. Variable responsiveness to clopidogrel and aspirin among patients with acute coronary syndrome as assessed by platelet function tests. Thromb Res 2008;122:336–45.

[124] Gurbel PA, Tantry US. Clopidogrel resistance? Thromb Res 1908;120:311–21.

[125] Muller-Schunk S, Linn J, Peters N, et al. Monitoring of clopidogrel-related platelet inhibition: correlation of nonresponse with clinical outcome in supraaortic stenting. AJNR Am J Neuroradiol 2008;29:786–91.

[126] Serebruany VL, Malinin AI, Pokov A, et al. Effects of clopidogrel and aspirin in combination versus aspirin alone on platelet activation and major receptor expression in diabetic patients: the Plavix use for treatment of diabetes (PLUTO-Diabetes) trial. Am Heart J 2008;155:93e.1–93e.7.

[127] Serebruany VL, Malinin AI, Ziai W, et al. Effects of clopidogrel and aspirin in combination versus aspirin alone on platelet activation and major receptor expression in patients after recent ischemic stroke: for the Plavix use for treatment of stroke (PLUTO-Stroke) trial. Stroke 2005;36:2289–92.

[128] Pfeffer MA, Jarcho JA. The charisma of subgroups and the subgroups of CHARISMA. N Engl J Med 2006;354:1744–6.

[129] Papp E, Havasi V, Bene J, et al. Does glycoprotein IIIa gene (PI(A)) polymorphism influence clopidogrel resistance?: a study in older patients. Drugs Aging 2007;24:345–50.

[130] Vilahur G, Choi B, Zafar M, et al. Normalization of platelet reactivity in clopidogrel-treated subjects. Journal of Thrombosis and Haemostasis 2007;5:82–90.

[131] Fukuuchi Y, Tohgi H, Okudera T, et al. A randomized, double-blind study comparing the safety and efficacy of clopidogrel versus ticlopidine in Japanese patients with non-cardioembolic cerebral infarction. Cerebrovasc Dis 2007;25:40–9.

[132] Zakarija A, Bandarenko N, Pandey DK, et al. An update of pharmacovigilance efforts conducted by independent researchers, pharmaceutical suppliers, and the food and drug administration. Stroke 2004;35:533–8.

[133] Bennett CL, Connors JM, Carwile MJ, et al. Thrombotic thrombocytopenic purpura associated with clopidogrel. N Engl J Med 2000;325:1371–2.

[134] Nara W, Ashley I, Rosner F. Thrombotic thrombocytopenic purpura associated with clopidogrel administration: case report and brief review. Am J Med Sci 2001;322:170–2.

[135] Trivier JM, Caron J, Mahieu M, et al. Fatal aplastic anaemia associated with clopidogrel. Lancet 2001;357:446.

[136] Ringleb PA, Bhatt DL, Hirsch AT, et al. Benefit of clopidogrel over aspirin is amplified in patients with a history of ischemic events. Stroke 2004;35:528–32.

[137] Bhatt DL, Chew DP, Hirsch AT, et al. Superiority of clopidogrel versus aspirin in patients with prior cardiac surgery. Circulation 2001;103:363–8.
[138] Bhatt DL, Marso SP, Hirsch AT, et al. Amplified benefit of clopidogrel versus aspirin in patients with diabetes mellitus. Am J Cardio 2002;90:625–8.
[139] Yusuf S, Zhao F, Mehta SR, et al. Effects of clopidogrel in addition to aspirin in patients with acute coronary syndromes without ST-segment elevation. N Engl J Med 2001;345:494–502.
[140] Yusuf S, Mehta SR, Zhao F, et al. Early and late effects of clopidogrel in patients with acute coronary syndromes. Circulation 2003;107:966–72.
[141] Hassan AE, Zacharatos H, Suri MF, et al. Drug evaluation of clopidogrel in patients with ischemic stroke. Expert Opin Pharmacother 2007;8:2825–38.
[142] Tantry US, Bliden KP, Gurbel PA. Prasugrel. Expert Opin Investig Drugs 2006;15: 1627–33.
[143] Jakubowski JA, Winters KJ, Naganuma H, et al. Prasugrel: a novel thienopyridine antiplatelet agent. A review of preclinical and clinical studies and the mechanistic basis for its distinct antiplatelet profile. Cardiovasc Res 2007;25:357–74.
[144] Frelinger AL III, Furman MI, Krueger LA, et al. Dissociation of glycoprotein IIb/IIIa antagonists from platelets does not result in fibrinogen binding or platelet aggregation. Circulation 2001;104:1374–9.
[145] Morel O, Ohlmanm P, Bareiss P. Platelet response to aspirin and clopidogrel. Biochemical evaluation, clinical impact, and pharmacological modulation. Arch Mal Coeur Vaiss 2007; 100:992–1002.
[146] Wiviott SD, Trenk D, Frelinger AL, et al. Prasugrel compared with high loading- and maintenance-dose clopidogrel in patients with planned percutaneous coronary intervention: the prasugrel in comparison to clopidogrel for inhibition of platelet activation and aggregation-thrombolysis in myocardial infarction 44 trial. Circulation 2007;116:2923–32.
[147] Wallentin L, Varenhorst C, James S, et al. Prasugrel achieves greater and faster P2Y12receptor-mediated platelet inhibition that clopidogrel due to more efficient generation of its active metabolite in aspirin-treated patients with coronary artery disease. Eur Heart J 2008;29:21–30.
[148] Jakubowski JA, Payne CD, Li YG, et al. A comparison of the antiplatelet effects of prasugrel and high-dose clopidogrel as assessed by VASP-phosphorylation and light transmission aggregometry. Thromb Haemost 2008;99:215–22.
[149] Wiviott SD, Braunwald E, McCabe CH, et al. Prasugrel versus clopidogrel in patients with acute coronary syndromes. N Engl J Med 2007;357:2001–15.
[150] Serbruany V, Midei M, Meilman H, et al. Rebound platelet activation after termination of prasugrel and aspirin therapy due to confirmed non-compliance in patient enrolled in the JUMBO Trial. Int J Clin Pract 2006;60:863–6.
[151] Cannon CP, Husted S, Harrington RA, et al. Safety, tolerability, and initial efficacy of AZD6140, the first reversible oral adenosine diphosphate receptor antagonist, compared with clopidogrel, in patients with non-ST-segment elevation acute coronary syndrome: primary results of the DISPERSE-2 trial. J Am Coll Cardiol 2007;50:1844–51.
[152] Bergamasco B, Benna P, Carolei A, et al. A randomized trial comparing ticlopidine hydrochloride with indobufen for the prevention of stroke in high-risk patients (TISS Study). Ticlopidine Indobufen Stroke Study. Funct Neurol 1997;12:33–43.
[153] Morocutti C, Amabile G, Fattapposta F, et al. Indobufen versus warfarin in the secondary prevention of major vascular events in nonrheumatic atrial fibrillation. SIFA (Studio Italiano Fibrillazione Atriale) investigators. Stroke 1997;28:1015–21.
[154] Lee BK, Lee SW, Park SW, et al. Effects of triple antiplatelet therapy (aspirin, clopidogrel, and cilostazol) on platelet aggregation and P-selection expression in patients undergoing coronary artery stent implantation. Am J Cardiol 2007;100:610–4.
[155] Lee SW, Park SW, Kim YH, et al. Comparison of triple versus dual antiplatelet therapy after drug-eluting stent implantation (from the DECLARE-Long Trial). Am J Cardiol 2007;100:1103–8.

[156] Ahn Y, Jeong MH, Jeong J, et al. Randomized comparison of cilostazol vs clopidogrel after drug-eluting stenting in diabetic patients—cilostazol for diabetic patient win drug-eluting stent (CIDES) trial. Circ J 2008;72:35–9.
[157] Gotoh F, Tohgi H, Hirai S. Cilostazol stroke prevention study: a placebo-controlled double-blind trial for secondary prevention of cerebral infarction. J Stroke Cerebrovasc Dis 2000;9:147–57.
[158] Matias-Guiu J, Ferro JM, Alvarez-Sabín J, et al. Comparison of triflusal and aspirin for prevention of vascular events in patients after cerebral infarction: the TACIP Study: a randomized, double-blind, multicenter trial. Stroke 2003;34:840–8.
[159] Topol EJ, Easton JD, Amarenco P, et al. Design of the blockade of the glycoprotein IIb/IIIa receptor to avoid vascular occlusion (BRAVO) trial. Am Heart J 2000;139:927–33.
[160] Cannon CP, McCabe CH, Wilcox RG, et al. Oral glycoprotein IIb/IIIa inhibition with orbofiban in patients with unstable coronary syndromes (OPUS-TIMI 16) trial. Circulation 2000;102:149–56.
[161] The SYMPHONY investigators comparison of sibrafiban with aspirin for prevention of cardiovascular events after acute coronary syndromes: a randomised trial. Lancet 2000; 355:337–45.
[162] Valencia R, Price MJ, Sawhney N, et al. Efficacy and safety of triple antiplatelet therapy with and without concomitant anticoagulation during elective percutaneous coronary intervention (the REMOVE Trial). Am J Cardiol 2007;100:1099–102.
[163] Johnson SG, Witt DM, Eddy TR, et al. Warfarin and antiplatelet combination use among commercially insured patients enrolled in an anticoagulation management service. Chest 2007;131:1500–7.
[164] Testa L, Zoccai GB, Porto I, et al. Adjusted indirect meta-analysis of aspirin plus warfarin at international normalized ratios 2 to 3 versus aspirin plus clopidogrel after acute coronary syndromes. Am J Cardiol 2007;99:1637–42.
[165] Nguyen M, Lim Y, Walton A, et al. Combining warfarin and antiplatelet therapy after coronary stenting in the global registry of acute coronary events: is it safe and effective to use just one antiplatelet agent? Eur Heart J 2007;28:1717–22.
[166] Khurram Z, Chou E, Minutello R, et al. Combination therapy with aspirin, clopidogrel and warfarin following coronary stenting is associated with a significant risk of bleeding. J Invasive Cardiol 2006;18:162–4.
[167] Delaney JA, Opatrny L, Brophy JM, et al. Drug-drug interactions between antithrombotic medications and the risk of gastrointestinal bleeding. CMAJ 2007;177:347–51.
[168] O'Connor CM, Gattis WA, Hellkamp AS, et al. Comparison of two aspirin doses on ischemic stroke in post-myocardial infarction patients in the warfarin (Coumadin) aspirin reinfarction study (CARS). Am J Cardio 2001;88:541–6.
[169] Pengo V, Palareti G, Cucchini U, et al. Low-intensity oral anticoagulant plus low-dose aspirin during the first six months versus standard-intensity oral anticoagulant therapy after mechanical heart valve replacement: a pilot study of low-intensity warfarin and aspirin in cardiac prostheses (LIWACAP). Clin Appl Thromb Hemost 2007;13:241–8.
[170] Massel D, Little SH. Risks and benefits of adding anti-platelet therapy to warfarin among patients with prosthetic heart valves: a meta-analysis. J Am Coll Cardiol 2001;37:569–78.
[171] Sullivan JM, Harken DE, Gorlin R. Pharmacologic control of thromboembolic complications of cardiac-valve replacement. N Engl J Med 1971;284:1391–4.
[172] Serebruany V, Malinin A, Ziai W, et al. Dipyridamole decreases protease-activated receptor and annexin-V binding on platelets of poststroke patients with aspirin non-responsiveness. Cerebrovasc Dis 2006;21:98–105.
[173] Tijssen JG. Low-dose and high-dose acetylsalicylic acid, with and without dipyridamole: a review of clinical trial results. Neurology 1998;51:S15–6.
[174] Wilterdink J, Easton J. Dipyridamole plus aspirin in cerebrovascular disease. Arch Neurol 1999;56:1087–92.

[175] Sivenius J, Riekkinen PJ, Laakso M, et al. European stroke prevention study (ESPS): antithrombotic therapy is also effective in the elderly. Acta Neurol Scand 1993;87: 111–4.
[176] Albers GW, Amarenco P, Easton JD, et al. Antithrombotic and thrombolytic therapy for ischemic stroke. The seventh ACCP Conference on antithrombotic and thrombolytic therapy. Chest 2004;126:483S–512S.
[177] Diener HC. The PRoFESS trial: future impact on secondary stroke prevention. Expert Rev Neurother 2007;9:1085–91.
[178] Kitahara H, Kobayashi Y, Fujimoto Y, et al. Late stent thrombosis in patients receiving ticlopidine and aspirin after sirolimus-eluting stent implantation. Circ J 2008;72:168–9.
[179] Serebruany V, Malinin A, Atar D. Combination antiplatelet therapy with aspirin and clopidogrel: the role of antecedent and concomitant doses of aspirin. An analysis of 711 patients. Cardiology 2007;107:307–12.
[180] Alstrom U, Tyden H, Oldgren J, et al. The platelet inhibiting effect of a clopidogrel bolus dose in patients on long-term acetylsalicylic acid treatment. Thromb Res 1908; 120:353–9.
[181] Diener H-C, Bogousslavsky J, Brass LM, et al. Aspirin and clopidogrel compared with clopidogrel alone after recent ischaemic stroke or transient ischaemic attack in high-risk patients (MATCH): randomised, double-blind, placebo-controlled trial. Lancet 2006; 364:331–7.
[182] Bhatt DL, Fox KAA, Hacke W, et al. Clopidogrel and aspirin versus aspirin alone for the prevention of atherothrombotic events. N Engl J Med 2006;354:1706–17.
[183] Markus HS, Droste DW, Kaps M, et al. Dual antiplatelet therapy with clopidogrel and aspirin in symptomatic carotid stenosis evaluated using Doppler embolic signal detection. Circulation 2006;111:2233–40.
[184] Bhatt DL, Flather MD, Hacke W, et al. Patients with prior myocardial infarction, stroke, or symptomatic peripheral arterial disease in the CHARISMA trial. J Am Coll Cardiol 2007;49:1982–8.
[185] Cooke GE, Goldschmidt-Clermont PJ. The safety and efficacy of aspirin and clopidogrel as a combination treatment in patients with coronary heart disease. Expert Opin Drug Saf 2006;5:815–26.
[186] Bartorelli AL, Tamburino C, Galassi A, et al. Comparison of two antiplatelet regimens (aspirin alone versus aspirin + ticlopidine or clopidogrel) after intracoronary implantation of a carbofilm-coated stent. Am J Cardiol 2007;99:1062–6.
[187] Fares RR, Lansing LS, Gallati CA, et al. Antiplatelet therapy with clopidogrel and aspirin in vascular diseases: clinical evidence for and against the combination. Expert Opin Pharmacother 2008;9:377–86.
[188] Helton T, Bavry A, Kumbhani D, et al. Incremental effect of clopidogrel on important outcomes in patients with cardiovascular disease: a meta-analysis of randomized trials. Am J Cardiovasc Drugs 2007;7:289–97.
[189] Keller TT, Squizzato A, Middeldorp S. Clopidogrel plus aspirin versus aspirin alone for preventing cardiovascular disease. Cochrane Database Syst Rev 2007;18:CD0051582007.
[190] The ACTIVE writing group on behalf of the ACTIVE, I. Clopidogrel plus aspirin versus oral anticoagulation for atrial fibrillation in the atrial fibrillation clopidogrel trial with Irbesartan for prevention of vascular events (ACTIVE W): a randomised controlled trial. Lancet 2006;367:1903–12.
[191] Hohnloser SH, Pajitnev D, Pogue J, et al. Incidence of stroke in paroxysmal versus sustained atrial fibrillation in patients taking oral anticoagulation or combined antiplatelet therapy: an ACTIVE w substudy. J Am Coll Cardiol 2007;50:2156–61.
[192] Adams RJ, Albers G, Alberts M, et al. Update to the AHA/ASA recommendations for the prevention of stroke in patients with stroke and transient ischemic attack. Stroke 2008;39: 1647–52.

ELSEVIER
SAUNDERS

Neurol Clin 26 (2008) 1079–1097

NEUROLOGIC
CLINICS

Endarterectomy for Symptomatic and Asymptomatic Carotid Stenosis

Peter M. Rothwell, MD, PhD, FRCP, FMedSci

Stroke Prevention Research Unit, University Department of Clinical Neurology, Level 6, West Wing, John Radcliffe Hospital, Headington, Oxford OX3 9DU, United Kingdom

Ipsilateral carotid stenosis of 50% or more is found in approximately 10% of carotid territory ischemic strokes and approximately 15% of transient ischemic attacks (TIAs) and is associated with a high risk of recurrent stroke [1,2]. This article considers the most appropriate use of carotid endarterectomy in recently symptomatic patients and in patients who are found to have an asymptomatic stenosis. Carotid stenting and effective medical treatment are reviewed elsewhere in this issue. Effective medical treatment is essential for several reasons. First, the risk of stroke in the days after the presenting event and before endarterectomy is high [1,2], particularly given the considerable delays to intervention that are often found in routine clinical practice [2]. Second, some patients decline endarterectomy or stenting or have disease that is not amenable to either intervention. Third, all patients with carotid disease are at high risk of stroke and acute ischemic events in other vascular territories.

Recent advances in surgical and anesthetic technique

Carotid endarterectomy (CEA) has been performed for more than 50 years, but the operation continues to evolve. Some recent advances are discussed in the following sections.

Operative technique

During traditional endarterectomy, the plaque is removed via a longitudinal arteriotomy. A plane of endarterectomy (somewhere in the media) is developed proximally, and the intima/media/plaque is transected and the

E-mail address: peter.rothwell@clneuro.ox.ac.uk

doi:10.1016/j.ncl.2008.09.013

plaque removed by extension of the endarterectomy plane until the lesion either feathers off or the intimal step is transected. One particular variation, eversion endarterectomy, which is becoming increasingly popular [3–6], involves first transecting the proximal internal carotid artery (ICA) at the bifurcation. A circumferential plane of endarterectomy is then developed in the distal ICA. The adventitia/residual media is everted and the tube of atheroma expelled as the dissection plane continues. Distal endarterectomy continues until the tube of atheroma feathers off. The distal common carotid artery is endarterectomized in the normal manner, and the bulb of the ICA is re-anastomosed to the bifurcation.

Advocates of eversion endarterectomy cite several advantages, including lower rates of late restenosis, no need to patch the artery, the ability to shorten any redundant segment of ICA to prevent kinking, and a shorter operation time. Disadvantages include the fact that the distal intimal step may not be clearly visualized and intimal flaps may be missed, the inability of the surgeon to insert a shunt until the plaque has been removed, and difficulty of surgery for plaques with distal extension. The main advantages of traditional endarterectomy include the fact that a shunt can be inserted from the outset, the distal intimal step is always visualized, and in the event that the surgeon encounters unexpected distal disease, further mobilization can be performed. Potential disadvantages of traditional endarterectomy include the fact that the procedure takes longer unless the artery is closed primarily, which is probably less preferable than patching (see later discussion), and the fact that traditional endarterectomy almost always produces a degree of functional elongation of the endarterectomy zone, which predisposes to rotation of the bifurcation or kinking of the distal ICA after restoration of flow and may promote early postoperative thrombosis.

A systematic review of five randomized controlled trials (2590 operations) compared eversion and conventional endarterectomy performed either with primary closure or patch angioplasty [5]. There was no significant difference in the rates of perioperative stroke, stroke, or death and local complication rates, but the absolute risks were rather low (risk of stroke or death = 1.7% with eversion versus 2.6% with conventional endarterectomy). Further data are required on the risks of restenosis during long-term follow-up.

Operative patch angioplasty

The reported rate of restenosis after endarterectomy varies enormously, depending mainly methodology and definition [7]. Recurrent atherothrombotic stenosis can occur, but usually not for some years, whereas early restenosis (within a year or so) is more likely to be caused by neointimal hyperplasia [8]. To reduce the risk of restenosis, many surgeons use a patch of autologous vein, or synthetic material, to close the artery and enlarge the lumen. Patching increases the surgery time, and there are potential complications, including rupture, which can cause a life-threatening neck hematoma, and infection if synthetic grafts are used, but a meta-analysis of several small, randomized trials of primary closure, vein patch, or synthetic patch (1127 patients undergoing 1307 operations) [9] showed that patch angioplasty was associated with approximately a 60% reduction in operative risks of stroke or death during the perioperative period ($P = .007$) and long-term follow-up ($P = .004$). Patching also was associated with an 85% reduction in risk of perioperative arterial occlusion ($P = .00004$) and an 80% reduction in risk of restenosis during long-term follow-up in five trials ($P < .00001$). Although the long-term risk of ischemic stroke ipsilateral to the operated artery is low (Fig. 1) [10], because the risks of a second endarterectomy are high [11], prevention of restenosis is important.

Some surgeons who use carotid patching favor using a patch made from an autologous vein, whereas others prefer to use synthetic materials. The most recent meta-analysis of randomized trials of different types of patch included data on 1480 operations [12]. During follow-up for more than 1 year, no difference was shown between the two types of patch for the risk of stroke, death, or arterial restenosis. The number of events was small, however. Based on 15 events in 776 patients in four trials, there were significantly fewer pseudoaneurysms associated with synthetic patches than vein (OR = 0.09, 0.02–0.49), but the clinical significance of this finding is uncertain [12].

Intraoperative shunting

In theory, it should be possible to prevent low cerebral blood flow during carotid clamping—and perhaps an ischemic stroke—by inserting a temporary intraluminal shunt from the common carotid artery to the ICA distal to the operation site. Some surgeons routinely shunt for this reason and

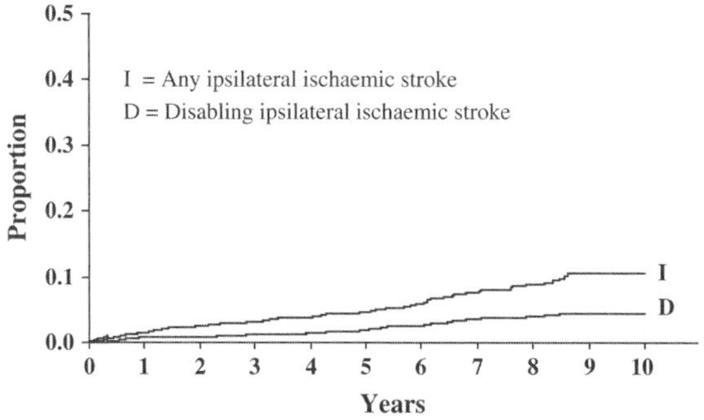

Fig. 1. The risk of stroke more than 30 days after successful carotid endarterectomy for recently symptomatic stenosis in patients randomized to surgery in the European Carotid Surgery Trial. (*Data from* Cunningham E, Bond R, Mehta Z, et al. Long-term durability of carotid endarterectomy in the European Carotid Surgery Trial. Stroke 2002;33:2659.)

to allow more time to teach trainees, but problems arise, including arterial dissection and transmission of emboli from thrombus in the common carotid artery and an increase in the duration of surgery and possibly local operation site complications. A compromise involves selectively shunting only patients likely to develop—or who actually experience—cerebral ischemia as a result of low flow. Efforts to identify patients who need shunting have been inconclusive, however [13,14], and there is considerable variation in routine practice [15]. Unfortunately, randomized trials of different shunting policies have been too small and too few to provide reliable answers [16]. As a result, there is no standard policy for either operative monitoring or use of shunts.

General versus local anesthesia

Surgery traditionally has been performed under general anesthesia (GA) rather than local anesthesia (LA), but surgery under LA is becoming more widespread. With LA, there is a much lower shunt rate because it is immediately obvious when a shunt is needed to restore blood flow distal to the carotid clamps, elaborate intraoperative monitoring is unnecessary, and hospital stays may be shorter. On the other hand, some patients do not tolerate the procedure and a quick change to GA may be required.

A systematic review of seven small randomized trials, involving 554 operations, showed that the use of LA was associated with a borderline statistically significant trend toward a reduced risk of operative death, but it showed no evidence of a reduction in risk of operative stroke [17]. A subsequent further small trial reported data that were also in favor of surgery under LA [18], but a large European multicenter randomized trial (GALA Trial) showed definitively that there is no major difference in operative risk of stroke and death combined. Patients with symptomatic or asymptomatic carotid stenosis from 95 centers in 24 countries were randomly assigned to GA or LA. The primary outcome (stroke, myocardial infarction, or death between randomization and 30 days after surgery) occurred in 84 of 1752 (4.8%) patients allocated GA and 80 of 1771 (4.5%) allocated LA (risk ratio = 0.94, 95% CI 0.70, 1.27). There were also no significant differences between the two treatments for quality of life or length of hospital stay.

Operative risks of carotid endarterectomy

CEA is associated with various potential complications [19,20]. Death within a few days of surgery occurs in approximately 1% to 2% of patients and is generally caused by stroke. Higher rates can be found in administrative data sets, which may be a more realistic reflection of routine practice than large randomized trials, but risk depends on case-mix, particularly the proportion of patients with asymptomatic stenosis who have a lower case fatality [11,21,22]. The reported risk of perioperative stroke ranges from an implausibly low rate of 1% or less to an unacceptably high rate of 10% or more [19,20,23,24]. This variation may be explained by differences in the definition of stroke, whether all strokes are detected, whether the study was prospective or based on retrospective medical record review, variation in case-mix, surgical and anesthetic skills, and publication bias [21]. A useful rule to consider is that no more than 20% of perioperative strokes should be fatal, based on the reliable follow-up from the large randomized controlled trials of surgery for symptomatic stenosis; reports in which a high proportion of operative strokes is fatal have probably undercounted mild strokes.

Most operative strokes are ischemic and ipsilateral to the operated carotid artery, but intracranial hemorrhage accounts for approximately 5% of perioperative strokes [20,25]. Hemorrhage may be caused by the increase in perfusion pressure and cerebral blood flow that occurs after removal of a severe ICA stenosis, particularly if cerebral autoregulation is defective as a consequence of a recent cerebral infarct [25]. Antithrombotic drugs and uncontrolled hypertension also may play a part. Transient cerebral hyperperfusion is common after CEA [26] and occasionally can cause ipsilateral transhemispheric cerebral edema, focal epileptic seizures and headache, and intracerebral hemorrhage.

It has been difficult to sort out whether there is a major systematic difference in operative risk between surgeons, partly because of differences in case-mix and chance effects caused by the inevitably small numbers operated on by each surgeon [27]. Surgeons who perform a high volume of operations might have lower operative risks than those who perform a low volume [28–33], but the data are inconclusive. Myocardial infarction occurs in 1% to 2% of patients during or soon after surgery [20], and cardiac failure, angina, and cardiac dysrhythmias are occasional complications [20,34,35]. Cranial or peripheral nerve injuries result from traction, pressure, or transection and occur in 5% to 20% of cases, depending on how hard one looks. These injuries seldom have any long-term consequences, however [36]. If a simultaneous or staged bilateral CEA is performed, then bilateral vocal cord paralysis or bilateral hypoglossal nerve damage is possible, either of which can cause airway obstruction. It is probably safer to perform the operations a few weeks apart. Local complications include infection, hematoma, and aneurysm formation weeks or years later. (Major hemorrhage caused by leakage or rupture of the arteriotomy or patch is rare but can be life threatening if it causes tracheal compression.)

Predicting operative risk

The operative risk of stroke and death depends on patient age and sex, the nature of the presenting event, and coexisting pathology. In a systematic review of 103 studies that stratified the risk of stroke and death caused by endartectomy by the nature of the presenting symptoms, the operative risk for symptomatic stenosis overall was higher than for asymptomatic stenosis (OR = 1.62, 95% CI = 1.45–1.81, $P < .00001$, 59 studies) but depended on the nature of the symptoms (Table 1) [11]. The operative risk in patients with ocular events only, for example, tended to be lower than that for asymptomatic stenosis (OR = 0.75, 0.50–1.14, 15 studies). Operative risk was the same for stroke and cerebral TIA (OR = 1.16, 0.99–1.35, $P = .08$, 23 studies) but higher for cerebral TIA than for ocular events only (OR = 2.31, 1.72–3.12, $P < .00001$, 19 studies).

In the randomized trials of CEA for symptomatic and asymptomatic carotid stenosis, benefit was decreased in women [37,38], partly because of a higher operative risk than in men, whereas operative risk in the trials was independent of age. In a systematic review of all publications reporting data on the association between age and/or sex and procedural risk of stroke and/or death from 1980–2004 [39], women had a higher rate of operative stroke and death (25 studies, OR = 1.31, 1.17–1.47, $P < .001$) than men but no increase in operative mortality (15 studies, 1.05, 0.81–0.86, $P = .78$).

The effects of increasing age on operative morbidity and mortality tend to be overestimated by clinicians. Compared with younger patients, operative mortality was increased at 75 years or older (20 studies, OR = 1.36, 1.07–1.68, $P = .02$) and at 80 years or older (15 studies, OR = 1.80, 1.26–2.45, $P < .001$) in the systematic review [39]. Operative risk of nonfatal stroke alone was not increased, however, and so the overall perioperative risk of stroke and death was only slightly increased at 75 years or older (21 studies, OR = 1.18, 0.94–1.44, $P = .06$) and at 80 years or older (10 studies, OR = 1.14, 0.92–1.36, $P = .34$). Operative risk of stroke is increased in women, and operative mortality—but not the risk of stroke—is increased in patients aged 75 years or more [39].

Only a few serious attempts have been made to sort out which other patient-related factors affect perioperative stroke risk. Risk factors almost

Table 1
The results of a systematic review of the studies reporting the operative risks of stroke or death due to carotid endarterectomy according to the nature of the presenting event

Presenting event	Number of studies	Number of operations	Absolute risk % & (95% CI)	$P_{heterogeneity}$
Symptomatic	95	36,482	5.1 (4.6–5.6)	< 0.001
Urgent	12	208	19.2 (10.7–27.8)	< 0.001
Stroke	50	7634	7.1 (6.1–8.1)	< 0.001
Cerebral TIA	24	8138	5.5 (4.7–6.3)	< 0.001
Ocular event	18	1784	2.8 (2.2–3.4)	< 0.001
Nonspecific	24	1751	4.2 (3.2–5.2)	< 0.001
Asymptomatic	60	14,399	2.8 (2.4–3.2)	< 0.001
Redo surgery	12	914	4.4 (2.4–6.4)	< 0.001

Data from Bond R, Rerkasem K, Rothwell PM. A systematic review of the risks of carotid endarterectomy in relation to the clinical indication and the timing of surgery. Stroke 2003;34:2293.

certainly include hypertension, peripheral vascular disease, contralateral ICA occlusion, and stenosis of the ipsilateral external carotid artery and carotid siphon [40]. The independent surgical risk factors for patients in the pooled analysis of data from European Carotid Surgery Trial (ECST) and the North American Symptomatic Carotid Endarterectomy Trial (NASCET) were female sex, presenting event diabetes, ulcerated plaque, and previous stroke [38]. Other predictors in the ECST that were not available from NASCET included systolic blood pressure and peripheral vascular disease [20].

Operative risk in relation to the timing of surgery

The optimal timing of surgery in patients with recently symptomatic stenosis has been controversial [41,42], but it is increasingly clear that surgery should be performed as soon as possible, given the high early risk of stroke during the first few days and weeks after the presenting TIA or stroke in patients with symptomatic carotid stenosis [1,2]. There has been concern that the operative risk may be increased if surgery is performed too early, particularly in patients with major cerebral infarction or stroke-in-evolution, but any increased operative risk caused by early surgery in stable patients with TIA or minor stroke is likely to be small and must be balanced against the substantial risk of stroke occurring before delayed surgery [2,43]. The pooled analyses of data from the randomized trials of endarterectomy for symptomatic carotid stenosis showed that benefit from surgery was greatest in patients randomized within 2 weeks after their last ischemic event and fell rapidly with increasing delay [38]. This trend was partly caused by the fact that the operative risk of endarterectomy was not increased in patients who underwent operation early—at least as close as 3 to 7 days after their last event [38,44].

A systematic review of all published surgical case series that reported data on operative risk by time since presenting event [11,45] also found no difference between early (first 3–4 weeks) and later surgery in stable patients (OR = 1.13, 0.79–1.62, $P = .62$, 11 studies). Emergency endarterectomy for patients with evolving symptoms (stroke-in-evolution, crescendo TIA, urgent cases) did have a higher operative risk of stroke and death (19.2%, 10.7–27.8) (Table 1) than surgery in patients with stable symptoms in the same studies, however (OR = 3.9, 2.7–5.7, $P < .001$, 13 studies). Some uncertainty exists in relation to the balance of risk and benefit of surgery within 24 to 72 hours of the presenting event, particularly in patients with minor stroke. A randomized trial of early versus delayed surgery during this time period would be ethical [45–47]. Delays to surgery in routine clinical practice in many countries currently can be measured in months, however [2,48–50], and so the question of "by how many hours should surgery be delayed" is of somewhat theoretic interest.

Who should have endarterectomy for recently symptomatic carotid stenosis?

The most reliable data on how the overall effect of endarterecomy relates to the degree of carotid stenosis come from a pooled analysis of data from the three largest randomized controlled trials of surgery for symptomatic carotid stenosis [51]. The overall operative mortality was 1.1% (95% CI 0.8–1.5) and the operative risk of stroke and death was 7.1% (95% CI 6.3–8.1), and both operative risks were independent of the degree of carotid stenosis. Based on the method of measurement of angiographic degree of stenosis used in the NASCET [52], endarterectomy reduced the 5-year absolute risk of any stroke or death in patients with 50% to 69% stenosis (absolute risk reduction [ARR] = 7.8%, 95% CI 3.1–12.5) and was highly beneficial in patients with 70% to 99% stenosis (ARR = 15.3%, 95% CI 9.8–20.7) but was of no benefit in patients with near occlusion. Qualitatively similar results were seen for disabling stroke.

With the exception of near occlusions, the degree of stenosis above which surgery is beneficial is 50% (equivalent to approximately 65% stenosis by the method of measurement used in the ECST [53]). The confidence intervals around the estimates of treatment effect in the near occlusions in the pooled analysis were wide, but the difference in the effect of surgery between this group and patients with 70% or more stenosis without near occlusion was highly statistically significant for each of the outcomes [51]. Some patients with near occlusion still may wish to undergo surgery, particularly if they experience recurrent TIAs. In the ECST [54], endarterectomy did reduce the risk of recurrent TIA in patients with near occlusion (ARR = 15%, P = .007). More work is required to assess the accuracy of noninvasive methods of carotid imaging in detecting near occlusion [55].

The degree of stenosis is a major determinant of benefit from endarterectomy, but several other clinical and angiographic characteristics might influence the risks and benefits of surgery. Subgroup analyses of pooled data from the large trials identified several clinically important interactions [38]. Sex (P = .003), age (P = .03), and time from the last symptomatic event to randomization (P = .009) each modified the effectiveness of surgery. Benefit from surgery was greatest in men, patients aged 75 years or older, and patients randomized within 2 weeks after their last ischemic event. For patients with 50% or more stenosis, the number needed to undergo surgery to prevent one ipsilateral stroke in 5 years was 9 for men versus 36 for women, 5 for age 75 or older versus 18 for younger than 65 years, and 5 for patients randomized within 2 weeks after their last ischemic event versus 125 for patients randomized more than 12 weeks. These observations were consistent across the 50% to 69% and 70% or more stenosis groups; similar trends were present in ECST and NASCET.

Women had a lower risk of ipsilateral ischemic stroke on medical treatment and a higher operative risk in comparison to men [38]. Surgery was clearly beneficial in women with 70% or more stenosis but not in women with 50% to 69% stenosis. In contrast, surgery reduced the 5-year absolute risk of stroke by 8% (3.4–12.5) in men with 50% to 69% stenosis. This sex difference was statistically significant even when the analysis of the interaction was confined to the 50% to 69% stenosis group. These same patterns were also shown in both of the large published trials of endarterectomy for asymptomatic carotid stenosis (see later discussion).

Benefit from endarterectomy increased with age in the pooled analysis of trials in patients with recently symptomatic stenosis, particularly in patients older than 75 years, mainly because of their high risk of stroke on medical treatment. Because there is no increase in the operative risk of stroke and death in patients older than 75 years operated outside the trials and only a small increase in operative mortality at 85 years or older [39], there is no justification for withholding treatment in older patients who are fit to undergo surgery. Benefit from surgery is probably also greatest in patients with stroke, intermediate in patients with cerebral TIA, and lowest in patients with retinal events [38]. There was also a trend in the trials toward greater benefit in patients with irregular plaque than smooth plaque [38].

The risk of stroke on medical treatment after a TIA or minor stroke in patients with carotid stenosis falls rapidly with time [38,56], possibly because of the "healing" of the unstable atheromatous plaque or an increase in collateral blood flow to the symptomatic hemisphere. The pooled analysis of data from the trials showed that benefit from endarterectomy was greatest in patients randomized within 2 weeks of their last event (Fig. 2), particularly in patients with 50% to 69% stenosis, whereas the reduction in the 5-year risk of stroke with surgery was considerable in patients who were randomized within 2 weeks of their last event (14.8%, 95% CI 6.2–23.4) but minimal in patients randomized later [38,44].

Effective prevention of stroke with endarterectomy or stenting is undermined in many health care systems by delays in investigation and intervention. For example, in a study of all patients undergoing carotid imaging for TIA or stroke in Oxfordshire, United Kingdom, during 2003 to 2004, 85 patients were found to have 50% to 99% symptomatic stenosis, of whom 49 had endarterectomy, but in only 3 patients (6%) was surgery performed within 2 weeks of their presenting event and only 21 (43%) had surgery within 12 weeks [2]. The reported risk of recurrent stroke before surgery in patients who would have been suitable for endarterectomy was approximately 20% during the 2 weeks after their presenting event. Other studies also underscored the high risk of stroke if endarterectomy is delayed [46].

The subgroup observations are of some help in clinical practice, but individual patients frequently have several important risk factors, each of which interact in a way that cannot be described using univariate subgroup analysis alone. One way in which clinicians can weigh the often-conflicting effects of the important characteristics of an individual patient on the likely benefit from treatment is to base decisions on the predicted absolute risks of a poor outcome with each treatment option using prognostic models [57].

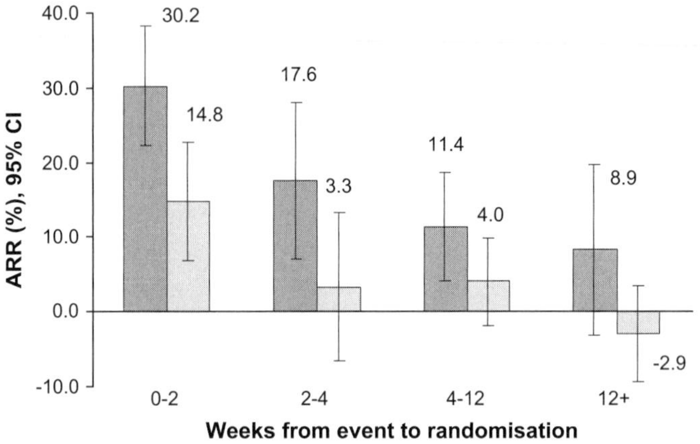

Fig. 2. Pooled analysis of data from randomized controlled trials of endarterectomy for symptomatic carotid stenosis shows the absolute reduction with surgery in the 5-year risk of ipsilateral carotid territory ischemic stroke and any stroke or death within 30 days after trial surgery in patients with 50% to 69% stenosis and 70% or more stenosis without near-occlusion stratified by the time from last symptomatic event to randomization. The numbers above the bars indicate the actual absolute risk reduction. ARR, absolute risk reduction. (*Data from* Rothwell PM, Eliasziw M, Gutnikov SA, et al, for the Carotid Endarterectomy Trialists Collaboration. Effect of endarterectomy for symptomatic carotid stenosis in relation to clinical subgroups and to the timing of surgery. Lancet 2004;363:923.)

A model for prediction of the risk of stroke on medical treatment in patients with recently symptomatic carotid stenosis was derived from the ECST (Table 2) [58,59]. The model (available at www.stroke.ox.ac.uk) was validated using data from NASCET and showed good agreement between predicted and observed medical risk ($P < .0001$) [59], reliably distinguishing between individuals with a 10% risk of ipsilateral ischemic stroke after 5 years follow-up and individuals with a risk of over 40% (Fig. 3). Importantly, the operative risk of stroke and death in patients who were randomized to surgery in NASCET was unrelated to the medical risk ($P = .32$). When the operative risk and the small additional residual risk of stroke after successful endarterectomy were taken into account, benefit from endarterectomy at 5 years varied significantly across the quintiles ($P = .001$) [59], with no benefit in patients in the lower three quintiles of predicted medical risk (ARR = 0–2%), moderate benefit in the fourth quintile (ARR = 10.8%, 95% CI 1.0–20.6), and substantial benefit in the highest quintile (ARR = 32%, 95% CI 21.9–42.1).

As an alternative to the computer model, color-coded risk tables allow a relatively small number of important variables to be considered and have the major advantage that they do not require the calculation of any score by the clinician or patient. A risk table for the 5-year risk of ipsilateral ischemic stroke in patients with recently symptomatic carotid stenosis on medical treatment has been derived from the ECST model [59] (also

Table 2
A multivariate analysis of predictors of ipsilateral ischemic stroke within 5 years in patients with recently symptomatic carotid stenosis randomized to medical treatment only in the European Carotid Surgery Trial

Risk factor	Hazard ratio (95% CI)	*P* value
Degree of stenosis (per 10%)	1.18 (1.10, 1.25)	< 0.0001
Near occlusion	0.49 (0.19, 1.24)	0.1309
Male sex	1.19 (0.81, 1.75)	0.3687
Age (per 10 years)	1.12 (0.89, 1.39)	0.3343
Time since last event (per 7 days)	0.96 (0.93, 0.99)	0.0039
Presenting event		
Ocular	1.00	—
Single TIA	1.41 (0.75, 2.66)	—
Multiple TIAs	2.05 (1.16, 3.60)	0.0067
Minor stroke	1.82 (0.99, 3.34)	—
Major stroke	2.54 (1.48, 4.35)	—
Diabetes	1.35 (0.86, 2.11)	0.1881
Previous myocardial infarction	1.57 (1.01, 2.45)	0.0471
Peripheral vascular disease	1.18 (0.78, 1.77)	0.4368
Treated hypertension	1.24 (0.88, 1.75)	0.2137
Irregular/ulcerated plaque	2.03 (1.31, 3.14)	0.0015

Data from Rothwell PM, Warlow CP, on behalf of the ECST Collaborators. Prediction of benefit from carotid endarterectomy in individual patients: a risk-modelling study. Lancet 1999;353:2105–10; and Rothwell PM, Z Mehta, Howard SC, et al. From subgroups to individuals: general principles and the example of carotid endartectomy. Lancet 2005;365;262.

available at www.stroke.ox.ac.uk). The table is based on the five variables that were significant predictors of risk in the ECST model and yielded clinically important subgroup treatment effect interactions in the analysis of pooled data from the relevant trials (sex, age, time since last symptomatic event, type of presenting event, and carotid plaque surface morphology). One potential problem with the ECST risk model is that it might overestimate risk in current patients because of improvements in medical treatment, such as the increased use of statins. Such improvements in treatment pose more problems for interpretation of the overall trial results than for the risk-modeling approach, however. For example, it would take only a relatively modest improvement in the effectiveness of medical treatment to erode the overall benefit of endarterectomy in patients with 50% to 69% stenosis. In contrast, major improvements in medical treatment would be required to significantly reduce the benefit from surgery in patients in the high predicted-risk quintile in Fig. 3.

Carotid endarterectomy for asymptomatic stenosis

The issue of endarterectomy for asymptomatic carotid stenosis arises when patients undergo imaging for some other indication—often a TIA or stroke in another arterial territory or before major surgery—or when

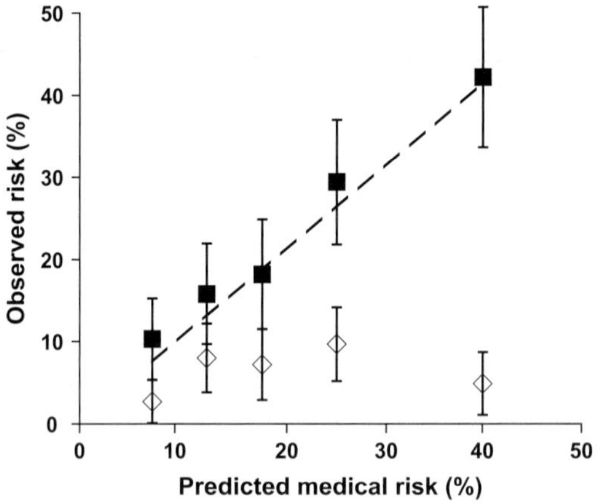

Fig. 3. Validation of the ECST model (see Table 1) for the 5-year risk of stroke on medical treatment in patients with 50% to 99% stenosis in NASCET. Predicted medical risk is plotted against observed risk of stroke in patients randomized to medial treatment in NASCET (*squares*) and against the observed operative risk of stroke and death in patients randomized to surgical treatment (*diamonds*). Groups are quintiles of predicted risk. Error bars represent 95% confidence intervals. (*Data from* Rothwell PM, Mehta Z, Howard SC, et al. From subgroups to individuals: general principles and the example of carotid endartectomy. Lancet 2005;365:259.)

a stenosis is found on screening. Guidelines on endarterectomy for asymptomatic stenosis are based on the results of the Asymptomatic Carotid Atherosclerosis Study (ACAS) [60], the Medical Research Council Asymptomatic Carotid Surgery Trial (ACST) [61], and a few previous smaller trials [62]. ACAS reported a 47% relative reduction in the risk of ipsilateral stroke and perioperative death in patients randomized to surgery despite a 5-year risk of ipsilateral stroke without the operation of only 11%. Although the number of endarterectomies performed for asymptomatic carotid stenosis in the United States each year subsequently increased to nearly 100,000 [63], in many other countries the finding in ACAS that 40 operations were needed to prevent one disabling or fatal stroke after 5 years was not felt to justify surgery, and rates remained low [48].

There was particular concern that the low operative risks in ACAS could not be matched in routine clinical practice. ACAS only accepted surgeons with an excellent safety record, rejecting 40% of initial applicants and subsequently barring from further participation some surgeons who had adverse operative outcomes during the trial [64]. A review compared the operative risks in ACAS with the results of a meta-analysis of the 46 surgical case series that published operative risks for asymptomatic stenosis during ACAS and the 5 years after publication [33]. Operative mortality was eight times higher than in ACAS (1.11% versus 0.14%, $P = .01$), and the risk of stroke and death was approximately three times higher among comparable studies in which outcome was assessed by a neurologist (4.3% versus 1.5%, $P < .001$).

The more pragmatic ACST probably produced more widely generalizable results [61]. Between 1993 and 2003, ACST randomized 3120 patients with more than 60% mainly asymptomatic carotid stenosis (12% had symptoms at least 6 months previously) to immediate endarterectomy plus medical treatment versus medical treatment alone or until the operation became necessary. Surgeons were required to provide evidence of an operative risk of 6% or less for their last 50 patients having an endarterectomy for asymptomatic stenosis, but none was excluded on the basis of his or her operative risk during the trial. Selection of patients was based on the "uncertainty principle," with few exclusion criteria. Stenosis was assessed by Doppler ultrasonography without central evaluation of the ultrasonographer's training or a centralized audit of his or her performance [65].

Despite the differences in methods of ACST and ACAS, the absolute reductions in 5-year risk of stroke with surgery were not different (5.3%, 95% CI 3%–7.8% versus 5.1%, 95% CI 0.9%–9.1%, respectively). Whereas ACAS reported only a nonsignificant 2.7% reduction ($P = .26$) in the absolute risk of disabling or fatal stroke with surgery, ACST reported a significant 2.5% (95% CI 0.8%–4.3%, $P = .004$) absolute reduction, although the number needed to undergo surgery to prevent one disabling or fatal stroke after 5 years remains approximately 40. The main differences between the trials were in the 30-day operative risks of death (0.14%, 95% CI 0–0.4% in ACAS versus 1.11%, 95% CI 0.6%–1.8% in ACST; $P = .02$) and in the combined operative risk of stroke and death (1.5%, 95% CI 0.6%–2.4% in ACAS versus 3%, 95% CI 2.1%–4.0% in ACST; $P = .04$). The operative risks in ACST were similar to risks reported in the recent systematic review of surgical case series [66] and risks reported after community-wide performance measurement and feedback in a study of data from 10 US states (1% mortality and 3.8% stroke and death) [67].

Neither ACST nor ACAS showed increasing benefit from surgery with increasing degree of stenosis within the 60% to 99% range [60,61], for which there are several potential reasons. First, ultrasound may be less accurate than catheter angiography in measuring the degree of stenosis. In ACAS, only patients randomized to surgery underwent catheter angiography, and in ACST all imaging was by Doppler ultrasound without any centralized audit [65]. The importance of the precise methods used to measure stenosis was highlighted in a study of patients randomized to the medical arm of the ECST, which demonstrated that angiographic measures of stenosis were most reliable in predicting recurrent stroke when selective carotid contrast injections were given, biplane views were available, and the mean of measurements made by two independent observers was used [68].

The second reason is that patients with carotid near-occlusion, which is not readily detectable on ultrasound, were not identified in the randomized trials of CEA for asymptomatic stenosis. In the ECST, for example, the proportion of near-occlusions was 0.6% at 60% to 69% stenosis, 2.3% at 70% to 79% stenosis, 9.2% at 80% to 89% stenosis, and 29.5% at 90% to 99% stenosis [69]. Only when near-occlusions were removed was the increased benefit of CEA with increasing stenosis between 70% and 99% clearly apparent. This issue is further complicated by the findings of recent study of 1115 patients with asymptomatic stenosis [70], in whom increasing stenosis on ultrasound was positively associated with risk of ipsilateral hemispheric ischemic events at mean 38 months' follow-up when stenosis was measured using ECST criteria but not when NASCET criteria were used.

The third reason is that the rate of stenosis progression may determine the risk of stroke in patients with asymptomatic stenosis [71]. This finding is potentially important considering the longer time frame over which strokes occur in patients with asymptomatic versus symptomatic stenosis. In the ECST, a strong association between the risk of ipsilateral stroke and the degree of carotid stenosis was only seen for strokes that occurred during the first year after randomization, and no relationship was seen between initial stenosis and strokes occurring more than 2 years later [53,56]. Although this finding could be partly caused by plaque "healing," it is conceivable that in some patients the degree of stenosis had progressed and the rate of this progression rather than the degree of stenosis at baseline was the important determinant of stroke risk.

Although some subgroup analyses were reported in ACAS, the trial had insufficient power to reliably analyze subgroup treatment effect interactions. Because of its larger sample size, ACST had greater power to evaluate subgroups, although no analyses were prespecified in the trial protocol [65]. ACST did perform some subgroup analyses but only reported results for the reduction in risk of non-perioperative stroke (ie, the benefit) and the perioperative risk (ie, the harm) separately [61]. The overall balance of hazard and benefit, which is of most importance to patients and clinicians, was not reported, although the data could be extracted from the Web tables that accompanied the ACST report [61]. ACAS reported a statistically borderline sex/treatment effect interaction, with reduced benefit from endarterecotmy in women [60]. The same trend was seen in ACST. A meta-analysis of the effect of endarterectomy on the 5-year risk of any stroke and perioperative death in ACAS and ACST (Fig. 4) [37] showed that benefit from surgery was greater in men than in women (pooled interaction $P = .01$). It remained uncertain whether there is any worthwhile benefit in women at 5 years' follow-up. Ten-year follow-up data, which are currently available from ACST, show that the small overall benefit seen at 5-year follow-up is maintained (10-year risk of any stroke including perioperative events = 18.3% with deferred surgery versus 14% with immediate surgery), but there is still little evidence of benefit in women. It is also worth noting that the overall 10-year benefit in men and women combined was limited for disabling or fatal stroke (10.1% with deferred surgery versus 8.6% with immediate surgery).

Subgroup	Events/Patients Surgical	Medical	OR	95% CI
Males				
ACST	51 /1021	97 /1023	0.50	0.35-0.72
ACAS	18 /544	38 /547	0.46	0.26-0.81
TOTAL	69 /1565	135 /1570	0.49	0.36-0.66
Females				
ACST	31 /539	34 /537	0.90	0.55-1.49
ACAS	15 /281	14 /287	1.10	0.52-1.82
TOTAL	46 /820	48 /824	0.96	0.63-1.45

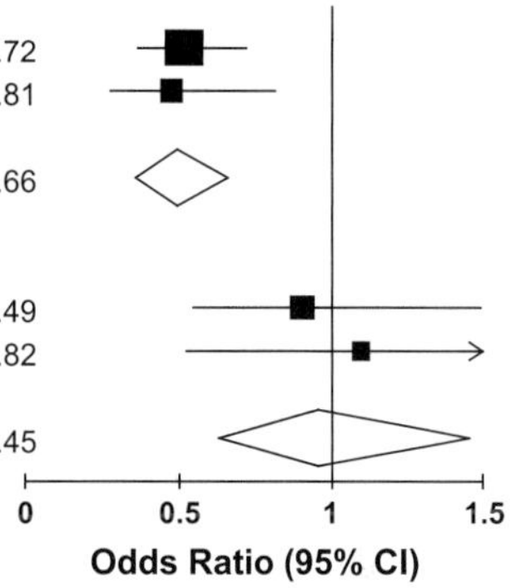

Fig. 4. The effect of carotid endarterectomy for asymptomatic stenosis on the risk of any stroke or operative death in the Asymptomatic Carotid Surgery Trial (ACST) and the Asymptomatic Carotid Atherosclerosis Study (ACAS) with results stratified by sex. (*Data from* Rothwell PM. ACST: which subgroups will benefit most from carotid endarterectomy? Lancet 2004;364:1123.)

Another subgroup of frequent clinical interest includes patients with asymptomatic stenosis and a contralateral carotid occlusion. A post-hoc subgroup analysis from ACAS found that patients with contralateral occlusion derived no long-term benefit from endarterectomy, largely because of a lower long-term risk on medical treatment [72], but this analysis was underpowered (163 patients) and there was no significant heterogeneity of benefit from surgery according to presence of contralateral occlusion in ACST [61].

Given the small absolute reductions in the risk of stroke with endarterectomy that were observed in ACST and ACAS, there is a need to identify which individual patients are at highest risk of stroke and which individuals are at such low risk of stroke that the risks of surgery cannot be justified. A similar risk-modeling approach to that used in symptomatic patients is required. Advances in other techniques, such as noninvasive imaging of plaque morphology and inflammation and the detection of microembolic signals, may help to risk stratify patients, but convincing data on clinical usefulness are lacking [73].

The need to target surgery for asymptomatic stenosis only at individuals at high risk of stroke without surgery is also highlighted by advances in medical treatment. Most patients in ACAS and ACST were not on what would currently be regarded as optimal medical treatment, and experts have argued that the results of these trials might no longer apply to current practice given the recent advances in medical treatment [74–76]. Although better medical treatment is unlikely to offset the large absolute benefit of early surgery for symptomatic carotid stenosis, the modest and gradually accruing benefits of endarterectomy for asymptomatic carotid stenosis might be reduced with the use of statins and other preventive treatments. In ACST, for example, most of the benefit from endarterectomy was confined to the 828 patients with a pre-randomization cholesterol levels of 6.5 mmol/L or more [61].

Summary

Recent research has helped to identify which patients are likely to benefit most from CEA and when the intervention is most effective in patients with symptomatic stenosis. Individual risk modeling is useful in selecting patients for endarterectomy for symptomatic stenosis, although timely surgery and optimal medical treatment are of equal importance. Long-term benefit from endarterectomy for asymptomatic carotid stenosis is limited, and further research is required to identify individuals with asymptomatic stenosis who have the most to gain from surgery.

References

[1] Lovett JK, Coull A, Rothwell PM, et al. Early risk of recurrent stroke by aetiological subtype: implications for stroke prevention. Neurology 2004;62:569–74.
[2] Fairhead JF, Mehta Z, Rothwell PM. Population-based study of delays in carotid imaging and surgery and the risk of recurrent stroke. Neurology 2005;65:371–5.
[3] Darling RC, Paty PSK, Shah DM, et al. Eversion endarterectomy of the internal carotid artery: technique and results in 449 procedures. Surgery 1996;120:635–9.
[4] Cao P, Giordano G, De Rango P, et al, Collaborators of the EVEREST Study Group. A randomised study on eversion versus standard carotid endarterectomy: study design and preliminary results: the Everest Trial. J Vasc Surg 1998;27:595–605.
[5] Cao P, De Rango P, Cieri E, et al. Eversion versus conventional endarterectomy. Semin Vasc Surg 2004;17:236–42.
[6] Brothers TE. Initial experience with eversion carotid endarterectomy: absence of a learning curve for the first 100 patients. J Vasc Surg 2005;42:429–34.
[7] Frericks H, Kievit J, van Baalen JM, et al. Carotid recurrent stenosis and risk of ipsilateral stroke: a systematic review of the literature. Stroke 1998;29:244–50.
[8] Hunter GC, Palmaz JC, Hayashi HH, et al. The aetiology of symptoms in patients with recurrent carotid stenosis. Arch Surg 1987;122:311–5.
[9] Bond R, Rerkasem K, Rothwell PM. Patch angioplasty versus primary closure for carotid endarterectomy. Cochrane Database Syst Rev 2004;2:CD000160.
[10] Cunningham E, Bond R, Mehta Z, et al. Long-term durability of carotid endarterectomy in the European Carotid Surgery Trial. Stroke 2002;33:2658–63.
[11] Bond R, Rerkasem K, Rothwell PM. A systematic review of the risks of carotid endarterectomy in relation to the clinical indication and the timing of surgery. Stroke 2003;34:2290–301.
[12] Bond R, Rerkasem K, Naylor R, et al. Patches of different types for carotid patch angioplasty. Cochrane Database Syst Rev 2004;2:CD000071.
[13] Naylor AR, Bell PRF, Ruckley CV. Monitoring and cerebral protection during carotid endarterectomy. Br J Surg 1992;79:735–41.

[14] Belardi P, Lucertini G, Ermirio D. Stump pressure and transcranial Doppler for predicting shunting in carotid endarterectomy. Eur J Vasc Endovasc Surg 2003;25:164–7.

[15] Bond R, Warlow CP, Naylor R, et al. Variation in surgical and anaesthetic technique and associations with operative risk in the European Carotid Surgery Trial: implications for trials of ancillary techniques. Eur J Vasc Endovasc Surg 2002;23:117–26.

[16] Bond R, Rerkasem K, Rothwell PM. Routine or selective carotid artery shunting for carotid endarterectomy. Cochrane Database Syst Rev 2002;2:CD000190.

[17] Rerkasem K, Bond R, Rothwell PM. Local versus general anaesthetic for carotid endarterectomy. Cochrane Database Syst Rev 2004;2:CD000126.

[18] Kasprzak PM, Altmeppen J, Angerer M, et al. General versus locoregional anesthesia in carotid surgery: a prospective randomised trial. VASA 2006;35:232–8.

[19] Naylor AR, Ruckley CV. Complications after carotid surgery. In: Campbell B, editor. Complications in arterial surgery: a practical approach to management. Oxford: Butterworth-Heinemann; 1996. p. 73–88.

[20] Bond R, Narayan S, Rothwell PM, et al. Clinical and radiological risk factors for operative stroke and death in the European Carotid Surgery Trial. Eur J Vasc Endovasc Surg 2002;23:108–16.

[21] Rothwell PM, Slattery J, Warlow CP. A systematic review of the risk of stroke and death due to endarterectomy for symptomatic carotid stenosis. Stroke 1996;27:260–5.

[22] Wennberg DE, Lucas FL, Birkmeyer JD, et al. Variation in carotid endarterectomy mortality in the medicare population: trial hospitals, volume, and patient characteristics. JAMA 1998;279:1278–81.

[23] Ferguson GG, Eliasziw M, Barr HWK, et al, for the North American Symptomatic Carotid Endarterectomy Trial (NASCET) Collaborators. The North American Symptomatic Carotid Endarterectomy Trial: surgical results in 1415 patients. Stroke 1999;30:1751–8.

[24] Bond R, Rerkasem K, Shearman CP, et al. Time trends in the published risks of stroke and death due to endarterectomy for symptomatic carotid stenosis. Cerebrovasc Dis 2004;18: 37–46.

[25] Ouriel K, Shortell CK, Illig KA, et al. Intracerebral haemorrhage after carotid endarterectomy: incidence, contribution to neurologic morbidity, and predictive factors. J Vasc Surg 1999;29:82–9.

[26] Adhiyaman V, Alexander S. Cerebral hyperperfusion syndrome following carotid endarterectomy. QJM 2007 Feb 16 [Epub ahead of print].

[27] Rothwell PM, Warlow CP, on behalf of the European Carotid Surgery Trialists' Collaborative Group. Interpretation of operative risks of individual surgeons. Lancet 1999;353:1325.

[28] Kucey DS, Bowyer B, Iron K, et al. Determinants of outcome after carotid endarterectomy. J Vasc Surg 1998;28:1051–8.

[29] Killeen SD, Andrews EJ, Redmond HP, et al. Provider volume and outcomes for abdominal aortic aneurysm repair, carotid endarterectomy, and lower extremity revascularization procedures. J Vasc Surg 2007;45:615–26.

[30] Wong JH, Findlay JM, Suarez-Almazor ME. Regional performance of carotid endarterectomy appropriateness, outcomes, and risk factors for complications. Stroke 1997;28:891–8.

[31] Naylor AR, Hayes PD, Allroggen H, et al. Reducing the risk of carotid surgery: a 7-year audit of the role of monitoring and quality control assessment. J Vasc Surg 2000;32:750–9.

[32] Brittenden J, Bradbury AW. Are we still performing inappropriate carotid endarterectomy? Eur J Vasc Endovasc Surg 2000;20:158–62.

[33] Rothwell PM, Slattery J, Warlow CP. A systematic comparison of the risks of stroke and death due to carotid endarterectomy for symptomatic and asymptomatic stenosis. Stroke 1996;27:266–9.

[34] Urbinati S, di Pasquale G, Andreoli A, et al. Preoperative noninvasive coronary risk stratification in candidates for carotid endarterectomy. Stroke 1994;25:2022–7.

[35] Paciaroni M, Eliasziw M, Kappelle LJ, et al, for the North American Symptomatic Carotid Endarterectomy Trial (NASCET) Collaborators. Medical complications associated with carotid endarterectomy. Stroke 1999;30:1759–63.

[36] Cunningham EJ, Bond R, Mayberg MR, et al. Risk of persistent cranial nerve injury after carotid endarterectomy. J Neurosurg 2004;101:455–8.
[37] Rothwell PM. ACST: which subgroups will benefit most from carotid endarterectomy? Lancet 2004;364:1122–3.
[38] Rothwell PM, Eliasziw M, Gutnikov SA, et al, for the Carotid Endarterectomy Trialists Collaboration. Effect of endarterectomy for symptomatic carotid stenosis in relation to clinical subgroups and to the timing of surgery. Lancet 2004;363:915–24.
[39] Bond R, Rerkasem K, Cuffe R, et al. A systematic review of the associations between age and sex and the operative risks of carotid endarterectomy. Cerebrovasc Dis 2005;20:69–77.
[40] Rothwell PM, Slattery J, Warlow CP. Clinical and angiographic predictors of stroke and death from carotid endarterectomy: systematic review. Br Med J 1997;315:1571–7.
[41] Pritz MB. Timing of carotid endarterectomy after stroke. Stroke 1997;28:2563–7.
[42] Eckstein H, Schumacher H, Klemm K, et al. Emergency carotid endarterectomy. Cerebrovasc Dis 1999;9:270–81.
[43] Blaser T, Hofmann K, Buerger T, et al. Risk of stroke, transient ischaemic attack, and vessel occlusion before endarterectomy in patients with symptomatic severe carotid stenosis. Stroke 2002;33:1057–62.
[44] Rothwell PM, Gutnikov SA, Eliasziw M, et al. Sex difference in effect of time from symptoms to surgery on benefit from endarterectomy for transient ischaemic attack and non-disabling stroke. Stroke 2004;35:2855–61.
[45] Fairhead JF, Rothwell PM. The need for urgency in identification and treatment of symptomatic carotid stenosis is already established. Cerebrovasc Dis 2005;19:355–8.
[46] Rantner B, Pavelka M, Posch L, et al. Carotid endarterectomy after ischemic stroke: is there a justification for delayed surgery? Eur J Vasc Endovasc Surg 2005;30:36–40.
[47] Welsh S, Mead G, Chant H, et al. Early carotid surgery in acute stroke: a multicentre randomized pilot study. Cerebrovasc Dis 2004;18:200–5.
[48] Pell JP, Slack R, Dennis M, et al. Improvements in carotid endarterectomy in Scotland: results of a national prospective survey. Scott Med J 2004;49:53–6.
[49] Rodgers H, Oliver SE, Dobson R, et al. A regional collaborative audit of the practice and outcome of carotid endarterectomy in the United Kingdom: Northern Regional Carotid Endarterectomy Audit Group. Eur J Vasc Endovasc Surg 2000;19:362–9.
[50] Turnbull RG, Taylor DC, Hsiang YN, et al. Assessment of patient waiting times for vascular surgery. Can J Surg 2000;43:105–11.
[51] Rothwell PM, Eliasziw M, Gutnikov SA, et al. Analysis of pooled data from the randomised controlled trials of endarterectomy for symptomatic carotid stenosis. Lancet 2003;361:107–16.
[52] North American Symptomatic Carotid Endarterectomy Trial Collaborators. Benefit of carotid endarterectomy in patients with symptomatic moderate or severe stenosis. N Engl J Med 1998;339:1415–25.
[53] European Carotid Surgery Trialists Collaborative Group. Randomised trial of endarterectomy for recently symptomatic carotid stenosis: final results of the MRC European Carotid Surgery Trial (ECST). Lancet 1998;351:1379–87.
[54] Rothwell PM, Gutnikov SA, Warlow CP. For the ECST: re-analysis of the final results of the European Carotid Surgery Trial. Stroke 2003;34:514–23.
[55] Ascher E, Markevich N, Hingorani A, et al. Pseudo-occlusions of the internal carotid artery: a rationale for treatment on the basis of a modified duplex scan protocol. J Vasc Surg 2002; 35:340–50.
[56] Rothwell PM, Gibson R, Warlow CP. The interrelation between plaque surface morphology, degree of stenosis and the risk of ischaemic stroke in patients with symptomatic carotid stenosis. Stroke 2000;31:615–21.
[57] Rothwell PM. Can overall results of clinical trials be applied to all patients? Lancet 1995;345: 1616–9.
[58] Rothwell PM, Warlow CP, on behalf of the ECST Collaborators. Prediction of benefit from carotid endarterectomy in individual patients: a risk-modelling study. Lancet 1999;353:2105–10.

[59] Rothwell PM, Mehta Z, Howard SC, et al. From subgroups to individuals: general principles and the example of carotid endartectomy. Lancet 2005;365:256–65.
[60] Executive Committee for the Asymptomatic Carotid Atherosclerosis Study. Endarterectomy for asymptomatic carotid artery stenosis. JAMA 1995;273:1421–8.
[61] Halliday A, Mansfield A, Marro J, et al, MRC Asymptomatic Carotid Surgery Trial (ACST) Collaborative Group. Prevention of disabling and fatal strokes by successful carotid endarterectomy in patients without recent neurological symptoms: randomised controlled trial. Lancet 2004;363:1491–502.
[62] Chambers BR, Donnan GA. Carotid endarterectomy for asymptomatic carotid stenosis. Cochrane Database Syst Rev 2005;(4):CD001923.
[63] Tu JV, Hannan EL, Anderson GM, et al. The fall and rise of carotid endarterectomy in the United States and Canada. N Engl J Med 1998;339:1441–7.
[64] Moore WS, Young B, Baker WH, et al. Surgical results: a justification of the surgeon selection process for the ACAS trial. J Vasc Surg 1996;23:323–38.
[65] Halliday AW, Thomas D, Mansfield A. The Asymptomatic Carotid Surgery Trial (ACST). Rationale and design. Eur J Vasc Surg 1994;8:703–10.
[66] Rothwell PM, Goldstein LB. Carotid endarterectomy for asymptomatic stenosis: Asymptomatic Carotid Surgery Trial. Stroke 2004;35:2425–7.
[67] Kresowik TF, Bratzler DW, Kresowik RA, et al. Multistate improvement in process and outcomes of carotid endarterectomy. J Vasc Surg 2004;39:372–80.
[68] Cuffe RL, Rothwell PM. Effect of non-optimal imaging on the relationship between the measured degree of symptomatic carotid stenosis and risk of ischemic stroke. Stroke 2006; 37:1785–91.
[69] Rothwell PM, Warlow CP. Low risk of ischaemic stroke in patients with collapse of the internal carotid artery distal to severe carotid stenosis: cerebral protection due to low post-stenotic flow? Stroke 2000;31:622–30.
[70] Nicolaides AN, Kakkos SK, Griffin M, et al. Severity of asymptomatic carotid stenosis and risk of ipsilateral hemispheric ischaemic events: results from the ACSRS study. Eur J Vasc Endovasc Surg 2005;30:275–84.
[71] Hennerici M, Hulsbomer HB, Hefter H, et al. Natural history of asymptomatic extracranial arterial disease: results of a long-term prospective study. Brain 1987;110(Pt 3):777–91.
[72] Baker WH, Howard VJ, Howard G, et al. Effect of contralateral occlusion on long-term efficacy of endarterectomy in the asymptomatic carotid atherosclerosis study (ACAS). ACAS Investigators. Stroke 2000;31:2330–4.
[73] Redgrave JN, Rothwell PM. Asymptomatic carotid stenosis: what to do. Curr Opin Neurol 2007;20:58–64.
[74] Chaturvedi S. Should the multicenter carotid endarterectomy trials be repeated? Arch Neurol 2003;60:774–5.
[75] Abbott AL, Bladin CF, Levi CR, et al. What should we do with asymptomatic carotid stenosis? Int J Stroke 2007;2:27–39.
[76] Abbott AL, Donnan GA. Does the high risk patient with asymptomatic carotid stenosis really exist? Eur J Vasc Endovasc Surg 2008;35:524–33.

ELSEVIER
SAUNDERS

Neurol Clin 26 (2008) 1099–1127

NEUROLOGIC
CLINICS

Endovascular Techniques for Stroke Prevention

Qasim Bashir, MD[a,*], Aamir Badruddin, MD[b], Victor Aletich, MD[a]

[a]*Neuroendovascular Division, Department of Neurosurgery, University of Illinois at Chicago, 912 South Wood Street, Chicago, IL 60612, USA*

[b]*Cerebrovascular and Neurological Critical Care Section, Department of Neurology and Rehabilitation, University of Illinois at Chicago, 912 South Wood Street, Chicago, IL 60612, USA*

Using their own experience and relying on clinical trials, the authors examine the various endovascular techniques for stroke prevention. These include embolic agents, devices, stents and antiplatelet drugs. They also examine the endovascular management of cerebral aneurysms, brain arteriovenous malformations, cervical internal carotid artery stenting and are optimistic about the safety of the endocervical treatment of a multitude of cerebrovascular diseases.

Endovascular treatment of cerebral aneurysms

Background

Intracranial cerebral aneurysms are thought by some investigators to result from a genetic or mutational predisposing defect arising during angiogenesis that modifies a vessel's response to stress in repair, regeneration, and maintenance of wall integrity. This propensity for degeneration, coupled with potential humoral, immune, and infectious triggers, and abnormal shear stress on the vascular wall, in time, induces vessel wall fatigue, allowing the development of an aneurysm [1]. The prevalence of cerebral aneurysms in the general population without specific risk factors (ie, family history of cerebral aneurysms, adult polycystic kidney disease) is estimated to be approximately 2.3%, and is positively associated with increasing age [2]. Autopsy studies have documented an estimated adult prevalence ranging

* Corresponding author.
E-mail address: bashir@uic.edu (Q. Bashir).

doi:10.1016/j.ncl.2008.09.014

from 0.2% to 9% [3,4], whereas only 0.5% to 1% have been discovered angiographically [5]. This article focuses on only congenital/acquired aneurysms.

Saccular aneurysms commonly develop at regions of major arterial branching, with most aneurysms (approximately 85%) involving the circle of Willis or middle cerebral artery (MCA) bifurcation, and are multiple in 15% to 20% of patients. The risk for rupture is directly related to size, following a bell curve of 4 to 25 mm, with most ruptured aneurysms presenting in clinical practice being less than 1 cm in size. The reasoning behind this paradox is that most aneurysms are small, and the percentage of rupture in this group outnumbers the higher percentage of rupture in large aneurysms, which are less common. In general, the incidence of subarachnoid hemorrhage (SAH) is between 6 and 12 per 100,000 population per year, translating into 15,000 to 30,000 new SAH patients annually [3,6–11], with most patients being younger than 55 years at the time of initial presentation [12]. At presentation, ruptured aneurysms are the cause in 85%, with the remainder a result of perimesencephalic hemorrhage (10%) and less common causes (5%), including inflammatory causes (eg, mycotic), noninflammatory causes (eg, dissection, arteriovenous malformations [AVMs], dural arteriovenous fistulas), spinal cord vascular lesions (eg, spinal AVMs, fistulas), sickle cell disease, coagulopathy, tumors, and drug abuse.

Precipitating factors leading to aneurysm rupture are complex, and some frequently quoted in the literature include blood pressure fluctuations and activities such as physical exercise, sexual intercourse, and straining [13,14]. Modifiable risk factors for SAH are hypertension, smoking, and excessive intake of alcohol, which can double the risk for SAH [15]. Patients who have a positive family history for cerebral aneurysms tend to present with SAH at a younger age and harbor multiple aneurysms, as compared with patients who have sporadic SAH [16–18]. Although most patients who have cerebral aneurysms present with SAH, other presentations include cranial nerve deficits, headache, seizures, transient ischemic attacks (TIAs) and infarction.

In population-based studies, the fatality rate following aneurysm rupture is approximately 50% [19], including a 10% to 15% mortality rate before reaching a hospital and an additional 25% mortality rate within 24 hours of rupture. [20]. Only one third of patients presenting with SAH have a functionally independent outcome [21–24]. Untreated ruptured aneurysms have a 48% to 78% morbidity and a 60% mortality at 6 months as a result of rerupture, stressing the need for urgent treatment [25–27].

Endovascular treatment of cerebral aneurysms had its beginning with Fedor A. Serbinenko in the 1970s, who first used detachable balloons to occlude the carotid and vertebral arteries harboring an aneurysm. In 1991, the introduction of the Guglielmi detachable coils (Boston Scientific/Target, Fremont, California) completely revolutionized the treatment of cerebral aneurysms [28,29] and has since been the mainstay of endovascular aneurysm treatment. Over the last decade, subsequent improvement in coil design and microcatheters and the development of adjunctive treatments such as the remodeling technique and stent-assisted coiling have continually increased the number of aneurysms amenable to endovascular techniques. Recently, the additions of new closed cell stents (stent grafts) and liquid embolic agents have been promising in further advancing the endovascular management of cerebral aneurysms.

Numerous studies, both prospective and retrospective, have been conducted over the years [26,30–53], the more prominent and controversial studies being the International Subarachnoid Aneurysm Trial (ISAT) [35,39,43,44] and the International Study of Unruptured Intracranial Aneurysms (ISUIA) [30,32].

In general, although controversies continue to exist, the endovascular management of cerebral aneurysms has been supported as a safe and effective treatment of ruptured and unruptured cerebral aneurysms.

Patient evaluation and selection

Cerebral aneurysms may present with SAH, with or without a parenchymal component or mass effect (ie, recurrent headaches, third nerve palsy, cavernous syndrome), or found as an incidental finding on noninvasive imaging studies obtained for other medical reasons. In cases based on noninvasive imaging where therapeutic decisions are difficult, a conventional cerebral angiogram is performed for definitive treatment planning. Selection criteria for surgical or endovascular treatment include, but are not limited to, aneurysm location, aneurysm geometry, patient age, associated medical comorbidities, coagulation status, Fischer CT grade and Hunt-Hess grade. In the authors' case, once all the clinically relevant information is obtained, patients who have unruptured aneurysms are reviewed and discussed at their weekly multidisciplinary neurovascular conference and the decision is made as to whether surgical clipping, endovascular treatment, or conservative management is the most appropriate course. Ruptured aneurysms are treated emergently, following consultation between the vascular neurosurgeon and the endovascular neurosurgeon.

Embolic agents and devices

Coils

Bare coils. Currently used coils consist of platinum, although in the past they were also composed of tungsten, and attached to a delivery microware or hypotube, with the detachment zone being variable as to the mode of detachment (mechanical, electrolytic, hydraulic, or low-temperature resistive heating). They come in various sizes and lengths and have varying degrees of stretch resistance, softness, and retained memory.

Bioactive coated coils. Biologically active surfaces or coated coils have been introduced primarily to address the issue of recanalization, which can occur with bare platinum coils. Polyglycolic-polylactic acid and expanding hydrogel are the only two bioactive agents currently available and are used by different coil manufacturers. A few investigators have compared bioactive coated coils with bare platinum coils [54–56] and found no significant difference in angiographic occlusion rates. Prospective studies are currently ongoing (Matrix And Platinum Science: A Prospective, Randomized, Multicenter Trial Investigating Matrix^2 [MAPS] and Guglielmi detachable coils for the treatment of intracranial saccular aneurysms).

Balloon-assisted coiling (the "remodeling technique")

Wide-necked aneurysms are defined as aneurysms with a dome-to-neck diameter ratio of less than 2 to 1, a neck diameter of greater than 4 mm, or a neck diameter greater than one half the diameter of the parent vessel. These aneurysms are difficult to treat successfully with coils alone [31,57]. To address this problem, Jacques Moret [58], in 1992, first described the "remodeling technique." This technique positions a compliant, nondetachable balloon in the parent artery straddling the aneurysm neck, which is inflated temporarily during coil placement by way of a second microcatheter. Various balloons are available, and the technique continues to be widely used in the treatment of cerebral aneurysms [31,59]. Although two or more microcatheters may be used with this technique, the "remodeling technique" does not increase periprocedural morbidity [31,60–62].

Intracranial stents

Similar to balloon remodeling, intracranial stents provide structural support during endovascular coiling; they were first reported as an adjunctive therapy in the treatment of cerebral aneurysms by Higashida and colleagues in 1997. Apart from providing structural support and preventing prolapse of coils into the parent artery, advantages suggested include disruption and flow diversion within the aneurysm, theoretically inducing further thrombosis/occlusion within the lumen of the aneurysm [63]; in addition, the presence of the stent scaffolding adjacent to the neck of the aneurysm may promote enhanced endothelial growth [64].

Currently available stents include

Neuroform stent (Boston Scientific, Freemont, CA), a hybrid cell design stent, first introduced in 2002 [65]. Limiting features include the inability to reposition once partially deployed; low radial force, which limits the ability to bear the coil mass effect, specifically with large aneurysms; and tracking difficulty through tortuous vessels.

Leo stent (Balt, Extrusion, France), a closed-cell design stent rendering high radial force and homogenous wall structure even in acute curvatures. Enhanced visibility of the stent length and diameter is achieved with two platinum wires. The Leo stent's high outward radial force and ability to be repositioned when up to 90% of the stent length is deployed offers a theoretic advantage over other self-expandable stents [66].

Enterprise stent (Cordis Neurovascular, Miami Lake, FL), which, similar to the Leo stent, is a closed-cell design with a near similar delivery mechanism. Unlike the Leo stent, the Enterprise stent is retrievable for repositioning when less than 70% of the total length of the stent is deployed.

Pipeline embolization device (Chestnut Medical, Menlo Park, CA), a self-expanding stent with 30% to 35% metal surface area compared with 6.5% to 9% metal surface area coverage provided by currently available self-expanding stents in the United States. The Pipeline stent reconstructs the entire segment of the parent vessel and has been proposed to overcome current endovascular aneurysm treatment limiting factors such as larger wide-necked aneurysms and the presence of intra-aneurismal thrombus. The recent Pipeline Intracranial Treatment of Aneurysms (PITA) trial demonstrated a 100% successful delivery rate, 6% procedural complication and complete angiographic occlusion of the aneurysm at 6 months in 28/30 aneurysms (93%).

Covered stents, although still in development for intracranial vasculature. Exclusion of the aneurysm with the use of stent grafts placed adjacent to the neck is feasible [67]. Recently, use of a new covered stent designed specifically for cerebral vasculature was reported for treating pseudoaneurysms [68].

Onyx

Onyx high density HD500 (eV3 Neurovascular, Irvine, CA) is a liquid embolic agent designed for endovascular treatment of cerebral aneurysms. It is an ethylene-vinyl-alcohol (EVOH) biocompatible copolymer used in conjunction with dimethyl sulfoxide (DMSO) as the solvent. To improve visualization under fluoroscopy, micronized tantalum powder is added to the mixture [69]. The technique involves placement of a DMSO-compatible balloon across the aneurysm neck and a second microcatheter into the aneurysm lumen. A seal test to evaluate the integrity of balloon occlusion at the aneurysm neck is performed and successful if stagnation of contrast occurs within the lumen of the aneurysm while the balloon is inflated. Onyx is then slowly delivered and precipitates as the mixture comes in contact with blood, which allows rapid diffusion of the DSMO, forming a spongy polymer cast. The material solidifies within 2 to 3 minutes, during which the balloon remains inflated. Complete solidification of the cast is achieved within 10 minutes. Durable aneurysm occlusion rates have been reported for small, large, and giant aneurysms [70,71].

A stent is essentially a metallic foreign body that will induce thrombus formation if adequate platelet inhibition is not achieved. Hence, antiplatelet drugs are an important part of the technique to prevent peri- or postembolization procedure. Coronary literature supports dual antiplatelet therapy efficacy over monotherapy [72]. An optimal antiplatelet therapy regimen does not exist and hence, subtle variations exist between physicians and institutions. In general, aspirin and Plavix are started 3 to 5 days before the scheduled procedure. In urgent situations, oral aspirin and Plavix loads can be administered. In emergent situations, intravenous glycoprotein IIb/IIIa inhibitor abciximab can be administered. The half-life of abciximab is between 10 and 30 minutes. Stent-assisted coil embolization is generally avoided in patients who have an acutely ruptured cerebral aneurysm.

Procedure

Endovascular treatment of aneurysms at the authors' institution is performed under general anesthesia with systemic heparinization, including recently ruptured aneurysms. A heparin bolus calculated by patient weight is administered to achieve an activated clotting time (ACT) between 200 and 250 seconds, and maintained by subsequent heparin administration throughout the remainder of the procedure. Flush lines are heparinized with 2000 units per liter normal saline.

Elective patients who have aneurysms that are anticipated to require a stent, or who are predetermined to have Onyx treatment of their aneurysm, are pretreated with a minimum of 81 mg aspirin per day and Plavix, 75 mg per day, 1 week before their scheduled procedure [72]. Emergent patients who have not been on antiplatelet medication and require a stent are treated with a weight-based Integrilin bolus and maintained on this medication until oral administration of aspirin and Plavix have been administered.

Post procedure, the heparin is typically reversed with protamine sulfate, 10 mg/1000 units heparin, administered at the end of the procedure, unless a technical or clinical complication has occurred that requires a more prolonged anticoagulation course. In patients in whom the "remodeling technique" has been performed, the systemic anticoagulation is not reversed but is allowed to be metabolized without replacement or continued for 24 hours, depending on the degree the balloon was used during the procedure.

Patients who have required a stent or had Onyx treatment of their aneurysm are maintained on oral aspirin, 81 mg/day, and Plavix, 75 mg/day, for a period of 3 to 6 months, at which time the Plavix may be discontinued and aspirin continued indefinitely.

Goals of embolization

The goal of endovascular treatment of cerebral aneurysms is the complete obliteration of the aneurysm lumen, eliminating the risk for subsequent growth or rupture with attendant sequelae.

Since the inception of endovascular treatment of cerebral aneurysms, controversy concerning the efficacy, safety, and durability of the endovascular approach to ruptured and unruptured aneurysms has persisted. Numerous reported case series and prospective studies have documented that treatment of cerebral aneurysms can be performed with minimal morbidity and mortality and, in the case of ruptured aneurysms, may be preferable to surgical clipping [44,57,73–75].

The durability of endovascular treatment of cerebral aneurysms, both ruptured and unruptured, remains a continual debate [76–84]. Prospective studies initiated even in the last 1 to 2 years cannot incorporate the rapidly changing technology in the endovascular treatment of cerebral aneurysms. Therefore, one must remain diligent in evaluating recent reports, case studies, and presentations to keep abreast of this ever-changing field.

Summary

The endovascular treatment of cerebral aneurysms has been shown to be a safe and effective treatment option to surgical management. Additionally, aneurysms previously considered untreatable are now being treated by an endovascular approach. Controversies concerning the durability of endovascular therapy of cerebral aneurysms persist, although technologic advancements in coil design, stents, liquid embolic agents, and innovative ideas such the endovascular clip system (eCLIPS) [85] may address these concerns and revolutionize the endovascular treatment of cerebral aneurysms.

Endovascular management of brain arteriovenous malformations

Background

Cerebral AVMs are proposed to result from a failure of the normal differentiation of primordial vascular channels into mature arteries, capillaries, and veins during embryogenesis [86]. They are characterized by direct connection of arterial feeders to the venous system, without an intervening capillary bed. This absence of a capillary bed results in direct transmission of arterial pressure to the venous system. AVMs can be present in the cerebrum or the brain stem/cerebellum and sizes can vary greatly, from a few millimeters to that involving an entire hemisphere.

Opinions vary greatly on the true prevalence of AVMs in the community. However, a systematic review published in 2001 estimated the prevalence of AVMs to be approximately 1 per 100,000 in unselected patients [87], and suggested them to be the leading cause of intracranial hemorrhages in young adults [88].

About 50% of patients present with intracranial hemorrhage, with the remaining patients presenting with seizures or headaches. Many AVMs are also found incidentally on imaging studies for other causes. The New York Islands AVM study reported the annual rupture risk for unruptured AVMs to be 1.2% per year [89]. However, the risk for rerupture in an intraparenchymal AVM carries an annual risk for SAH or intraparenchymal hemorrhage of between 3% and 4%, and a cumulative long-term risk of 30% to 40%. This risk may be slightly higher in the first year after an initial hemorrhage but remains constant from that point for the remainder of patient's life, with hemorrhage in many patients occurring years to decades following the initial diagnosis [90]. Stapf and colleagues [91] reported the annual rupture risk of an unruptured AVM to be 1.3%, whereas the rerupture risk is 5.9% annually.

Although general agreement exists about treating ruptured AVMs, given the high rehemorrhage rate, whether or not to treat unruptured AVMs has become a controversial topic. A few authors [92] have recently argued that, because the risk for hemorrhage for unruptured AVMs is only 1.2% per year and the risk for morbidity with intervention, whether surgical, endovascular, radiation, or combination, is around 10%, invasive treatment of an unruptured AVM cannot be justified. This argument led to the launch of A Randomized trial of Unruptured Brain AVMs (ARUBA) in 2006. The study plans enrollment of 800 patients who have unruptured AVMs randomized to invasive treatment (surgical, endovascular, radiation, or combination) or conservative management. A 5-year follow-up is planned.

The authors disagree with the conservative management of AVMs because the premise of the ARUBA study is based on low annual risk for rupture. This risk is derived from the Columbia AVM database, which has a mean follow-up of less than 3 years, and complication rates with endovascular treatment are quoted for initial experience with new embolic material. These rates may change with operator experience, new agents, and more refined techniques. Given the cumulative risk for rupture throughout the expected lifetime of a patient, an upfront risk of treatment may be acceptable to some physicians and patients.

A multidisciplinary approach to AVM treatment is widely accepted. AVMs may be treated with embolization as an adjunctive treatment before surgical resection or radiosurgery to reduce the arterial shunt and decrease the nidus size. Embolization before radiation has been performed; however, some studies have shown that a lower obliteration rate was achieved in AVMs that had undergone embolization before radiation, compared with those treated with radiation alone [93,94]. Several factors may account for this observed reduction in obliteration rate. Because AVM size is the most significant determinant of the outcome and it is likely that larger AVMs were selected for preradiation embolization, these AVMs may have been less susceptible to obliteration with radiation alone, and the study results may have been impacted by selection bias. It has also been shown that embolized portions of the AVM may recanalize, based on the embolic agent used, which may also account for lower obliteration rates achieved with radiation in AVMs pretreated with embolization [93]. These data have not been validated in more recent studies. In addition, newer embolic agents may provide a decreased recanalization rate and a more successful obliteration rate with combined endovascular and radiation therapy.

More recently, several centers have performed endovascular embolization of the AVM as the only therapy and often intended as a curative measure. AVMs of Spetzler-Martin grade IV to V have higher surgical risk, and endovascular treatment may be the only feasible approach. However, lower-grade lesions have also been targeted for curative embolization because new embolization materials have shown initial promise of durability [95].

Patient evaluation and selection

Intracranial hemorrhage is the most common presentation of an AVM. Noninvasive modalities such as MR and CT angiography have increasingly diagnosed AVMs for neurologic presentations such as headache or seizures, or as an incidental finding. Multiple factors are considered in the approach to cerebral AVMs. The foremost is whether treatment can, or should, be offered to the patient; if yes, then decisions concerning the forms of treatment to be offered should be individualized to maximize the chance of cure. This primary decision making involves a comparison between the natural history and the risks of the various treatment options. In addition, other factors to consider include the patient's age, the angioarchitecture of the AVM, coexisting medical problems, and current clinical status. The individual treatment recommendation may be best approached through a multidisciplinary consensus among neurologists, neurosurgeons, and endovascular neurosurgeons.

Noninvasive imaging can be used to plan an endovascular approach. A CT scan with contrast injection can be diagnostic for an AVM. A typical CT image of a cerebral AVM is an isodense brain region that enhances after intravenous contrast infusion, and demonstrates serpentine enhancement radiating from the lesion.

In MRI, the regions of high-velocity intravascular blood flow within the AVM are seen as a network of flow voids on T1- and T2-weighted images. The detailed anatomy of the AVM, the nidus, and its relationship to the surrounding brain are most clearly demonstrated by MR imaging.

Angiography remains indispensable in AVM treatment planning. MR and CT angiography provide important information about the feeding vessels and the draining veins; however, they have not been able to replace conventional angiography as a tool for fully evaluating the angioarchitecture of cerebral AVMs. Selective and superselective cerebral angiography remains the gold standard for the pretreatment assessment of all AVMs. A complete, four-vessel cerebral angiography can provide precise information of feeding arteries, draining veins, and nidus size (Fig. 1). Any associated aneurysms, fistulae, or venous anomalies can also be confirmed. In the authors' experience, the presence of associated aneurysms (congenital, flow related, or intranidal) with AVMs has been 46%, intranidal fistulae 31%, venous stenosis 12%, and venous aneurysms 5% [96]. The presence of any of these findings may be crucial in selecting the initial vessels to be embolized.

Angiography and angioarchitecture

The appearance of a draining vein during the arterial phase of a conventional angiogram is the sine qua non of AVM. Feeding arteries may arise

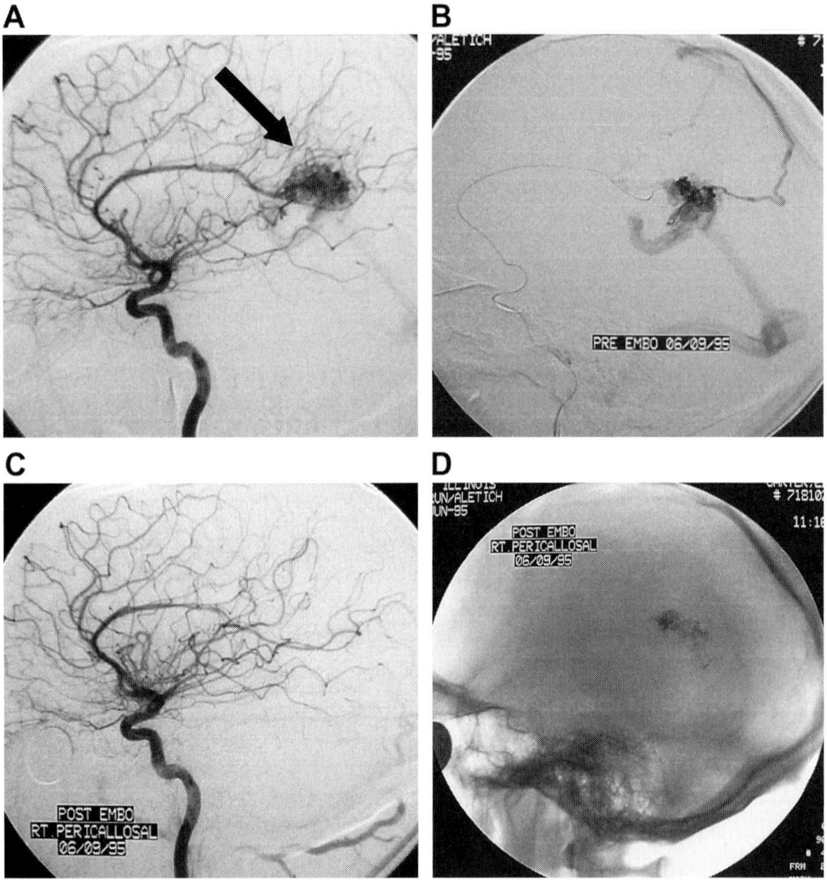

Fig. 1. (*A*) AVM nidus at the end of the pericallosal artery (*arrow*). (*B*) Draining veins for the same AVM. (*C*) Angiogram showing obliteration of the AVM after embolization. (*D*) A cast of the embolic material.

from the terminus of a large-caliber native vessel or may come off as small feeder arteries "en passage." Arterial feeders connect directly to the draining veins without an intervening capillary bed, resulting in high-flow arteriovenous shunts. Histologically, these vessels may vary from well-differentiated arteries with muscular layers to thin-walled veins, and some vessels are identifiable as neither [97]. These vessels form dilated loops, similar to a bag of worms, and this "bag" is called the nidus (from the Latin for "nest"). No intervening functional brain has been identified in between these blood vessels, lending credence to the theory that these malformations form during the antenatal period, displacing the normal brain on the periphery. The nidus is readily identifiable as a tangle of vessels and may sometimes give an appearance of moyamoya. Venous drainage may be through cortical veins, or dural sinuses for more superficial AVMs. For large or deep AVMs, deep venous drainage is usually present. The presence of more than one draining vein is the rule. Identification of all feeding arteries and their pedicles, number, and pattern of draining venous structures, and associated aneurysms, intranidal fistulae, and venous outflow anomalies, are the objectives of angiography.

Embolic agents

Various techniques are used for embolization of brain AVMs. Particulate agents are used primarily as a presurgical procedure because subsequent long-term recanalization is common. These agents include polyvinyl alcohol, balloons, coils, and silk thread, or a combination of these agents, with balloons and silk thread being mostly of historical interest [98–103]. The liquid agents, including alcohol, n - butyl cyanoacrylate, and its precursor, isobutyl 2 cyanoacrylate, provide more chance of permanent occlusion [104]. Recently, other variants of acrylic-based glues, such as 2-hexyl cyanoacrylate (neuracryl M) [105] in humans and Eudragit (copolymer of methyl and butyl methacrylate and dimethylaminoethyl methacrylate) [106] and 2-poly-hydroxyethyl-methacrylate [107] in animals have been used but have failed to gain popularity. The two most commonly used liquid embolic agents are described below.

N-butyl cyanoacrylate

Cyanoacrylate is a liquid acrylic resin that polymerizes and sets quickly when contact is made with an ionic solution. It has been used for medical purposes since the 1960s, and the first reports of its use in the treatment of cerebral AVMs were published in the early 1980s. Several variants of cyanoacrylate have different polymerization times and quality of cast, although, at present, only n-butyl cyanoacrylate (NBCA) has been approved for medical use. It has a slightly longer polymerization time compared with other cyanoacrylate compounds, and the polymerization time can be adjusted by mixing with Ethiodol, which also allows visualization under fluoroscopy [108]. Some neurointerventionalists add tantalum powder to this mixture to enhance the radio-opacity. NBCA, once injected into the AVM, will set in the nidus and obstruct blood flow. It also triggers an inflammatory reaction and fibrotic growth, which facilitate permanent obliteration. Once the AVM is filled, the occlusion is likely durable [104,109].

Ethylene vinyl alcohol copolymer (Onyx)

Ethylene vinyl alcohol copolymer (EVOH) is a nonadhesive liquid embolic agent that is dissolved in DMSO. Tantalum powder is added to make the compound radio-opaque. EVOH is naturally a cohesive compound; however, it remains liquid when dissolved in DMSO and only aggregates into a sponge-like substance when DMSO is allowed to diffuse in blood or any hydrophilic environment. It solidifies from the outside as the operator injects more embolic material and can be visualized as oozing lava with a cool top crust while the molten lava underneath continues to flow forward. This advantage has enabled the interventionalist to embolize large portions of AVMs while engaged in a single pedicle.

EVOH comes in concentrations of 6% and 8%. EVOH 6% is less viscous and is better suited for distal embolization. EVOH 8% is effective for high-flow shunts. DMSO is angiotoxic and may result in vasculitis, vascular necrosis, and hemorrhage [110]; however, when infused at less than 0.25 mL/90 s, it has been shown to be safe [111]. DMSO is a potent solvent and may dissolve the catheter through which it is injected; hence, only specially designed catheters can be used for its delivery. Although EVOH was first used in 1990, it was not commercially available until 2005 [112]. Data on durability and long-term follow-up are limited, although several more recent series have demonstrated near-complete to complete obliteration of the AVM nidus and low recanalization or recurrence rates in short-term follow-up [95,113,114].

Goals of embolization and procedural aspects

At the author's institution, once the patient's history, imaging reports, and other details are collected, the case is discussed at a weekly multidisciplinary conference with representatives present from neurology, neurosurgery, endovascular neurosurgery, and neuroradiology services.

The diagnostic angiogram is reviewed and the presence of associated aneurysms, high-flow fistulas, venous ectasia, and draining vein stenosis is ascertained. Once a patient has been determined to be eligible for treatment, the authors' current strategy is to perform staged embolization for large AVMs with subsequent surgical resection or radiosurgery. Smaller AVMs, especially in younger patients, may undergo direct surgical resection, unless the lesion is within, or adjacent to, the basal ganglia/thalamus or brainstem. In these cases, endovascular embolization may be considered in selected cases [115].

The authors' approach in the initial embolization of AVMs is to treat the most threatening feature, such as associated aneurysms or intranidal fistulae, which may minimize subsequent rupture. This treatment may require a staged approach over several sessions. In the case of feeding vessel aneurysms that are in close proximity to the AVM nidus, and intranidal aneurysms, the vessel harboring the aneurysm is the first vessel selected for embolization and, if possible, the aneurysm is included in the glue or Onyx cast. The presence of a feeding vessel aneurysm that is not in close proximity to the AVM nidus poses a dilemma. Embolization in the proximal trunk of the feeding vessel carries high risk for embolizing normal parenchymal branches. In this circumstance, more distal embolization of the AVM compartment fed by the feeder is performed to diminish the shunt through the AVM, with hopes that the flow-related aneurysm will regress.

In AVMs that are associated with marked venous ectasia or venous outflow stenosis, the initial embolization is aimed at diminishing the flow through the compartment draining through the stenosed or ectatic vein. In other cases, the largest feeding vessels are selected for embolization because these vessels are the easiest to catheterize and provide the best access to the AVM nidus. Collateral circulations are avoided because direct access to the AVM nidus may be difficult, if not impossible. Once the target vessels are determined, the access vessel is evaluated (carotid or vertebral artery) for concomitant disease, such as arteriosclerotic changes and tortuosity, which aids in the selection and shaping of the guide catheter to be used in the procedure.

At the authors' center, embolization procedures are performed under general anesthesia and systemic anticoagulation with heparin based on weight. An ACT is maintained between 200 and 250 seconds. Heparin reversal is achieved with protamine sulfate at the end of the session. The mean arterial blood pressure is maintained at approximately 10% to 15% below baseline to minimize the risk for normal pressure breakthrough phenomena, and a tapering dose of steroids may be instituted if a large amount of NBCA was used to reduce posttreatment inflammatory response to the embolic agent.

The goal of embolization is to reduce the size and diminish the anomalous flow of the vascular malformation. In 10% to 15% of cases, embolization alone may cure the anomaly, and in most of the remaining cases, effective reduction of nidus size or reduced flow allows for adjunctive surgery or radiosurgery to be performed with reduced morbidity and mortality [100]. The two primary approaches to the endovascular embolization of cerebral AVMs are feeding artery embolization and nidus embolization.

Feeding artery embolization uses a microcatheter placed within the feeding arterial pedicle of the AVM proximal to the nidus for delivery of the embolic agent. The embolic material, usually a particulate, flows to the AVM nidus. Occasionally, the feeding artery itself is intentionally occluded just proximal to the nidus.

Nidus embolization, as the name implies, requires placement of the microcatheter at, or within, the interstices of the nidus for the delivery of the embolic agent, which is usually NBCA or EVOH. The microcatheter should be in a wedged position to prevent reflux along it and to allow the operator optimal control of the embolic material progression into the nidus [87,116,117].

Both techniques are performed routinely in the embolization of cerebral AVMs; however, the goals and risks of particulate embolization differ from NBCA embolization.

1. It is the authors' opinion that embolization with solid particles should be viewed as an adjunctive, preoperative procedure only because the agents do not typically provide permanent occlusion. Incomplete occlusion of the AVM nidus and proximal feeder occlusion alone allow for subsequent recruitment of secondary feeders and collaterals, and permit nidus recanalization [118,119]. Although recanalization of the nidus

after embolization with NBCA is controversial, several reports suggest that complete casting of the interstices of the AVM nidus with cyanoacrylate glue embolization leads to permanent occlusion [104,110,120–122]. The possibility of nidus recanalization following feeding artery embolization limits the use and effectiveness of subsequent radiosurgery because the curative effects of radiosurgery may not be observed for up to 2 to 3 years. However, because the portion of the nidus that has been well casted with cyanoacrylic glue (and possibly EVOH) may be permanently occluded, it may not need to be included in the irradiated volume during radiosurgery, decreasing the associated treatment morbidity.

2. NBCA and EVOH embolizations may be curative without adjunctive surgical resection or radiosurgery in selected cases. These AVMs are typically small, with few feeding arteries and draining veins [121,123–125]. Additionally, these agents may obliterate any collateral circulation at the periphery of the dominant compartment of the AVM. For example, a parietal lobe nidus with predominant arterial feeding arteries by MCA branches and collateral circulation from anterior cerebral artery branches at the mesial edge of the AVM may be cured by embolizing the MCA feeders alone.
3. Solid particles require larger delivery systems that are stiffer and require the use of guiding wires, which significantly increase the risk for vascular damage during catheter advancement, as compared with the flow-directed microcatheters used with cyanoacrylates. Additionally, because of their larger size and increased stiffness, catheters used in particulate embolization are difficult to place in close proximity to the AVM nidus, thereby increasing the risk for the embolic agent to reflux into normal cerebral vasculature.

Complications

The major complications of endovascular embolization are delayed hemorrhage by venous outflow obstruction causing normal pressure breakthrough, embolization of normal parenchyma, vessel rupture, and microcatheter retention.

Venous outflow obstruction is the most common cause of delayed postembolization hemorrhage [116,121] because of normal pressure breakthrough. A complete understanding of the angioarchitecture of the AVM and embolic agent used for embolization is necessary to minimize migration of embolic material into the venous outflow of the AVM. In addition, staged procedures, where less than 30% to 35% of the AVM nidus is occluded per session, may minimize the risk for hemorrhage from normal pressure breakthrough, unless the entire nidus can be obliterated in one session.

Embolization leading to infarction of normal parenchyma can be minimized if nidus rather than feeder embolization is performed.

Microcatheter retention can occur with cyanoacrylate and EVOH, and is typically caused by entrapment of the microcatheter tip in embolic material that has migrated proximally. It can also be caused by vasospasm, even if no embolic material has been injected. This complication may be reduced by diluting the cyanoacrylate mixture and obtaining a wedge position in the nidus or distal feeding artery. Additionally, flow-guided microcatheters are preferable, as they minimize vasospasm during microcatheter manipulation.

Microcatheter retention is infrequent and in most instances does not result in any long-term clinical sequelae.

Risk for embolic material migration to the draining vein and pulmonary embolism has been reported [126,127]. Thus, the flow of the embolic agent should be controlled, to avoid filling the draining vein. A detailed review article on complications of AVM embolization has been published by Jayaraman and colleagues [128].

Outcomes

With the advent of newer embolic agents, catheters, and techniques and increased experience, endovascular embolization and obliteration rates are increasing. Recent obliteration rates have been reported at between 16% and 53.9% [95,110] and endovascular cerebral AVM treatment is increasingly being used by some as the only modality of treatment [95]. However, long-term durability data with newer agents are lacking.

Summary

Cerebral AVM is a common cause of intracranial hemorrhage, and asymptomatic AVMs are increasingly being diagnosed with modern imaging techniques. Although the treatment of unruptured AVMs has recently been questioned, treatment decisions should be individualized, given the long-term risk.

Cerebral AVM obliteration rates have increased with the advent of newer embolic agents and techniques. Complications of AVM embolization are related to the angioarchitecture of the AVM, the type of embolic agents used, and the operator experience. Therefore, a multidisciplinary approach with combination therapy, such as embolization followed by surgical resection or radiosurgery, should be used. This approach should minimize morbidity and mortality during embolization.

Intracranial stenting and angioplasty

Background

Intracranial atherosclerotic disease accounts for about 5% to 10% of all ischemic strokes [129,130]. Recurrent stroke risk has been estimated to be 7% to 40% annually, and disease progression is common [131–134]. Ischemic stroke causes in patients who have intracranial atherosclerotic disease may include hypoperfusion, acute occlusion due to plaque rupture, distal thromboembolism, or associated small penetrating artery occlusion. The management of a patient who has symptomatic intracranial atherosclerotic disease remains a dilemma of modern-day medicine. The GESICA study followed 102 patients who had symptomatic intracranial stenosis (50%–99%) treated with antithrombotic therapy for up to 36 months [135]. In 27.4% of the patients, the stenoses had clinical hemodynamic characteristics. During a mean follow-up of 23.4 months, 38.2% of the patients had a cerebrovascular event (TIA 24.5% and ischemic stroke 13.7%). Patients who had clinical hemodynamic features had a 60.7% recurrent stroke or TIA rate in the territory of the stenotic artery. In the Warfarin versus Aspirin for Symptomatic Intracranial Disease (WASID) study, the 2-year risk for stroke in the territory of the stenotic artery in patients who had greater than or equal to 70% stenosis was 19%, and 10% in patients who had less than 70% stenosis [136]. Most of these strokes occurred within the first year. A similar finding was reported by Kim and colleagues [137], suggesting an 11% ipsilateral stroke risk in the first year, and more than double that if the stenosis was 70% or more. In WASID, increasing blood pressure and low-density lipoprotein levels predicted recurrent stroke during follow-up, despite nearly all patients receiving treatment with statins by the end of the study [138]. Considering the disappointingly high recurrent stroke risk despite medical therapy, interest in endovascular treatment with intracranial balloon angioplasty and stenting has been increasing.

In 1964, Dotter and Judkins recorded the earliest description of percutaneous transluminal angioplasty (PTA) of the peripheral vascular system. Since 1977, when Andreas R. Gruentzig performed the first successful human coronary artery angioplasty in Zurich, Switzerland, the field of endovascular intervention has gone through a revolutionary technical transformation. The introduction of more flexible stents and delivery systems has made stent-assisted angioplasty a feasible approach to medically refractory symptomatic intracranial stenoses [139,140]. Concurrently, advancements in neuroendovascular technology, such as three-dimensional angiography, high-resolution and high-speed angiography, biplane road mapping, and three-dimensional road mapping have improved the safety and precise deployment of bioimplants. After successful reports by Sundt and colleagues [141] of balloon angioplasty in two patients who had medically refractory basilar stenosis, numerous studies have reported technical success with angioplasty, with or without stenting [142–147]. The procedure is thought to improve cerebral blood flow through the affected area. It also prevents platelet activation secondary to high shear within the stenotic segment, promotes a smooth neointimal growth across the lesion, and prevents plaque rupture and platelet adherence.

Patient evaluation and selection

In the authors' practice, symptomatic patients who have greater than 50% stenosis of a major intracranial vessel are offered intracranial angioplasty and stenting if they have been refractory to medical therapy, cerebrovascular reserve is impaired, and the anatomy suggests the procedure is feasible with reasonable safety. Additionally, patients who have chronic occlusion, severe neurologic impairment from a stroke distal to the lesion, a major stroke within the last 6 weeks, or contraindication to dual antiplatelet agents are not considered candidates.

In intracranial vessels, the stenosis is calculated as $(1 - [D_{stenosis}/D_{normal}]) \times 100$, where $D_{stenosis}$ is the diameter of the artery at the site of the most severe stenosis and D_{normal} is the diameter of the proximal normal artery [148]. Classification systems such as Location, Morphology and Access [144] and Mori's classification (morphologic features) [149] have been associated with technical success, procedural risk, and restenosis.

The procedure is generally performed on an elective basis at least 4 to 6 weeks after ischemic stroke, unless the patient is experiencing crescendo TIAs attributable to the lesion or has evidence of hemodynamically sensitive symptoms or acute rethrombosis, in which case emergent treatment may be necessary. Patients undergoing elective angioplasty and stenting are pretreated with aspirin, 325 mg daily, and clopidogrel, 75 mg daily for 5 days. Ticlopidine, 250 mg twice daily, or cilostazol, 100 mg twice daily, may be used if clopidogrel cannot be tolerated. If done urgently, aspirin 325 mg, and clopidogrel, 300 to 450 mg, loading may be done 6 hours before the procedure, or intravenous glycoprotein IIb/IIIa agents such as abciximab (0.20 mg/kg bolus followed by 0.125 μg/kg/min up to 10 μg/min for 12 hours afterward) or eptifibatide (2 μg/kg/min up to 15 mg/h for 12 hours) may be used. Intravenous heparin is infused during the procedure to maintain an ACT greater than 200 (<180 if intravenous antiplatelet agents are concomitantly used).

Techniques and devices

Low-profile, flexible percutaneous transluminal angioplasty over-the-wire balloons

No prospective studies of intracranial PTA without stenting have, thus far, been reported. Although technical success, defined as reduction in stenosis to less than 50%, can be achieved in most patients, the reported 30-day stroke or death rates range from 4% and 40% in published series (see Refs. [142,143,146,147,150–155]). Additionally, the restenosis rate after PTA without stenting ranges from 24% to 40% [143,146], and restenosis has been linked to Mori's morphologic classification [156] with technical success and 1-year restenosis rates of 92% and 0% for type A lesions, 82% and 33% for type B lesions, and 33% and 100% for type C lesions.

Unlike the coronary or peripheral arterial system, intracranial PTA carries a higher procedural complication rate because of an absence of surrounding supportive tissue and weaker vessel wall composition. Outcomes and periprocedural morbidity and mortality are related to selection of

PTA balloon (size/length), inflation pressure, speed, and duration of inflation.

Percutaneous transluminal angioplasty with stenting

The term "stent" was coined after an English dentist, Charles Stent (1845–1901), developed a mold that was used to form teeth and oral cavity impressions. Thereafter, it was used in association with a device that held a skin graft in position. More recently, the term has been used for an endovascular scaffolding to relieve and prevent vascular obstruction [157]. Stenting was developed to ameliorate the high short-term recoil rates, incomplete dilation, procedural dissection, and late restenosis associated with PTA alone.

The Stenting of Symptomatic atherosclerotic Lesions in the Vertebral or Intracranial Arteries (SSYLVIA) trial was a nonrandomized, multicenter study to evaluate the safety and performance of primary stenting with bare-metal balloon-expandable stents in 43 patients [158]. Technical success was achieved in 95% and the 30-day stroke rate was 7.2%, with no mortality. Angiographically confirmed recurrent stenosis greater than or equal to 50% at 6 months was seen in 18 of 51 patients (35%). The combined 1-year and procedural stroke rate was 10.9%. The SSYLVIA study revealed factors that were associated with restenosis, such as diabetes, postprocedure stenosis diameter greater than 30%, and smaller vessel caliber.

Jiang and colleagues [159] reported a 7.2% 1-year stroke risk with intracranial stenting for 126 patients who had severe intracranial atherosclerotic stenosis greater than or equal to 70%. The same investigators reported the results of another study, of 46 patients who had 50% or greater symptomatic stenosis treated with the Apollo stent (Microport Medical, Shanghai, China). Only 3 of 46 patients had a stroke within 30 days and only 1 patient had a target-lesion stroke beyond 30 days. Restenosis occurred in 28% [160]. Frietas and colleagues [161] reported an observational study of 33 patients who had greater than 50% symptomatic intracranial atherostenosis and underwent stenting with a novel balloon expandable stent (Pharos, Biotronik, AG, Bülach, Switzerland) not currently available in the United States performed in six Latin American centers. Stroke did not recur during a mean follow-up of 10.2 months, and restenosis 50% or greater was seen in only 8.7%. Technical success was achieved in 31 of 33 patients.

Because restenosis rates due to myointimal hyperplasia have been reported ranging from 10% to 40% at 6 to 12 months after intracranial stenting, some interventionalists have been prompted to use the coronary drug-eluting stents [162]. Paclitaxel, a microtubule inhibitor, and sirolimus (rapamycin), an antifungal agent, have been shown to prevent neointimal proliferation and restenosis in the coronary vasculature but have not been approved for the intracranial circulation. Therefore, the number of such stents deployed for intracranial stenosis remains too low to date to comment on performance data and safety [163,164]. In sharp contrast to earlier findings on the prevention of neointimal proliferation shown by the use of drug-eluting stents, the more recent reports of late-stent thrombosis and increased risk for myocardial infarction or even death might limit their use in the intracranial vasculature [165].

The first bare-metal self-expanding stent (Wingspan, Boston Scientific, Freeport, California) specifically designed for intracranial stenosis was approved by the Food and Drug Administration (FDA) in 2005 as a humanitarian device exemption category for patients who have 50% to 99% symptomatic intracranial stenosis and are refractory to medical therapy. The United States Wingspan stent registry enrolled 129 consecutive patients who had 70% to 99% intracranial stenosis who were treated with the Wingspan stent at 16 centers [166]. Technical success was achieved in 96.7%, with a mean residual stenosis of 20%. Within 30 days, any stroke or death occurred in 9.6%, and 4.4% of patients had a stroke in the territory of the target lesion between 30 days and 6 months of treatment. Among 52 patients who underwent repeat angiography, 25% had restenosis at a mean 4.8 months after stenting.

The procedural approach may depend on the vascular and lesional anatomy and operator experience to manipulate microwires and microcatheters across the stenotic segment. Different approaches have potential advantages and disadvantages and no consensus exists as to which is preferred. Primary stenting without predilatation is frequently feasible. Only severely stenotic and long lesions may require predilatation for safe stent placement [167].

Summary

Despite considerable progress in understanding the natural history of symptomatic intracranial atherosclerotic disease [168], our understanding of the appropriate treatment of these lesions has not progressed at the same pace. It is to be hoped that the results of recently launched and future randomized clinical trials will clarify the role of intracranial PTA and stenting.

Cervical internal carotid artery stenting

Background

Atherosclerotic cervical internal carotid artery stenosis is present in 5% to 10% of adults older than 65 [169] and can be found in up to 10% of patients who have ischemic stroke [170]. Perhaps the most widely used endovascular treatment of stroke prevention has been PTA and stenting of cervical internal carotid artery stenosis. Carotid artery stenting (CAS) was developed as a less invasive alternative to carotid endarterectomy (CEA). However, CAS failed to perform to the established standard set by CEA in earlier trials [171]. The advent of distal protection devices has been integral to reducing one of the primary procedural causes of morbidity and mortality, stroke due to distal embolization. These devices and improved stent structure and composition, such as nitinol, have renewed enthusiasm for CAS. The role of CEA for stroke prevention is discussed in detail elsewhere in this issue.

Indications and patient selection for carotid artery stenting

More recent clinical trials have helped clarify the current role of CAS. The Stenting and Angioplasty with Protection in Patients at High Risk for Endarterectomy (SAPPHIRE) trial enrolled 747 patients who had clinically significant cardiac disease, severe pulmonary disease, contralateral carotid occlusion, contralateral laryngeal palsy, previous radical neck surgery or radiation therapy, recurrent stenosis after CEA, or age older than 80 years [172]. Symptomatic patients who had greater than 50% atherosclerotic cervical internal carotid stenosis and asymptomatic patients who had greater than 80% stenosis were eligible. After review by a local multidisciplinary team at each site, 413 patients were deemed ineligible for one procedure or the other and entered into a registry (406 received CAS and 7 received CEA). The remaining 334 patients were randomized to receive CAS with distal protection using a self-expanding nitinol stent, or CEA. Technical success was achieved in 95.6% of patients assigned to CAS. The primary end point of stroke, myocardial infarction, or death within 30 days (4.4% CAS versus 9.9% CEA; $P = .06$) and ipsilateral stroke or neurologic death from 30 days to 1 year occurred in 12% of patients receiving a stent compared with 20.1% of those receiving CEA ($P = .05$), with significantly fewer procedurally related cranial nerve palsies in the stent group. The mean length of stay was 1 day shorter for the CAS group compared with the CEA group (1.84 days CAS versus 2.85 days CEA; $P = .002$). Subgroup analysis of patients enrolled on the basis of symptomatic carotid artery stenosis revealed no significant differences in the 1-year primary end point between the CAS and CEA groups. The 1-year primary end points occurred in 9.9% of asymptomatic patients receiving CAS and in 21.5% of those receiving CEA ($P = .02$).

The results of the SAPPHIRE trial have led to FDA approval of CAS with distal protection for patients who have a high risk for CEA and symptomatic cervical internal artery stenosis 50% or greater. CAS with distal protection has not yet been approved for patients who have asymptomatic stenosis because the natural history of asymptomatic SAPPHIRE-eligible patients is unknown.

The Endarterectomy Versus Angioplasty in Patients with Symptomatic Severe Carotid Stenosis (EVA-3S) study was a multicenter trial of 520 patients within 120 days of symptoms attributable to an atherosclerotic cervical internal carotid artery stenosis 60% 99% randomized to CAS or CEA [173]. Patients who had high surgical risk were excluded. Multiple stent types were used and 92% used distal protection with various available devices. The study was halted prematurely after 9.6% of patients who received CAS suffered a stroke or death by 30 days compared with 3.9% of those who received CEA ($P = .01$). However, from 30 days until the 4-year follow-up, recurrent stroke events were similar between the groups [174].

In the Stent-Protected Angioplasty versus Carotid Endarterectomy (SPACE) trial, ipsilateral stroke or death within 30 days occurred in 6.8% of 599 patients randomized to CAS and in 6.3% of 584 patients randomized to CEA [175]. At 2 years, ipsilateral stroke and periprocedural stroke or death was 9.5% in the CAS group compared with 8.8% in the CEA group (hazard ratio 1.10, CI 0.75–1.61; $P = .62$) [176]. Increasing age was found to be a significant risk factor for stroke or death within 30 days in the CAS group but not in the CEA group [177].

At present, CAS has not been proved to be superior to CEA in symptomatic patients who do not have a high risk for CEA. Additional data with technologic advances and improved operator skill are needed before CAS can be recommended as a first-line treatment in these patients.

Summary

CAS with distal protection is FDA approved for symptomatic patients at high-risk for CEA. It is not approved for asymptomatic patients and symptomatic patients who do not have a high risk for CEA. Endovascular technology continues to evolve rapidly. The disappointing results of previous trials have failed to temper enthusiasm for CAS. Results from large, ongoing, randomized trials of CAS versus CEA, such as the Carotid Revascularization Endarterectomy versus Stent Trial (CREST) [178] and the International Carotid Stenting Study (ICSS) [179], are eagerly awaited.

References

[1] Aneurysmal vasculopathy: segmental vulnerability Surgical neuroangiography. In: Lasjaurias P, ter Brugge KG, Berenstein A, editors. Berlin: Springer-Verlag; 2004. p. 375–380.
[2] Rinkel GJ, et al. Prevalence and risk of rupture of intracranial aneurysms: a systematic review. Stroke 1998;29(1):251–6.
[3] Inagawa T, Hirano A. Autopsy study of unruptured incidental intracranial aneurysms. Surg Neurol 1990;34(6):361–5.
[4] McCormick WF, Nofzinger JD. Saccular intracranial aneurysms: an autopsy study. J Neurosurg 1965;22:155–9.
[5] Atkinson JL, et al. Angiographic frequency of anterior circulation intracranial aneurysms. J Neurosurg 1989;70(4):551–5.
[6] Bederson JB, et al. Recommendations for the management of patients with unruptured intracranial aneurysms: a statement for healthcare professionals from the Stroke Council of the American Heart Association. Stroke 2000;31(11):2742–50.
[7] Ingall TJ, et al. Has there been a decline in subarachnoid hemorrhage mortality? Stroke 1989;20(6):718–24.
[8] Kassell NF, Drake CG. Timing of aneurysm surgery. Neurosurgery 1982;10(4):514–9.
[9] Mayberg MR, et al. Guidelines for the management of aneurysmal subarachnoid hemorrhage. A statement for healthcare professionals from a special writing group of the Stroke Council, American Heart Association. Circulation 1994;90(5):2592–605.

[10] Phillips LH 2nd, et al. The unchanging pattern of subarachnoid hemorrhage in a community. Neurology 1980;30(10):1034–40.
[11] van Gijn J, Rinkel GJ. Subarachnoid haemorrhage: diagnosis, causes and management. Brain 2001;124(Pt 2):249–78.
[12] Epidemiology of aneurysmal subarachnoid hemorrhage in Australia and New Zealand: incidence and case fatality from the Australasian Cooperative Research on Subarachnoid Hemorrhage Study (ACROSS). Stroke 2000;31(8):1843–50.
[13] Fann JR, et al. Physical activity and subarachnoid haemorrhage: a population based case-control study. J Neurol Neurosurg Psychiatry 2000;69(6):768–72.
[14] Anderson C, et al. Triggers of subarachnoid hemorrhage: role of physical exertion, smoking, and alcohol in the Australasian Cooperative Research on Subarachnoid Hemorrhage Study (ACROSS). Stroke 2003;34(7):1771–6.
[15] Feigin VL, et al. Risk factors for subarachnoid hemorrhage: an updated systematic review of epidemiological studies. Stroke 2005;36(12):2773–80.
[16] Bromberg JE, et al. Subarachnoid haemorrhage in first and second degree relatives of patients with subarachnoid haemorrhage. BMJ 1995;311(7000):288–9.
[17] Ronkainen A, Hernesniemi J, Ryynanen M. Familial subarachnoid hemorrhage in east Finland, 1977–1990. Neurosurgery 1993;33(5):787–96 [discussion: 796–7].
[18] Ruigrok YM, et al. Characteristics of intracranial aneurysms in patients with familial subarachnoid hemorrhage. Neurology 2004;62(6):891–4.
[19] Stegmayr B, Eriksson M, Asplund K. Declining mortality from subarachnoid hemorrhage: changes in incidence and case fatality from 1985 through 2000. Stroke 2004; 35(9):2059–63.
[20] Hop JW, et al. Case-fatality rates and functional outcome after subarachnoid hemorrhage: a systematic review. Stroke 1997;28(3):660–4.
[21] Kassell NF, Torner JC. The International Cooperative Study on Timing of Aneurysm Surgery–an update. Stroke 1984;15(3):566–70.
[22] Locksley HB. Natural history of subarachnoid hemorrhage, intracranial aneurysms and arteriovenous malformations. J Neurosurg 1966;25(3):321–68.
[23] Locksley HB. Natural history of subarachnoid hemorrhage, intracranial aneurysms and arteriovenous malformations. Based on 6368 cases in the cooperative study. J Neurosurg 1966;25(2):219–39.
[24] Suzuki J, Hori S, Sakurai Y. Intracranial aneurysms in the neurosurgical clinics in Japan. J Neurosurg 1971;35(1):34–9.
[25] Nishioka H, et al. Cooperative study of intracranial aneurysms and subarachnoid hemorrhage: a long-term prognostic study. II. Ruptured intracranial aneurysms managed conservatively. Arch Neurol 1984;41(11):1142–6.
[26] Kassell NF, Torner JC. Aneurysmal rebleeding: a preliminary report from the Cooperative Aneurysm Study. Neurosurgery 1983;13(5):479–81.
[27] Jane JA, Winn HR, Richardson AE. The natural history of intracranial aneurysms: rebleeding rates during the acute and long term period and implication for surgical management. Clin Neurosurg 1977;24:176–84.
[28] Guglielmi G, et al. Electrothrombosis of saccular aneurysms via endovascular approach. Part 2: preliminary clinical experience. J Neurosurg 1991;75(1):8–14.
[29] Guglielmi G, et al. Electrothrombosis of saccular aneurysms via endovascular approach. Part 1: electrochemical basis, technique, and experimental results. J Neurosurg 1991; 75(1):1–7.
[30] Unruptured intracranial aneurysms–risk of rupture and risks of surgical intervention. International Study of Unruptured Intracranial Aneurysms Investigators. N Engl J Med 1998;339(24):1725–33.
[31] Aletich VA, et al. The remodeling technique of balloon-assisted Guglielmi detachable coil placement in wide-necked aneurysms: experience at the University of Illinois at Chicago. J Neurosurg 2000;93(3):388–96.

[32] Ausman JI. The New England Journal of Medicine report on unruptured intracranial aneurysms: a critique. Surg Neurol 1999;51(2):227–9.
[33] Barker FG 2nd, et al. Age-dependent differences in short-term outcome after surgical or endovascular treatment of unruptured intracranial aneurysms in the United States, 1996–2000. Neurosurgery 2004;54(1):18–28 [discussion: 28–30].
[34] Barker FG 2nd, et al. In-hospital mortality and morbidity after surgical treatment of unruptured intracranial aneurysms in the United States, 1996–2000: the effect of hospital and surgeon volume. Neurosurgery 2003;52(5):995–1007 [discussion: 1007–9].
[35] Barrow DL. Bad science ISAT: the impact on neurosurgical practice. Clin Neurosurg 2004; 51:126–31.
[36] Cross DT 3rd, et al. Mortality rates after subarachnoid hemorrhage: variations according to hospital case volume in 18 states. J Neurosurg 2003;99(5):810–7.
[37] Dickey P, Kailasnath P. The diameter-cube hypothesis: a new biophysical model of aneurysm rupture. Surg Neurol 2002;58(3–4):166–73 [discussion: 173–80].
[38] Dippel DW, Habbema JD. Natural history of unruptured aneurysms. J Neurosurg 1994; 80(4):772–4.
[39] Diringer MN. To clip or to coil acutely ruptured intracranial aneurysms: update on the debate. Curr Opin Crit Care 2005;11(2):121–5.
[40] Hoh BL, et al. In-hospital morbidity and mortality after endovascular treatment of unruptured intracranial aneurysms in the United States, 1996–2000: effect of hospital and physician volume. AJNR Am J Neuroradiol 2003;24(7):1409–20.
[41] Juvela S, Porras M, Heiskanen O. Natural history of unruptured intracranial aneurysms: a long-term follow-up study. J Neurosurg 1993;79(2):174–82.
[42] Juvela S, Porras M, Poussa K. Natural history of unruptured intracranial aneurysms: probability of and risk factors for aneurysm rupture. J Neurosurg 2000;93(3):379–87.
[43] Molyneux A, et al. International Subarachnoid Aneurysm Trial (ISAT) of neurosurgical clipping versus endovascular coiling in 2143 patients with ruptured intracranial aneurysms: a randomised trial. Lancet 2002;360(9342):1267–74.
[44] Molyneux AJ, et al. International Subarachnoid Aneurysm Trial (ISAT) of neurosurgical clipping versus endovascular coiling in 2143 patients with ruptured intracranial aneurysms: a randomised comparison of effects on survival, dependency, seizures, rebleeding, subgroups, and aneurysm occlusion. Lancet 2005;366(9488):809–17.
[45] Nakagawa T, Hashi K. The incidence and treatment of asymptomatic, unruptured cerebral aneurysms. J Neurosurg 1994;80(2):217–23.
[46] Tomasello F, et al. Asymptomatic aneurysms. Literature meta-analysis and indications for treatment. J Neurosurg Sci 1998;42(1 Suppl 1):47–51.
[47] Ujiie H, et al. Clinical analysis of incidentally discovered unruptured aneurysms. Stroke 1993;24(12):1850–6.
[48] van der Schaaf I, et al. Endovascular coiling versus neurosurgical clipping for patients with aneurysmal subarachnoid haemorrhage. Cochrane Database Syst Rev 2005;(4):CD003085.
[49] van der Schaaf IC, et al. Quality of life, anxiety, and depression in patients with an untreated intracranial aneurysm or arteriovenous malformation. Stroke 2002;33(2):440–3.
[50] Wiebers DO, et al. Unruptured intracranial aneurysms: natural history, clinical outcome, and risks of surgical and endovascular treatment. Lancet 2003;362(9378):103–10.
[51] Winn HR, et al. Prevalence of asymptomatic incidental aneurysms: review of 4568 arteriograms. J Neurosurg 2002;96(1):43–9.
[52] Winn HR, Richardson AE, Jane JA. The long-term prognosis in untreated cerebral aneurysms: I. The incidence of late hemorrhage in cerebral aneurysm: a 10-year evaluation of 364 patients. Ann Neurol 1977;1(4):358–70.
[53] Yasui N, et al. Long-term follow-up study of unruptured intracranial aneurysms. Neurosurgery 1997;40(6):1155–9 [discussion: 1159–60].

[54] Butteriss D, et al. Single-center experience of cerecyte coils in the treatment of intracranial aneurysms: initial experience and early follow-up results. AJNR Am J Neuroradiol 2008;29(1):53–6.

[55] Cloft HJ. HydroCoil for Endovascular Aneurysm Occlusion (HEAL) study: 3–6 month angiographic follow-up results. AJNR Am J Neuroradiol 2007;28(1):152–4.

[56] White PM, et al. HydroCoil Endovascular Aneurysm Occlusion and Packing Study (HELPS trial): procedural safety and operator-assessed efficacy results. AJNR Am J Neuroradiol 2008;29(2):217–23.

[57] Debrun GM, et al. Selection of cerebral aneurysms for treatment using Guglielmi detachable coils: the preliminary University of Illinois at Chicago experience. Neurosurgery 1998;43(6):1281–95 [discussion: 1296–7].

[58] Moret J, et al. [Reconstruction technique in the treatment of wide-neck intracranial aneurysms. Long-term angiographic and clinical results. Apropos of 56 cases]). J Neuroradiol 1997;24(1):30–44.

[59] Spelle L, et al. Saccular intracranial aneurysms: endovascular treatment - devices, techniques and strategies, management of complications, results. Neuroimaging Clin N Am 2006;16(3):413–51, viii.

[60] Lefkowitz MA, et al. Balloon-assisted Guglielmi detachable coiling of wide-necked aneurysms: Part II–clinical results. Neurosurgery 1999;45(3):531–7 [discussion: 537–8].

[61] Malek AM, et al. Balloon-assist technique for endovascular coil embolization of geometrically difficult intracranial aneurysms. Neurosurgery 2000;46(6):1397–406 [discussion: 1406–7].

[62] Nelson PK, Levy DI. Balloon-assisted coil embolization of wide-necked aneurysms of the internal carotid artery: medium-term angiographic and clinical follow-up in 22 patients. AJNR Am J Neuroradiol 2001;22(1):19–26.

[63] Canton G, et al. Flow changes caused by the sequential placement of stents across the neck of sidewall cerebral aneurysms. J Neurosurg 2005;103(5):891–902.

[64] Horowitz MB, Purdy PD. The use of stents in the management of neurovascular disease: a review of historical and present status. Neurosurgery 2000;46(6):1335–42 [discussion: 1342–3].

[65] Fiorella D, et al. Preliminary experience using the Neuroform stent for the treatment of cerebral aneurysms. Neurosurgery 2004;54(1):6–16 [discussion: 16–7].

[66] Lubicz B, et al. Retractable self-expandable stent for endovascular treatment of wide-necked intracranial aneurysms: preliminary experience. Neurosurgery 2006;58(3):451–7 [discussion: 451–7].

[67] Saatci I, et al. Treatment of internal carotid artery aneurysms with a covered stent: experience in 24 patients with mid-term follow-up results. AJNR Am J Neuroradiol 2004;25(10):1742–9.

[68] Li MH, et al. A new covered stent designed for intracranial vasculature: application in the management of pseudoaneurysms of the cranial internal carotid artery. AJNR Am J Neuroradiol 2007;28(8):1579–85.

[69] Struffert T, et al. Onyx in an experimental aneurysm model: histological and angiographic results. J Neurosurg 2008;109(1):77–82.

[70] Cekirge HS, et al. Late angiographic and clinical follow-up results of 100 consecutive aneurysms treated with Onyx reconstruction: largest single-center experience. Neuroradiology 2006;48(2):113–26.

[71] Cekirge HS, et al. Intrasaccular combination of metallic coils and onyx liquid embolic agent for the endovascular treatment of cerebral aneurysms. J Neurosurg 2006;105(5):706–12.

[72] Leon MB, et al. A clinical trial comparing three antithrombotic-drug regimens after coronary-artery stenting. Stent Anticoagulation Restenosis Study Investigators. N Engl J Med 1998;339(23):1665–71.

[73] Byrne JV, et al. Five-year experience in using coil embolization for ruptured intracranial aneurysms: outcomes and incidence of late rebleeding. J Neurosurg 1999;90(4):656–63.

[74] Murayama Y, et al. Guglielmi detachable coil embolization of cerebral aneurysms: 11 years' experience. J Neurosurg 2003;98(5):959–66.

[75] Vinuela F, Duckwiler G, Mawad M. Guglielmi detachable coil embolization of acute intracranial aneurysm: perioperative anatomical and clinical outcome in 403 patients. J Neurosurg 1997;86(3):475–82.

[76] CARAT Investigators. Rates of delayed rebleeding from intracranial aneurysms are low after surgical and endovascular treatment. Stroke 2006;37(6):1437–42.

[77] Cognard C, et al. Long-term angiographic follow-up of 169 intracranial berry aneurysms occluded with detachable coils. Radiology 1999;212(2):348–56.

[78] Gallas S, et al. A multicenter study of 705 ruptured intracranial aneurysms treated with Guglielmi detachable coils. AJNR Am J Neuroradiol 2005;26(7):1723–31.

[79] Johnston SC, et al. Predictors of rehemorrhage after treatment of ruptured intracranial aneurysms: the Cerebral Aneurysm Rerupture After Treatment (CARAT) study. Stroke 2008;39(1):120–5.

[80] Raymond J, et al. Long-term angiographic recurrences after selective endovascular treatment of aneurysms with detachable coils. Stroke 2003;34(6):1398–403.

[81] Rivet DJ, et al. Single-institution experience with matrix coils in the treatment of intracranial aneurysms: comparison with same-center outcomes with the use of platinum coils. AJNR Am J Neuroradiol 2007;28(9):1736–42.

[82] Sluzewski M, et al. Late rebleeding of ruptured intracranial aneurysms treated with detachable coils. AJNR Am J Neuroradiol 2005;26(10):2542–9.

[83] Thornton J, et al. What percentage of surgically clipped intracranial aneurysms have residual necks? Neurosurgery 2000;46(6):1294–8 [discussion: 1298–300].

[84] Thornton J, et al. Follow-up angiography of intracranial aneurysms treated with endovascular placement of Guglielmi detachable coils. Neurosurgery 2002;50(2):239–49 [discussion: 249–50].

[85] Marotta TR, et al. A novel endovascular clip system for the treatment of intracranial aneurysms: technology, concept, and initial experimental results. Laboratory investigation. J Neurosurg 2008;108(6):1230–40.

[86] Marin-Padilla M. Embryology. In: Yasargil MG, editor. Microneurosurgery, vol 3ANew York: Thieme; 1987. p. 23–47.

[87] Al-Shahi R, Warlow C. A systematic review of the frequency and prognosis of arteriovenous malformations of the brain in adults. Brain 2001;124(Pt 10):1900–26.

[88] Choi JH, Mohr JP. Brain arteriovenous malformations in adults. Lancet Neurol 2005;4: 299–308.

[89] Stapf C, Mast H, Sciacca RR, et al, New York Islands AVM Study Collaborators. The New York Islands AVM Study: design, study progress, and initial results. Stroke 2003;34(5): e29–33.

[90] Ondra SL, Troupp H, George ED, et al. The natural history of symptomatic arteriovenous malformations of the brain: a 24 year follow up assessment. J Neurosurg 1990;73:387–91.

[91] Stapf C, Mast H, Sciacca RR, et al. Predictors of hemorrhage in patients with untreated brain arteriovenous malformation. Neurology 2006;66(9):1350–5.

[92] Stapf C, Mohr JP. Unruptured brain arteriovenous malformations should be treated conservatively: yes. Stroke 2007;38(12):3308–9.

[93] Gobin YP, Laurent A, Merienne L, et al. Treatment of brain arteriovenous malformations by embolization and radiosurgery. J Neurosurg 1996;85(1):19–28.

[94] Izawa M, Chernov M, Hayashi M, et al. Combined management of intracranial arteriovenous malformations with embolization and Gamma Knife radiosurgery: comparative evaluation of the long-term results. Surg Neurol. 2008 Feb 19 [Epub ahead of print].

[95] Katsaridis V, Papagiannaki C, Aimar E. Curative embolization of cerebral arteriovenous malformations (AVMs) with Onyx in 101 patients. Neuroradiology 2008;50(7):589–97.

[96] Aletich VA, Debrun G, Charbel F, Ausman J. Incidence and endovascular approach to BAVMs with associated true intranidal fistulas, associated aneurysms, and venous outflow

anomalies. Abstract Presented at the Joint Meeting of the AANS/CNS Section on Cerebrovascular Surgery & American Society of Interventional and Therapeutic Neuroradiology Nashville TN, Jan 31-Feb 3 1999.
[97] Weigele John B, Robert Hurst W, et al. Endovascular management of brain arteriovenous malformations. Interventional neuroradiology. In: Rosenwasser Robert H, editor. New York: Informa Healthcare; 2007.
[98] Sorimachi T, Koike T, Takeuchi S, et al. Embolization of cerebral arteriovenous malformations achieved with polyvinyl alcohol particles: angiographic reappearance and complications. AJNR Am J Neuroradiol. 1999;20(7):1323–8.
[99] Dehdashti AR, Muster M, Reverdin A, et al. Preoperative silk suture embolization of cerebral and dural arteriovenous malformations. Neurosurg Focus. 2001;11(5):e6.
[100] Deruty R, Pelissou-Guyotat I, Mottolese C, et al. The combined management of cerebral arteriovenous malformations. Experience with 100 cases and review of the literature. Acta Neurochir (Wien) 1993;123:101–12.
[101] Duong H, Tampieri D, TerBrugge KG, et al. Transcranial Doppler ultrasonographic changes after embolization of cerebral arteriovenous malformations. Can Assoc Radiol J 1994;45:447–51.
[102] Fournier D, TerBrugge KG, Willinsky R, et al. Endovascular treatment of intracerebral arteriovenous malformations: experience in 49 cases. J Neurosurg 1991;75:228–33.
[103] Aj Pelz DM, Lee DH. Arteriovenous malformations of the brain: recent results of endovascular therapy. Radiology 1990;177:51–7.
[104] Wikholm G. Occlusion of cerebral arteriovenous malformations with N-butyl cyanoacrylate is permanent. AJNR Am J Neuroradiol. 1995;16(3):479–82.
[105] Komotar RJ, Ransom ER, Wilson DA, et al. 2-Hexyl cyanoacrylate (neuracryl M) embolization of cerebral arteriovenous malformations. Neurosurgery 2006;59.
[106] Arakawa H, Murayama Y, Davis CR, et al. Endovascular embolization of the swine rete mirabile with Eudragit-E 100 polymer. AJNR Am J Neuroradiol. 2007;28(6): 1191–6.
[107] Klisch J, Yin L, Requejo F, et al. Liquid 2-poly-hydroxyethyl-methacrylate embolization of experimental arteriovenous malformations: feasibility study. AJNR Am J Neuroradiol. 2002;23(3):422–9.
[108] Brothers MF, Kaufmann JCE, Fox AJ, et al. N-butyl 2-cyanoacrylate - substitute for IBCA in interventional neuroradiology: histopathologic and polymerization time study. AJNR Am J Neuroradiol 1989;10:777–86.
[109] Yu SC, Chan MS, Lam JM, et al. Complete obliteration of intracranial arteriovenous malformation with endovascular cyanoacrylate embolization: initial success and rate of permanent cure. AJNR Am J Neuroradiol 2004;25(7):1139–43.
[110] Chaloupka JC, Viñuela F, Vinters HV, et al. Technical feasibility and histopathologic studies of ethylene vinyl copolymer (EVAL) using a swine endovascular embolization model. AJNR Am J Neuroradiol. 1994;15(6):1107–15.
[111] Murayama Y, Viñuela F, Ulhoa A, et al. Nonadhesive liquid embolic agent for cerebral arteriovenous malformations: preliminary histopathological studies in swine rete mirabile. Neurosurgery 1998;43(5):1164–75.
[112] Taki W, Yonekawa Y, Iwata H, et al. A new liquid material for embolization of arteriovenous malformations. AJNR Am J Neuroradiol. 1990;11(1):163–8.
[113] van Rooij WJ, Sluzewski M, Beute GN. Brain AVM embolization with Onyx. AJNR Am J Neuroradiol. 2007;28(1):172–7.
[114] Weber W, Kis B, Siekmann R, et al. Preoperative embolization of intracranial arteriovenous malformations with Onyx. Neurosurgery 2007;61(2):244–52.
[115] Hurst RW, Berenstein A, Kupersmith MJ, et al. Deep central arteriovenous malformations of the brain: the role of endovascular treatment. J Neurosurg 1995;82:190–5.
[116] Debrun GM, Aletich V, Ausman JI, et al. Embolization of the nidus of brain arteriovenous malformations with N-butyl-cyanoacrylate. Neurosurgery 1997;40(1):112–20.

[117] Aletich VA, Debrun GM, Koenigsberg R, et al. AVM nidus catheterization with the Terumo 0.010 hydrophilic wire and Balt magic catheter: a technical report. AJNR 1997; Vol 18:929–35.

[118] Berthelsen B, Lofgren J, Svendsen P. Embolization of cerebral arteriovenous malformations with bucrylate: experience in a first series of 29 patients. Acta Radiol 1990;31:13–21.

[119] Dion JE, Duckwiler GR, Lylyk P, et al. Progressive Suppleness Pursil Catheter: a new tool for superselective angiography and embolization. AJNR Am J Neuroradiol 1989;10: 1068–70.

[120] Dion JE, Mathis JM. Cranial arteriovenous malformations. The role of embolization and stereotactic surgery. Neurosurg Clin N Am 1994;5:459–74.

[121] Duckwiler GR, Dion JE, Vinuela F, et al. Delayed venous occlusion following embolotherapy of vascular malformations in the brain. AJNR Am J Neuroradiol 1992;13:1571–9.

[122] Fournier D, Ter Brugge K, Rodesch G, et al. Revascularization of brain arteriovenous malformations after embolization with bucrylate. AJNR Am J Neuroradiol 1990;32:497–501.

[123] Chaloupka JC, Vinuela F, Robert J, et al. An in vivo arteriovenous malformation model in swine: preliminary feasibility and natural history study. AJNR Am J Neuroradiol 1994;15: 945–50.

[124] Ezura M, Takahashi A, Yoshimoto T. Successful treatment of an arteriovenous malformation by chemical embolization with estrogen followed by conventional radiotherapy. Neurosurgery 1992;31:1105–7 [discussion: 1107].

[125] Germano IM, Davis RL, Wilson CB, et al. Histopathological follow-up study of 66 cerebral arteriovenous malformations after therapeutic embolization with polyvinyl alcohol. J Neurosurg 1992;76:607–14.

[126] Kline JN, Ryals TJ, Galvin JR, et al. Pulmonary embolization and infarction. An iatrogenic complication of transcatheter embolization of a cerebral arteriovenous malformation with polyvinyl alcohol sponge. Chest 1993;103:1293–5.

[127] Pelz DM, Lownie SP, Fox AJ, et al. Symptomatic pulmonary complications from liquid acrylate embolization of brain arteriovenous malformations. AJNR Am J Neuroradiol 1995;16:19–26.

[128] Jayaraman MV, Marcellus ML, Hamilton S, et al. Neurologic complications of arteriovenous malformation embolization using liquid embolic agents. AJNR Am J Neuroradiol. 2008;29(2):242–6.

[129] Klijn CJ, et al. Outcome in patients with symptomatic occlusion of the internal carotid artery or intracranial arterial lesions: a meta-analysis of the role of baseline characteristics and type of antithrombotic treatment. Cerebrovasc Dis 2001;12(3):228–34.

[130] Wong KS, Li H. Long-term mortality and recurrent stroke risk among Chinese stroke patients with predominant intracranial atherosclerosis. Stroke 2003;34(10):2361–6.

[131] Thijs VN, Albers GW. Symptomatic intracranial atherosclerosis: outcome of patients who fail antithrombotic therapy. Neurology 2000;55(4):490–7.

[132] Akins PT, et al. Natural history of stenosis from intracranial atherosclerosis by serial angiography. Stroke 1998;29(2):433–8.

[133] Moufarrij NA, et al. Basilar and distal vertebral artery stenosis: long-term follow-up. Stroke 1986;17(5):938–42.

[134] Qureshi AI, et al. Stroke-free survival and its determinants in patients with symptomatic vertebrobasilar stenosis: a multicenter study. Neurosurgery 2003;52(5):1033–9 [discussion: 1039–40].

[135] Mazighi M, et al. Prospective study of symptomatic atherothrombotic intracranial stenoses: the GESICA study. Neurology 2006;66(8):1187–91.

[136] Kasner SE, et al. Warfarin vs aspirin for symptomatic intracranial stenosis: subgroup analyses from WASID. Neurology 2006;67(7):1275–8.

[137] Kim JK, et al. Elective stenting for symptomatic middle cerebral artery stenosis presenting as transient ischaemic deficits or stroke attacks: short term arteriographical and clinical outcome. J Neurol Neurosurg Psychiatry 2004;75(6):847–51.

[138] Derdeyn CP, Chimowitz MI. Angioplasty and stenting for atherosclerotic intracranial stenosis: rationale for a randomized clinical trial. Neuroimaging Clin N Am 2007;17(3): 355–63, viii-ix.

[139] Al-Mubarak N, et al. Stenting of symptomatic stenosis of the intracranial internal carotid artery. AJNR Am J Neuroradiol 1998;19(10):1949–51.

[140] Mori T, Kazita K, Mori K. Cerebral angioplasty and stenting for intracranial vertebral atherosclerotic stenosis. AJNR Am J Neuroradiol 1999;20(5):787–9.

[141] Sundt TM Jr, et al. Transluminal angioplasty for basilar artery stenosis. Mayo Clin Proc 1980;55(11):673–80.

[142] Alazzaz A, et al. Intracranial percutaneous transluminal angioplasty for arteriosclerotic stenosis. Arch Neurol 2000;57(11):1625–30.

[143] Connors JJ 3rd, Wojak JC. Percutaneous transluminal angioplasty for intracranial atherosclerotic lesions: evolution of technique and short-term results. J Neurosurg 1999;91(3): 415–23.

[144] Jiang WJ, et al. Stenting of symptomatic M1 stenosis of middle cerebral artery: an initial experience of 40 patients. Stroke 2004;35(6):1375–80.

[145] Levy EI, et al. Comparison of periprocedure complications resulting from direct stent placement compared with those due to conventional and staged stent placement in the basilar artery. J Neurosurg 2003;99(4):653–60.

[146] Marks MP, et al. Angioplasty for symptomatic intracranial stenosis: clinical outcome. Stroke 2006;37(4):1016–20.

[147] Takis C, et al. Intracranial angioplasty: experience and complications. AJNR Am J Neuroradiol 1997;18(9):1661–8.

[148] Samuels OB, et al. A standardized method for measuring intracranial arterial stenosis. AJNR Am J Neuroradiol 2000;21(4):643–6.

[149] Mori T, et al. Percutaneous transluminal cerebral angioplasty: serial angiographic follow-up after successful dilatation. Neuroradiology 1997;39(2):111–6.

[150] Clark WM, et al. Safety and efficacy of percutaneous transluminal angioplasty for intracranial atherosclerotic stenosis. Stroke 1995;26(7):1200–4.

[151] Gress DR, et al. Angioplasty for intracranial symptomatic vertebrobasilar ischemia-Neurosurgery 2002;51(1):23–7 [discussion: 27–9].

[152] Gupta R, et al. Urgent endovascular revascularization for symptomatic intracranial atherosclerotic stenosis. Neurology 2003;61(12):1729–35.

[153] Higashida RT, et al. Transluminal angioplasty for atherosclerotic disease of the vertebral and basilar arteries. J Neurosurg 1993;78(2):192–8.

[154] Marks MP, et al. Outcome of angioplasty for atherosclerotic intracranial stenosis. Stroke 1999;30(5):1065–9.

[155] Nahser HC, et al. Intracranial vertebrobasilar stenosis: angioplasty and follow-up. AJNR Am J Neuroradiol 2000;21(7):1293–301.

[156] Mori T, et al. Follow-up study after intracranial percutaneous transluminal cerebral balloon angioplasty. AJNR Am J Neuroradiol 1998;19(8):1525–33.

[157] Dorland's illustrated medical dictionary. 28th edition. Philadelphia: WB Saunders Co.; 1994.

[158] Stenting of Symptomatic Atherosclerotic Lesions in the Vertebral or Intracranial Arteries (SSYLVIA): study results. Stroke 2004;35(6):1388–92.

[159] Jiang WJ, et al. Comparison of elective stenting of severe vs moderate intracranial atherosclerotic stenosis. Neurology 2007;68(6):420–6.

[160] Jiang WJ, et al. Apollo stent for symptomatic atherosclerotic intracranial stenosis: study results. AJNR Am J Neuroradiol 2007;28(5):830–4.

[161] Freitas JM, et al. Intracranial arterial stenting for symptomatic stenoses: a Latin American experience. Surg Neurol 2007;68(4):378–86.

[162] Stone GW, et al. A polymer-based, paclitaxel-eluting stent in patients with coronary artery disease. N Engl J Med 2004;350(3):221–31.

[163] Abou-Chebl A, Bashir Q, Yadav JS. Drug-eluting stents for the treatment of intracranial atherosclerosis: initial experience and midterm angiographic follow-up. Stroke 2005; 36(12):e165–8.

[164] Gupta R, et al. Safety, feasibility, and short-term follow-up of drug-eluting stent placement in the intracranial and extracranial circulation. Stroke 2006;37(10):2562–6.

[165] Iakovou I, et al. Incidence, predictors, and outcome of thrombosis after successful implantation of drug-eluting stents. JAMA 2005;293(17):2126–30.

[166] Zaidat OO, Klucznik R, Alexander MJ, et al. The NIH registry on use of the Wingspan stent for symptomatic 70–99% intracranial stenosis. Neurology 2008;70:1518–24.

[167] Lylyk P, et al. Endovascular reconstruction by means of stent placement in symptomatic intracranial atherosclerotic stenosis. Neurol Res 2005;27(Suppl 1):S84–8.

[168] Chimowitz MI, et al. Comparison of warfarin and aspirin for symptomatic intracranial arterial stenosis. N Engl J Med 2005;352(13):1305–16.

[169] Fine-Edelstein JS, et al. Precursors of extracranial carotid atherosclerosis in the Framingham study. Neurology 1994;44(6):1046–50.

[170] Lovett JK, Coull A, Rothwell PM. Early risk of recurrence by subtype of ischemic stroke in population-based incidence studies. Neurology 2004;62(4):569–73.

[171] Coward LJ, Feaherstone RL, Brown MM, et al. Safety and efficacy of endovascular treatment of carotid artery stenosis compared with carotid endarterectomy: a Cochrane systematic review of the randomized evidence. Stroke 2005;36:905–11.

[172] Yadav JS, Wholey MH, Kuntz RE, et al. Protected carotid-artery stenting versus endarterectomy in high-risk patients. N Engl J Med 2004;351:1493–501.

[173] Mas JL, Chatellier G, Beyssen B, et al. Endarterectomy versus stenting in patients with symptomatic severe carotid stenosis. N Engl J Med 2006;355:1660–71.

[174] Mas JL, Trinquart L, Leys D, et al. Endarterectomy versus angioplasty in patients with symptomatic severe stenosis (EVA 3S) trial: results up to 4 years from a randomised, multicentre trial. Lancet Neurol 2008;7:885–92.

[175] The SPACE Collaborative Group. 30-day results from the SPACE trial of stent-protected angioplasty versus carotid endarterectomy in symptomatic patients: a randomised, non-inferiority trial. Lancet 2006;368:1239–47.

[176] Eckstein HH, Ringleb P, Allenburg JR, et al. Results of the Stent-protected Angioplasty Versus Carotid Endarterectomy (SPACE) study to treat symptomatic stenosis at 2 years: a multinational, prospective, randomised trial. Lancet Neurol 2008;7:893–902.

[177] Stingele R, Burger J, Alfke K, et al. Clinical and angiographic risk factors for stroke and death within 30 days after carotid endarterectomy and stent-protected angioplasty: a subanalysis of the SPACE study. Lancet Neurol 2008;7:216–22.

[178] Carotid Revascularization Endarterectomy versus Stenting Trial. Available at: www.clinicaltrials.gov.

[179] Featherstone RL, Brown MM, Coward LJ, et al. The international carotid stenting study: protocol for a randomised clinical trial comparing carotid stenting with endarterectomy in symptomatic carotid artery stenosis. Cerebrovasc Dis 2004;18(1):69–74.

ELSEVIER
SAUNDERS

Neurol Clin 26 (2008) 1129–1160

NEUROLOGIC
CLINICS

Stroke Prevention in Atrial Fibrillation and Other Major Cardiac Sources of Embolism

William D. Freeman, MD[a,*], Maria I. Aguilar, MD[b]

[a]*Departments of Neurology and Critical Care, Mayo Clinic, Cannaday 2 East, 4500 San Pablo Road, Jacksonville, FL 32224, USA*
[b]*Department of Neurology, Mayo Clinic, 5777 East Mayo Boulevard, Phoenix, AZ 85054, USA*

Cardiac embolism and stroke

Cardioembolic stroke accounts for 20% of all ischemic strokes [1], and its frequency has increased over time, likely reflecting improvement in cardiac imaging [2]. Cardioembolic stroke can be caused by different cardiac disorders, but occurs most commonly from atrial fibrillation in adults (50%) (Fig. 1) [2–4]. Other important causes include ventricular thrombus (20%), structural heart defects or tumors (15%) and valvular heart disease (15%) (Table 1) [4–7]. Although the aortic arch is not a cardiac structure, it is usually considered under sources of cardiac embolism and is reviewed in this article.

Cardioembolic stroke is therefore a syndrome with diverse causes and not a single disease entity. A systematic approach, including a detailed history, physical examination, and review of neuroimaging, ECG, and echocardiographic data, may disclose the cause of cardioembolic stroke. However, echocardiography sometimes fails to disclose the cardioembolic source despite a suggestive history (eg, palpitations or valsalva before stroke). The authors endorse the diagnostic approach recommended in the American Heart Association (AHA) ischemic stroke guidelines, but also describe newer diagnostic approaches in cardioembolic stroke patients who have negative echocardiograms [8,9].

Dr. Freeman acknowledges research funding provided in part by the Robert H. and Clarice Smith/M.L. Simpson Foundation Trust. Dr. Aguilar chairs the Event Adjudication Committee for the NINDS-sponsored SPS3 trial.

* Corresponding author.
E-mail address: freeman.william1@mayo.edu (W.D. Freeman).

doi:10.1016/j.ncl.2008.07.001 *neurologic.theclinics.com*

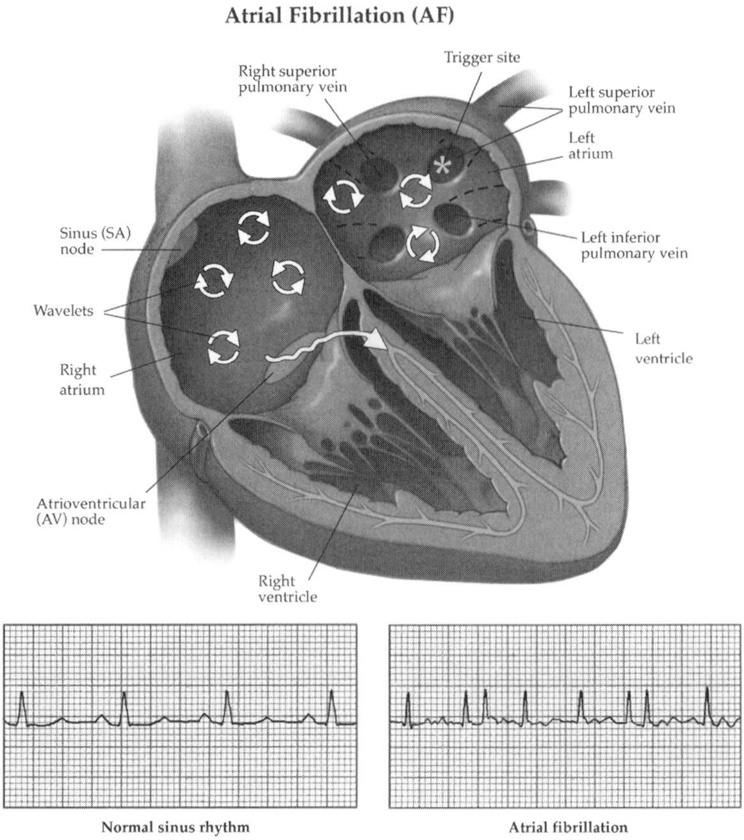

Fig. 1. Atrial fibrillation. Diagram depicts the abnormal electrical activity within the atria, which may lead to uncoordinated contraction of the atria, stagnant blood, and thrombus formation, and an irregular heart rhythm. (*Courtesy of* the Mayo Clinic and Foundation for Medical Education and Research, Rochester, MN; with permission.)

Overall, cardiac embolism as the cause of stroke is diagnosed in the absence of a large artery stenosis or occlusion, a clinical syndrome or radiographic appearance of a lacunar stroke, and unusual causes of stroke (eg, vasculitis, drug abuse). However, approximately 15% of patients who have lacunar syndromes would also have risk factors for cardioembolism [10,11]. The stroke mechanism (defined by the standard stroke evaluation) dictates optimal intervention and preventative strategies, which are discussed.

Diagnostic approach to cardioembolic stroke

A systematic approach is fundamental to diagnose patients who have experienced cardioembolic stroke. For example, the clinical history may

Table 1
Major etiologies of cardioembolic stroke

Cause of cardioembolism	Cardioembolic stroke (%)
Atrial fibrillation (see Fig. 1)	50 [2–4,29,31–43]
Ventricular thrombus	20 [76–80]
Congestive heart failure/cardiomyopathy	—
Myocardial infarction	—
Structural heart defects or tumors	15 [5–7]
Patent foramen ovale, ventricular septal defect, atrial septal defect or aneurysm, atrial myxoma, fibroelastoma	[6,28]
Valvular heart disease	15 [100–107,111–117,122]
Prosthetic valves, rheumatic mitral or aortic valve disease, endocarditis vegetations, noninfectious endocarditis vegetations, aortic stenosis (calcific disease), mitral valve disease (myxomatous prolapse or calcific annulus)	—

provide clues to a cardioembolic source. Patients may have a history of palpitations (eg, mitral valve disease, atrial fibrillation), episodic or sustained tachycardia (eg, arrhythmia or atrial fibrillation with rapid ventricular response), angina or dyspnea (eg, myocardial infarction or heart failure), or stroke symptoms after valsalva (eg, cough, sneeze, bowel movement), which may suggest an intracardiac shunt or other possible source of embolism (eg, large patent foramen ovale with atrial septal aneurysm).

Onset of cardioembolic stroke is typically sudden and involves a large intracranial artery territory (eg, 3-mm arterial diameter in the middle cerebral artery [12] M1 segment) with corresponding major or minor clinical deficits. Nonsudden onset may occur, however, with progressive or stuttering neurologic deficit pattern, which has been posited to represent migration of embolism to more distal arterial channels [13,14].

Although the clinical presentation of cardioembolic stroke is considered typical, neurologic features are insufficiently predictive to establish the stroke mechanism, and neuroimaging and cardiac studies are needed to confirm diagnosis. Transient ischemic attacks (TIAs) are less frequent predecessors of cardioembolic stroke than stroke because of large-vessel atherosclerosis [15]. Sudden onset of neurologic symptoms has low specificity for cardioembolism, because this also occurs as a result of other mechanisms in most (>60%) stroke cases [15,16]. Rapid improvement of neurologic deficit [13], maximal deficit from onset [15,17], simultaneous strokes in different vascular territories (Fig. 2), hemorrhagic transformation of an ischemic infarct (Fig. 3), and early arterial recanalization may suggest a cardiac source of embolism [18].

A cardiovascular examination, along with cardiac enzyme tests (eg, creatine kinase, the myocardial isoform of creatine kinase, or troponin), and 12-lead ECG should then be performed in all stroke patients [19]. Other blood

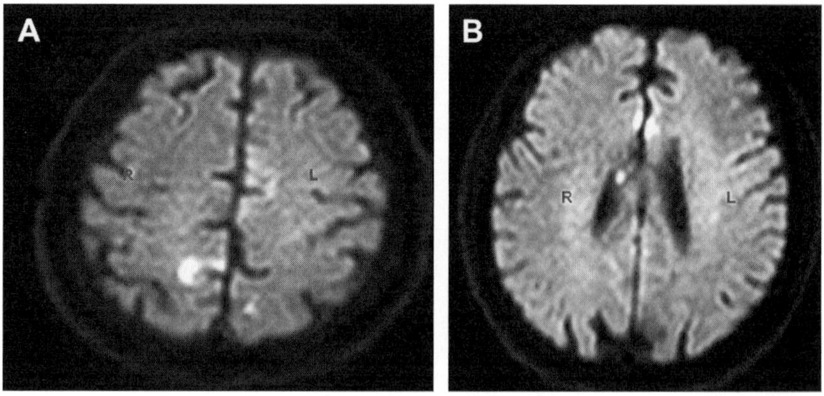

Fig. 2. Simultaneous acute ischemic strokes in different vascular territories. Diffusion-weighted imaging restriction at right parasagittal parietal cortex (*A*) and the frontal parasagittal cortex bilaterally (*B*) in a 64-year-old man presenting with bilateral leg weakness. He was found to have paroxysmal atrial fibrillation and nonischemic dilated cardiomyopathy. R, right; L, left.

work obtained at admission includes a complete blood cell count (CBC) with platelets, prothrombin time (PT), and activated thromboplastin time (aPTT). Young patients who experience cardioembolic events may require a prothrombotic workup for GP20210 (prothrombin gene) mutation, factor

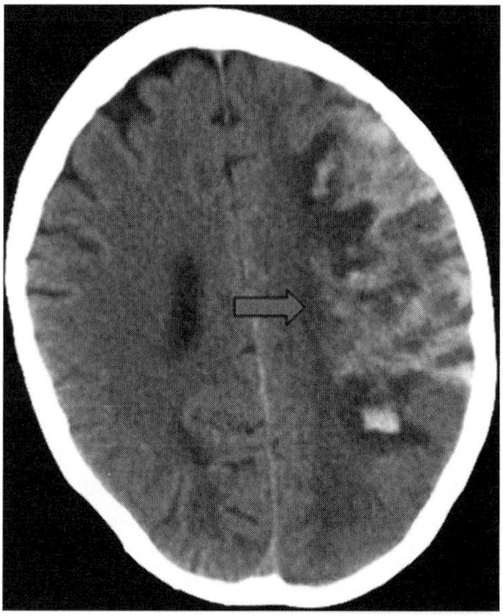

Fig. 3. Hemorrhagic transformation of an ischemic stroke. CT head study showing hemorrhagic transformation of an ischemic stroke (*arrows*) affecting the left middle cerebellar artery territory. This patient presented 10 hours after the onset of right-sided hemiparesis and did not undergo thrombolytic therapy. She also had an acute myocardial infarction with anterior wall hypokinesis and depressed ejection fraction (12%).

V Leiden mutation, protein C or S deficiency, antithrombin III deficiency, antiphospholipid antibodies, or lupus anticoagulant. Deep venous thrombosis (DVT) screening with lower extremity Doppler ultrasound should be considered when paradoxical embolism and cryptogenic stroke are suspected. Other considerations include air and fat emboli syndromes, and insoluble material injected intravenously by street-drug users.

All stroke patients should be admitted to a hospital unit with cardiac monitoring, because atrial fibrillation and other arrhythmias may be transient and missed by the initial 12-lead ECG (eg, paroxysmal atrial fibrillation). The AHA previously recommended chest radiography as part of the standard acute ischemic stroke diagnostic workup, but recently made it optional because of a low yield of information leading to actual changes in clinical management.

Echocardiography, especially transesophageal echocardiography (TEE), remains the diagnostic standard to evaluate for cardioembolic sources of stroke [8,19,20]. TEE is superior to transthoracic echocardiography (TTE) in detecting cardioembolic sources [21]. Some clinicians prefer to perform TTE first and, if negative for identification of a cardioembolic source, follow with TEE. TEE may be problematic in patients who have an extremely sensitive gag reflex despite topical anesthetics, cannot be sedated for medical reasons (eg, end-stage cardiopulmonary disease), or raised intracranial pressure. TTE and TEE sensitivity for right-to-left shunting can be roughly doubled by intravenous injection of saline mixed with air (ie, saline bubble study), which allows visualization of microbubbles in the chambers of the left side of the heart that would otherwise be filtered by lung capillaries. Another sensitive test that detects right-to-left shunting is bubble-contrast transcranial Doppler ultrasonography, in which intravenous microbubbles are detected as they pass through the middle cerebral artery segment (M1). Transcranial Doppler bubble contrast studies may provide similar accuracy to TEE [22].

Neuroimaging data typically show a cortical or cortical–subcortical pattern of ischemia corresponding with the arterial territory, which is usually the middle cerebral artery (M1, M2, or even M3 branches) or posterior cerebral artery territories. In contradistinction, vascular territory ischemic events such as lacunar or branch penetrating disease (arteriolar vessel diameter of 100 μm) typically suggest in situ small vessel occlusion associated with hypertension or diabetes, rather than cardioembolic events. Furthermore, hemorrhagic infarctions may occur after transient large intracranial artery occlusion, with subsequent spontaneous recanalization, or after cardioembolism, with leakage of erythrocytes through the damaged blood–brain barrier and ischemic reperfusion injury. Also, recurrent cardioembolic events may be associated with transient neurologic deficits which, for example, alternate from one brain hemisphere to the other. Cardioembolic stroke may affect the posterior circulation [23], accounting for up to 25% of posterior circulation ischemic events in some registries [24–27]. Posterior inferior cerebellar artery and posterior cerebral artery territories are particularly prone to cardiac emboli [28,29].

Other newer technologies include multidetector CT for left atrial thrombi [8,30] and MRI [8,9]. Limitations of cardiac MRI include lack of widespread availability, limited physician knowledge about this technology and when it is indicated, and poor reimbursement. Current indications and guidelines for cardiac MRI are as follows [8,9]:

- TTE study is questionable for the presence of left ventricular thrombus
- Cardiac mass suspected on TTE and requires further evaluation
- Patient cannot tolerate TEE and/or cannot undergo TEE secondary to medical reasons
- TEE study was inconclusive
- Suspected false-negative TEE results, where CMR can adequately image potentially missed sources of embolus, such as left ventricular thrombus, cardiac masses, aortic plaque, or left atrial appendage thrombus

The authors suggest that clinicians classify stroke mechanism using the modified Trial of Org 10172 in Acute Stroke Treatment (TOAST) criteria, which subdivide the cause of stroke into five subtypes based on clinical features and the results of diagnostic tests: (1) large-artery atherosclerosis, (2) cardioembolism, (3) small-vessel occlusion, (4) stroke of other known cause, and (5) stroke of unknown cause (cryptogenic). A mechanistic classification is clinically practical because it may coincide with evidence-based treatment recommendations.

Stroke prevention in atrial fibrillation

Systemic embolization is a potential complication of any form of atrial fibrillation, and it can occur in patients with acute atrial fibrillation lasting as little as 72 hours [12]. The forms of atrial fibrillation proposed by the American College of Cardiology/AHA/ European Society of Cardiology are as follows [32,33]:

- Paroxysmal: self-terminating atrial fibrillation, in which episodes generally last less than 7 days and usually less than 24 hours; it may be recurrent
- Persistent: fails to self-terminate and lasts longer than 7 days
- Permanent: lasts for more than 1 year
- Lone: paroxysmal, persistent, or permanent atrial fibrillation in the absence of structural heart disease. This term was coined before echocardiography became widely available, and most cardiologists consider it now outdated. Whether left atrial enlargement and hypertensive heart disease fall under the definition of *structural heart disease* is unclear
- Nonvalvular: cases without rheumatic mitral valve disease, prosthetic heart valve, or valve repair

Nonvalvular or nonrheumatic atrial fibrillation is a common cardiac arrhythmia, affecting approximately 0.7% of the general population and increasing in prevalence with age [34,35]. The incidence of stroke associated with atrial fibrillation also increases with age (Fig. 4) [36,37].

Not every patient who has paroxysmal atrial fibrillation must be anticoagulated. When considering long-term anticoagulation, the risk for stroke should be addressed and balanced with the potential risk for hemorrhagic complication.

Multiple risk stratification schemes exist. The Atrial Fibrillation Investigators (AFI) systematically pooled data from five randomized trials evaluating atrial fibrillation in stroke prevention (The Boston Area Anticoagulation Trial of Atrial Fibrillation Investigators (BAATAF) [38], Stroke Prevention in Nonrheumatic Atrial Fibrillation (SPINAF) [39], Copenhagen Atrial Fibrillation, Aspirin, and Anticoagulation Study (AFASAK) [40], Canadian Atrial Fibrillation Anticoagulation study (CAFA) [41], and Stroke Prevention in Atrial Fibrillation [SPAF] [42]), identifying the following independent risk factors for embolism in atrial fibrillation: age older than 65 years, history of stroke or transient ischemic attack (TIA), diabetes mellitus, and history of systemic hypertension.

In 2000, Pearce and colleagues [43] compared three stroke risk stratification schemes (AFI [44], American College of Chest Physicians (ACCP) [45], SPAF [46]) in nonvalvular atrial fibrillation. They concluded that these

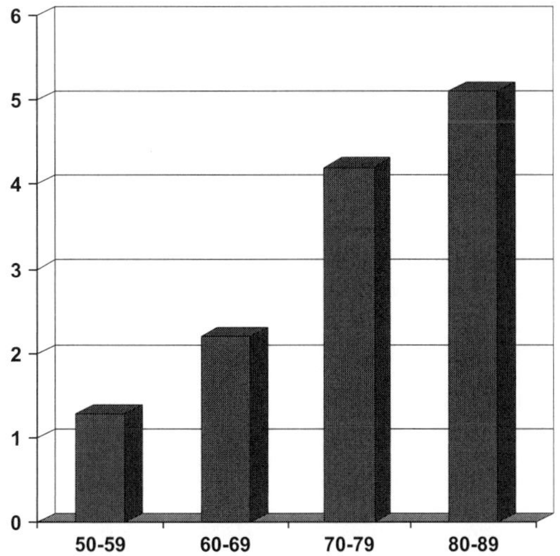

Fig. 4. Incidence of cardioembolic stroke caused by atrial fibrillation according to age. Stroke rate (*y* axis) presented as stroke incidence per 100 patients per year. Age (by decades) is presented on the *x* axis. These subjects are diagnosed with atrial fibrillation and have no prior history of stroke [36,37].

risk-stratification schemes successfully identified patients who had low rates of ischemic stroke (low-risk atrial fibrillation), but less consistently identified high-risk patients. The CHADS2 score (Table 2) was then implemented [3], taking into consideration risk factors identified by the AFI [45] and SPAF [46] (C, congestive heart failure [1 point]; H, hypertension [1 point]; A, age older than 75 years [1 point]; D, diabetes mellitus [1 point]; S2, history of stroke or TIA [2 points]).

Table 2 shows the estimated risk for stroke per year based on the CHADS2 score.

Table 2
Cardioembolic stroke etiology and stroke rate

Cardioembolic etiology	Stroke rate (95% CI)
AF	[3]
CHADS2 score[a]	
0	1.9 (1.2–3.0)
1	2.8 (2.0–3.8)
2	4.0 (3.1–5.1)
3	5.9 (4.6–7.3)
4	8.5 (6.3–11.1)
5	12.5 (8.2–7.5)
6	18.2 (10.5–27.4)
Cardiomyopathy	[3,92]
LVEF >35%	Without AF, 2%–4%/y[21,34,80] With AF 2%–18%/y[73]
Reduced LVEF (<35%)	1.6%/y
AMI	1%–3% any AMI 2%–6% anterior wall MI
Left ventricular thrombus	15% within 3 mo
Valvular disease	
Mitral: rheumatic	5%/y
Mitral: prolapse	1%
Endocarditis	12%–40%
Prosthetic valves	
Mitral: bioprosthetic	0.4%–1.9%/y
Mitral: mechanical	22%/y
Aortic: bioprosthetic	—
Aortic: mechanical	12%/y
Valvular strands	
Lambl's excrescence	1%–2%/y
Nonbacterial thrombotic endocarditis	42% [99]
PFO	0%–4%/y dependent on size and echo characteristics
PFO + ASA	14% in cryptogenic stroke patients aged <55 years

Abbreviations: AF, Atrial fibrillation; AMI, Acute myocardial infarction; ASA, Atrial septal aneurysm; INR, International normalized ratio; MI, Myocardial infarction.

[a] C, Congestive heart failure; H, Hypertension; A, Age older than 75 years; D, Diabetes mellitus; S, Stroke or TIA. All letters are counted 1 point except for stroke/TIA counted 2 points [3].

Modified from Sila CA. Neurological therapeutics: principles and practice. Cardioembolic Stroke 2003;1; with permission.

Antithrombotic strategies

Before the late 1980s, antithrombotic therapy for stroke prevention in atrial fibrillation was limited to those who had rheumatic heart disease or prosthetic heart valves [37]. Between 1989 and 2007, 29 randomized trials were published, evaluating the efficacy and safety of antithrombotic agents for stroke prevention in atrial fibrillation [47]. These studies included 28,044 patients.

Adjusted-Dose Warfarin Versus Placebo or no Treatment

Six randomized trials (AFASAK I [40], SPAF I [42], BAATAF [38], CAFA [41], SPINAF [48], and European Atrial Fibrillation Trial (EAFT) [49]), including 2900 participants, have addressed this clinical question. A meta-analysis [47,50] showed that the absolute risk reduction in all strokes with use of warfarin was 2.7% per year for primary prevention (the number needed to treat [NNT] for 1 year to prevent one stroke was 37) and 8.4% per year for secondary prevention (NNT, 12). When only ischemic strokes were considered, adjusted-dose warfarin was associated with a 67% relative risk reduction (95% CI, 54%–77%).

Antiplatelet Therapy Versus Placebo or no Treatment

Eight trials (AFASAK I [40], SPAF I [42], EAFT [49], European Stroke Prevention Study II (ESPS II) [51], United Kingdom Transient Ischemic Attack (UK-TIA) [52], Low dose Aspirin Atrial Fibrillation study (LASAF) [53], Japan Atrial Fibrillation Stroke Trial (JAST) [54], Swedish Atrial Fibrillation Trial (SAFT) [55] included 4876 participants. The intervention varied as follows: five trials studied aspirin versus placebo (AFASAK I [40], SPAF I [42], EAFT [49], ESPS II [51], UK-TIA [52]), two aspirin versus no treatment (LASAF [53], JAST [54]), one aspirin plus low-dose warfarin versus control (SAFT [55]), one dipyridamole versus placebo (ESPS II [51]). and one dipyridamole plus aspirin versus placebo (ESPS II [51]).

In a meta-analysis [47] comparing aspirin alone with placebo or no treatment in 3990 participants in seven trials, aspirin was associated with a 19% reduction in incidence of stroke (95% CI, 1%–35%). Absolute risk reductions of 0.8% (NNT, 125) and 2.5% (NNT, 40) per year were seen for primary and secondary prevention trials, respectively. When only ischemic strokes are considered, aspirin results in a 21% reduction in strokes (95% CI, 1%–38%). When considering all eight trials, antiplatelet therapy reduced stroke by 22% (95% CI, 6%–35%).

Adjusted-Dose Warfarin Versus Antiplatelet Therapy

Interventions using warfarin and other vitamin K antagonists varied, with eight trials (AFASAK I [40], SPAF II [56], EAFT [49], AFASAK II [57], Prevention of Arterial Thromboembolism in Atrial Fibrillation

[PATAF] [58], Vemmos and colleagues [59], Chinese Antithrombotics in Atrial Fibrillation Study [ATAFS] [60], and Warfarin versus Aspirin for Stroke Prevention in Octogenarians [WASPO] [61]) comparing this treatment with various dosages of aspirin, three trials comparing it with other antiplatelet agents (Studio Italiano Fibrillazione Atriale [SIFA] [62], National Study for Prevention of Embolism in Atrial Fibrillation [NASPEAF] [63], and Atrial fibrillation Clopidogrel Trial with Irbesartan for prevention of Vascular Events [ACTIVE-W] [64]), and two comparing it with aspirin combined with low fixed-dose warfarin in two trials (SPAF III [65], AFASAK II [57]).

For the 11 trials comparing adjusted-dose warfarin with antiplatelet therapy alone, warfarin was associated with a 37% reduction in strokes (95% CI, 23%–48%). In ACTIVE-W [64], anticoagulation therapy was superior to the combination clopidogrel plus aspirin (relative risk reduction, 40%; 95% CI, 18%–56%).

In meta-analysis of the 29 trials mentioned earlier, the risk for intracranial hemorrhage was doubled with adjusted-dose warfarin compared with aspirin. The absolute risk increase, however, was small (0.2% per year).

Solid evidence supports the use of antithrombotic therapy for most patients who have atrial fibrillation (Table 3). Oral anticoagulants reduce stroke in patients who have atrial fibrillation more effectively than antiplatelet agents. The threshold of absolute benefit warranting anticoagulation instead of antiplatelet therapy remains controversial and depends on the estimated risk for stroke, patient preference, and availability of optimal anticoagulation monitoring. No evidence favors one dosage of aspirin over another. Adding clopidogrel to aspirin provides no major benefit in patients who have atrial fibrillation.

Patent foramen ovale

Patent foramen ovale (PFO) is a flap-like defect in the interatrial septum (Fig. 5) and a common finding (25%) in the general population. In utero, PFO allows oxygenated blood from the mother to bypass the lungs and go directly into fetal systemic circulation (by way of the right to left atria pathway). At birth, the lungs expand from breathing air, which fills the lungs with deoxygenated blood that enters the right atrium, the right ventricle, and the lung capillary beds. Blood is oxygenated before entering the left atrium and left ventricle, which subsequently distributes freshly oxygenated blood into the systemic circulation. This flap-like opening, the PFO, closes in most infants at birth, but fails to close (lack of fusion between the primum and secundum septae) in approximately one of three to four infants.

PFO may also be associated with other cardiac defects, including atrial septal aneurysm (ASA), in which the septum has an aneurysmal appearance (tissue bulges into either right or left atrium); atrial septal defect, which is similar to PFO in that a hole is present between the right and left atria; Ebstein's

Table 3
Cardioembolic stroke therapy

Cardioembolic etiology	Therapy and evidence level
AF	Aspirin therapy: 22% relative risk reduction Warfarin: 54%–77% relative risk reduction [47] and superior to aspirin [33,50,57]; level I–II
Reduced LVEF (<35%) Stroke risk increases 18% for each LVEF decrease of 5 percentage points [6] (relative risk, 1.18; 95% CI, 1.02–1.36; $P = .03$); stroke risk when LVEF ≤28% is double LVEF ≥35% [84] Women who have reduced LVEF are at higher risk than men with reduced LVEF (Studies of Left Ventricular Dysfunction [SOLVD] [21])	Aspirin provides a 56% relative risk reduction in patients who have reduced ejection fraction with no AF or other embolic risk factors; level II [85,93,98] Warfarin reduces risk for stroke for patients who have reduced LVEF and AF, embolic events, or left ventricular thrombus and effect only slightly inferior to aspirin (level II–III) [82,85,92]
Acute myocardial infarction	Anticoagulation,[a] level II [68]
Left ventricular thrombus	Anticoagulation,[a] level II [68,82]
Valvular disease	
Mitral: rheumatic	Aspirin, anticoagulation [a] or valve repair level II [68,82]
Mitral: prolapse	None, antiplatelet,[b] unless AF then anticoagulation,[a] level II [68,82]
Endocarditis	Antibiotics, level II Controversy regarding antiplatelet[b] or anticoagulation[a],[22,102,112–117]
Prosthetic valves	Level II [68,108]
Mitral: bioprosthetic	Dependent on valve type and AF
Mitral: mechanical	INR 2.5–3.5 and 81–100 mg aspirin
Aortic: bioprosthetic	Antiplatelet[b]
Aortic: mechanical	Anticoagulation[a] INR 2.5–3.5 (most valves). Ball in cage (higher INR)
Valvular strands	Unclear if therapy needed; level V [82]
Nonbacterial thrombotic endocarditis	Heparin; level IV [102]
PFO and cryptogenic stroke	Aspirin for TIA/stroke; level I–II [5–7,69–71]
PFO + ASA and cryptogenic stroke	Aspirin first, anticoagulation[a] if antiplatelet[b] fails; level I–II [5–7,69–71]

Abbreviations: AF, atrial fibrillation; LVEF, left ventricular ejection fraction.
[a] Anticoagulation: heparin [short-term], warfarin [long-term].
[b] Antiplatelet: aspirin, aspirin-dipyramidole combination, clopidogrel, or ticlopidine.

anomaly, in which the tricuspid valve is malformed and positioned lower than normal; and other complex cardiac defects associated with cyanosis (eg, transposition of the great vessels). This article's focus is on PFO with or without ASA, which is a common echocardiographic finding.

The relationship of PFO and ischemic stroke remains an area of considerable debate (see Table 2) [5–7]. The high prevalence of PFO seen on echocardiography in stroke patients makes proving causality of PFO in ischemic stroke initially problematic. Previous retrospective studies did

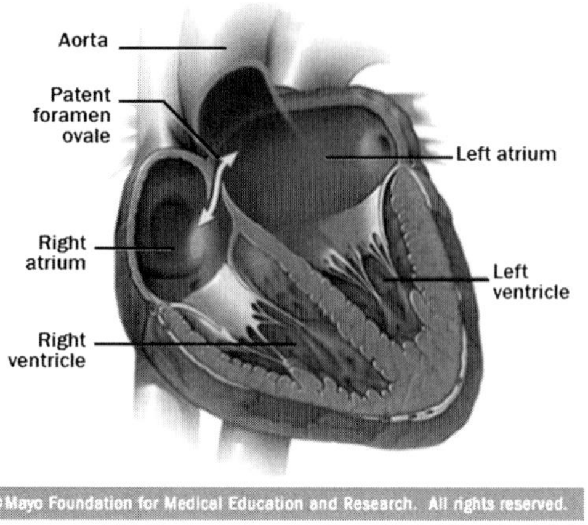

Fig. 5. Patent foramen ovale. PFO is a defect between the two upper chambers of the heart (right and left atria) allowing blood to pass from right to left (systemic circulation). (*Courtesy of* the Mayo Clinic and Foundation for Medical Education and Research, Rochester, MN; with permission.)

not control for all echocardiographic findings, such as ASA, size of PFO, presence of right to left shunt with valsalva maneuver, use of bubble studies, or different treatments (eg, aspirin or warfarin) [7]. However, recent prospective data have elucidated PFO in relation to cryptogenic stroke [5–7].

The mechanism through which PFO causes ischemic stroke remains speculative. The prevailing hypothesis is that PFO-mediated stroke results from "paradoxical" (right to left) embolism caused by clots originating in the right side of the venous circulation proximal to the PFO that then travel into the left atrium and the systemic circulation. Clinical observations of patients who have PFO, documented DVT and simultaneous pulmonary embolism (PE), and ischemic stroke support a right-sided to left-sided, or "paradoxical," circulatory mechanism for stroke. However, most patients who experience cryptogenic stroke and PFO have an unremarkable diagnostic workup for typical venous sources of (eg, DVT) of paradoxical embolus. Cryptogenic embolism is not synonymous with paradoxical embolism, and cryptogenic stroke may in fact coexist with PFO or occur separately.

Another hypothesis about PFO-mediated stroke is that vasoactive substances (eg, serotonin) normally deactivated in the pulmonary circulation cross into the systemic circulation and lead to ischemic stroke. The latter hypothesis is weakly supported by the finding of patients who have PFO and experience migraines who improve after PFO closure. The results from a recent systematic review of the literature suggested PFO closure seemed to affect migraine patterns favorably, but a low grade of evidence (level III) was available to provide definitive conclusions [66].

Regardless of hypothetical mechanism, prospective studies show that PFO is found more commonly in patients who have a cryptogenic stroke mechanism in both younger and older adults [5,7]. Other studies suggest that the size of the PFO defect is important, with a large PFO ($\geq$2 mm) more likely to be associated with an embolic stroke than a small PFO (<2 mm) [67]. Therefore, PFO may act as a potential primary source of cardioembolism (ie, in situ thrombus formation and right to left embolization) or simply as a potential paradoxical embolic passageway.

The combination of PFO with atrial septal aneurysm may explain how clot forms near the PFO hole and crosses through. An ASA is a sustained 15-mm segmental bowing of the interatrial septal membrane in the fossa ovalis of at least 11 to 15 mm beyond the plane of the interatrial septum, or may be a phasic excursion to either side of the same distance [6]. Therefore, an ASA may be the substrate for in situ thrombus to form, which later passes through the PFO (right- to left-sided circulation).

This theory is supported by a prospective multicenter study of 581 patients aged 18 to 55 years who experienced symptomatic cryptogenic stroke treated with 300 mg/d of aspirin followed up over 4 years [7]. The presence of PFO alone had a 2.3% risk of recurrent stroke compared with 4.2% in the absence of PFO [7]. However, the risk for recurrent stroke over 4 years on aspirin was 15.2% when both PFO and ASA were present on echocardiography (Table 4). No stroke recurrences occurred among patients who had ASA alone taking aspirin. The presence of both PFO and ASA predicted a significant increased risk for recurrent stroke (hazard ratio for both PFO and ASA versus absence of both abnormalities, 4.17; 95% CI, 1.47–11.84).

Furthermore, the study showed that in patients 18 to 55 years of age who had isolated PFO and cryptogenic stroke started on aspirin, regardless of PFO size, were not at higher risk for recurrent stroke [7] compared with patients in prior studies. This study may not have been adequately powered, however, to account for shunt degree and ASA severity. Because patients who had both PFO and ASA had recurrent cryptogenic strokes despite aspirin therapy, randomized trials comparing aspirin versus warfarin were performed and are discussed under medical therapy.

In another prospective study of 503 patients who experienced stroke [5], PFO or PFO-ASA was detected in 34% and 14% of the patients classified with cryptogenic stroke by TOAST criteria, versus 12% and 4%, respectively, with stroke of known type ($P<.001$). The study also compared 131 younger patients (<55 years) with 372 older patients (>55 years) and found that the PFO-ASA combination was strongly associated with cryptogenic

Table 4
Echocardiographic findings and risk for recurrent stroke for patients experiencing initial cryptogenic stroke at age 18 to 55 years [6,7]

Echocardiographic finding	Risk for recurrent stroke
No PFO or ASA	4.2% (95% CI, 1.8%–6.6%)
PFO without ASA	2.3% (95% CI, 0.3%–4.3%)
PFO with ASA	15.2% (95 CI, 1.8%–28.6 %)

stroke in younger ($P < .049$) and older patients ($P < .001$) compared with patients who had known stroke subtype.

Medical therapy

Studies investigating medical therapy for PFO are largely retrospective and do not show any advantage of warfarin over aspirin (see Table 3). Most of these studies, however, have been limited by insufficient power to compare aspirin with warfarin, nonrandomized treatment allocation or non-masked treatment, or allocation, crossover, or unblinded ascertainment of end points [6].

In the PFO in Cryptogenic Stroke Study (PICCS), patients were randomized to warfarin (international normalized ratio [INR] target, 1.4–2.8) or aspirin (325 mg daily) as part of the Warfarin-Aspirin Recurrent Stroke Study (WARSS) [69], and compared for 2-year outcome end points of stroke, death, and bleeding (203 in the PFO group versus 398 in the non-PFO group). The study confirmed PFO was associated with cryptogenic stroke subtype, but echocardiographic findings of PFO (including varying size) compared with the combined PFO and ASA group did not show a statistically significant difference in stroke end points by 2 years. Minor bleeding was more common with warfarin than aspirin treatment, but major bleeding did not differ significantly.

This study included a broad range of patient ages (30–85 years) compared with the New England Studies, which split patients into those younger or older than 55 years of age [5–7]. The PICCS study also compared patients who had cryptogenic and noncryptogenic stroke subtypes. Finally, the study used a lower target INR of 1.4 to 2.8, which is lower than that used for atrial fibrillation stroke prevention. The study concluded that evidence was insufficient to determine if warfarin was superior to aspirin in preventing recurrent stroke or death in patients who had PFO (with or without ASA).

Despite current evidence and guidelines [70,71], the authors consider warfarin therapy for young patients who experienced cryptogenic stroke with PFO who have a history of stroke during valsalva, have large PFO with right to left shunt seen on valsalva/echocardiographic bubble study, or have PFO-ASA on echocardiography. Although current guidelines [70,71] suggest that young patients who experience cryptogenic stroke with PFO who have a history of stroke during valsalva, have a large PFO with right-to-left shunt seen on valsalva/echocardiographic bubble study, or have PFO-ASA on echocardiography may be considered for warfarin if aspirin fails, they do not support PFO surgical/endovascular closure.

Surgical and endovascular closure for patent foramen ovale

Recent methods to repair PFO using endovascular means have been developed within the past decade (Fig. 6) [67] and allow this anatomic defect to be

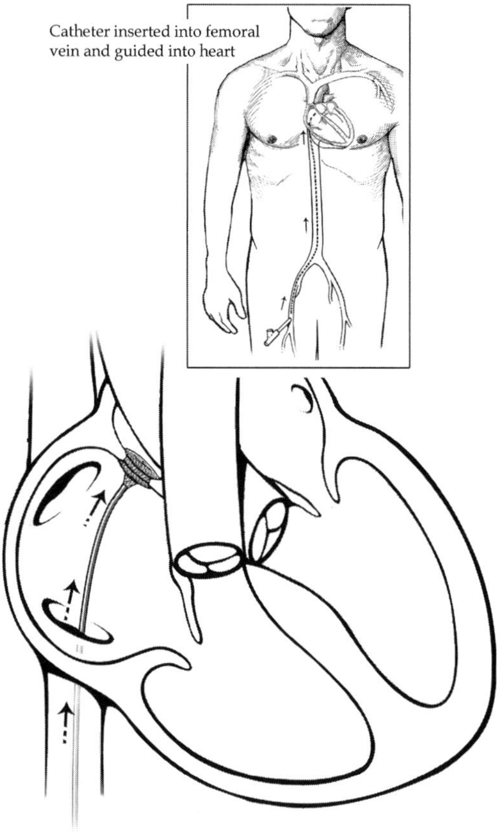

Fig. 6. Patent foramen ovale endovascular occluder. The device is inserted through the right femoral artery and placed in the PFO to seal the defect. (*Courtesy of* the Mayo Clinic and Foundation for Medical Education and Research, Rochester, MN; with permission.)

treated less invasively [6,67]. Given the association of PFO in cryptogenic stroke, repair of the defect is a logical target for subsequent stroke prevention. However, no randomized trial has been completed, despite five ongoing studies recruiting patients for PFO closure in cryptogenic stroke (www.clinicaltrials.gov identifiers, NCT00557479, NCT00196040m, NCT00562289, NCT00201461, and NCT00166257). Unfortunately, enrollment has been slow in these studies. For example, the Randomized Evaluation of Recurrent Stroke Comparing PFO Closure to Established Current Standard of Care Treatment (RESPECT) trial enrolled 359 patients as of September 2007, with a goal of 500 patients, although it began enrollment in 2003 with 60 trial centers. Similarly, the Patent Foramen Ovale and Cryptogenic Embolism study started enrolling patients in 2000 and had only 314 patients enrolled as of October 2006, with 26 centers and a goal of 450 patients.

Because of the lack of randomized trial data comparing PFO closure to standard medical therapy, the American Academy of Neurology issued practice parameters concluding insufficient evidence to recommend routine percutaneous closure of PFOs in patients experiencing cryptogenic stroke [71]. Until further randomized controlled data are available, the authors recommend following the AAN guidelines on PFO closure.

In some circumstances, the authors consider PFO closure in young patients experiencing cryptogenic stroke in whom antiplatelet therapy failed and the lifelong treatment risks associated with warfarin versus those of short-term PFO closure are weighed. However, the aforementioned evidence and guidelines discussed earlier make this a low level of evidence (level V) recommendation. Additional patients considered for PFO closure include those at high risk for bleeding complications with long-term warfarin therapy, if aspirin therapy fails and no other cause for stroke can be found despite an exhaustive workup (level V). Other considerations in these difficult cases include the experience and complication rate of the cardiothoracic surgeon or endovascular interventionalist in relation to a patient's long-term stroke risk and other comorbidities.

Many patients who undergo PFO closure will be placed on warfarin for 3 to 6 months before endovascular closure and switched to aspirin or another antiplatelet agent 3 months after the procedure. The pre- and postprocedure anticoagulation period depends largely on the preference of the surgeon or interventional specialist. These recommendations have a low level of evidence (level V), represent the authors' opinions, and could be incorrect and subject to change given future PFO closure evidence. Clinicians should use their best judgment based on all available evidence.

Aortic arch disease

An overlooked but a potentially serious source of embolic stroke is the aortic arch, especially when proximal aortic atheromatous disease is present [72]. Aortic embolic events may be misclassified as cryptogenic unless adequate transesophageal echocardiography of the aorta is performed. Aortic embolic disease manifests in different forms, including mobile and ulcerated plaques, aortic dissection, and aneurysms (Fig. 7). Patients who have ascending aorta or proximal arch plaques of 4 mm thickness are up to seven times more likely to have cerebral infarction than controls (14.4% versus 2%; $P<.001$) [72,73].

The authors have observed mobile or unstable aortic atheromatous plaques in some patients after coronary artery bypass, cerebral angiography, cardiac catheterization, and intra-aortic balloon pump placement when consulted for stroke (level V evidence). Whether the aortic plaque formed de novo after the procedure or was present preprocedure remains unknown, because most did not have a preprocedure aortic evaluation and multiple atherosclerotic risk factors.

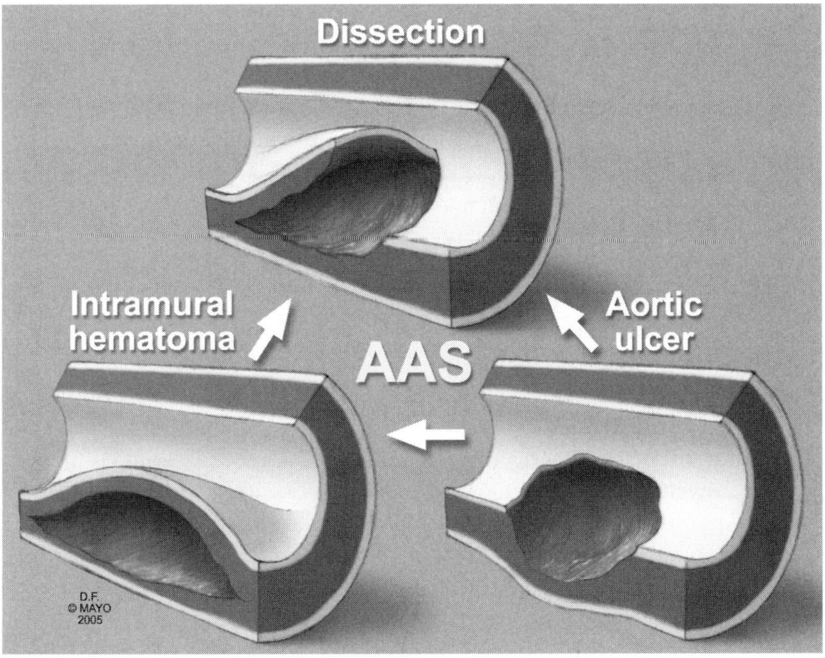

Fig. 7. Aortic atherosclerosis. Aortic atherosclerosis (AAS) mechanisms, including aortic ulcer (*bottom right*), followed by intramural hematoma (*bottom left*), which is a raised structure creating reduced caliber to the aortic lumen. Similarly, although not shown, aortic atheroma narrow the aortic lumen and may lead to local thrombus formation and embolization. The top shows aortic luminal dissection. (*Courtesy of* the Mayo Clinic and Foundation for Medical Education and Research, Rochester, MN; with permission.)

For nonmobile aortic plaque, statin therapy may be protective in preventing stroke (level II evidence [74]), whereas uncertainty remains about whether aspirin or warfarin is the optimal antithrombotic, [74]. However, mobile aortic plaques may be treated with warfarin anticoagulation (target INR, 2–3; 45% versus 5%; $P = .006$) [75]. The dimensions of the mobile atheroma may not predict stroke risk; only the presence or absence of the mobile component predicts this risk. Surgical resection of large mobile atheroma with potential high risk for embolization are reported, but the morbidity and mortality with the surgery is substantial [71]. Descending aortic arch atheroma do not pose cerebral embolic risk, as does ascending and proximal arch disease, but poses risk for embolization to the viscera and peripheral limbs.

Myocardial infarction, left ventricular dysfunction, and heart failure

Myocardial infarction, its associated ventricular wall immobility, and subsequent dilated cardiomyopathy may lead to left ventricular thrombus formation and cardioembolic stroke [76–81]. Cardioembolic strokes may occur within 1 day of myocardial infarction, and approximately half occur within the first week, although stroke risk remains high up to 3 months and then decreases gradually [76–81]. Anterior wall myocardial infarction carries a higher risk for stroke than inferior wall myocardial infarction (25% versus 5%). Treating patients who have experienced myocardial infarction with heparin for coronary disease helps reduce the risk for ventricular wall thrombus formation [82]. TTE is the preferred test for detecting left ventricular wall and apical thrombi. However, TEE may be used if TTE has a suboptimal transthoracic view.

Patients who experience anterior wall myocardial infarction and are found to have ventricular wall thrombus should be placed on warfarin, with the goal of attaining an INR of 2.0 to 3.0 for up to 6 months [68]. Thereafter, aspirin therapy may be used. Prolonged anticoagulation decreased stroke risk up to 40% over 3 years in the Anticoagulants in the Secondary Prevention of Events in Coronary Thrombosis (ASPECT) trial, although major bleeding complications were increased [78]. If atrial fibrillation develops after myocardial infarction, anticoagulation may be considered indefinitely depending on other ischemic stroke risk factors, such as age older than 70 years, hypertension, heart failure, diabetes, and stroke [3].

Reduced left ventricular ejection fraction

Among patients older than 55 years, 3.9% have heart failure [83]. When heart failure occurs, stroke risk increases almost threefold by 5 years [84]. The Survival and Ventricular Enlargement (SAVE) trial [85] showed every decrease of five percentage points in left ventricular ejection fraction (LVEF) was accompanied by an 18% increase in stroke risk. More than 50 years ago, experts discovered that warfarin reduced the risk for pulmonary embolism, which was a major cause of death in patients who had heart failure [86–88]. However, these patients also had a high prevalence of atrial fibrillation and more DVT-PE risks. Patients who had an LVEF of 28% or less had almost double the risk for stroke compared with those who had an LVEF greater than 35%.

Cerebrovascular reactivity also decreases linearly with decreasing LVEF [89], and reduced regional cerebral blood flow foci seen in patients who had heart failure [90] may be a factor predisposing to stroke. Reduced cerebrovascular reactivity and regional cerebral blood flow in these patients may also signify intracranial atherosclerotic disease, which also may be a risk factor. Both warfarin and aspirin are effective in reducing stroke risk, but warfarin is associated with more bleeding complications, especially when used with aspirin. However, decreasing LVEF is associated with increased stroke risk [31,84,91]. Whether antiplatelet or anticoagulant therapy is more beneficial for stroke prevention in patients who have heart failure remains uncertain.

Dilated cardiomyopathy

Dilated cardiomyopathy is associated with various different etiologies (ischemic and nonischemic, infectious and infiltrative). The Study of Left Ventricular Dysfunction (SOLVD) [92] clarified the relation between embolic stroke risk and worsening ventricular function. Increased stroke risk was seen only in women (2.4 events per 100 patient-years compared with 1.8 events per 100 patient-years in men). In this study, warfarin and aspirin were associated with a lower rate of death or hospitalization for heart failure than aspirin, but only warfarin reduced death from worsening heart failure.

Although embolic stroke risk doubles when LVEF declines below 28% compared with 35%, patients also benefit from aspirin alone (56% relative risk reduction in SAVE [85]), without the bleeding complications. Although controlled studies of patients who have left ventricular dysfunction and anticoagulation are lacking [82], oral anticoagulation (INR intensity, 2.0–3.0) is recommended in those who have atrial fibrillation, previous episodes of thromboembolism (stroke or systemic or pulmonary embolism), or documented left ventricular thrombus [93]. For patients who do not have these risk factors, controversy exists about whether antiplatelet or anticoagulation therapy should be used [85,92,94–96].

The Warfarin and Aspirin Therapy in Heart Failure trial (WATCH) [97] was designed to compare aspirin 160 mg/d, clopidogrel 75 mg/d, and warfarin (INR, 2.5–3.0) in 4500 patients who had poor left ventricular function. However, the trial was terminated 18 months prematurely (June 2003) by the VA Cooperative Study Program because of poor enrollment. Results presented in 2004 [98] showed that warfarin reduced nonfatal stroke compared with aspirin and clopidogrel ($P = .05$), but the combined end point of nonfatal myocardial infarction or stroke and death did not reach statistical significance ($P = .21$). The Warfarin Versus Aspirin in Patients With Reduced Cardiac Ejection Fraction (WARCEF trial) [99] is a randomized, double-blind, multi-center trial studying the efficacy of warfarin (INR, 2.5–3.0; target, 2.75) versus aspirin (325 mg/d) on all-cause mortality and stroke (both ischemic and hemorrhagic) in patients who have LVEF of 35% or less. As of February 2008, the study, which began in 2002, had 1644 patients enrolled of its goal of 3201. The results of this study will be useful in determining optimal medical therapy in patients who have heart failure within sinus rhythm.

Valvular heart disease

Aortic Stenosis

Clinically symptomatic cerebral embolic events are uncommon in calcific aortic valve disease (Fig. 8) [100–104] unless concomitant atrial fibrillation, reduced LVEF, or mitral valve disease is present. Calcific emboli to the retina (ie, asymptomatic emboli) or after valvuloplasty are reported [102,105].

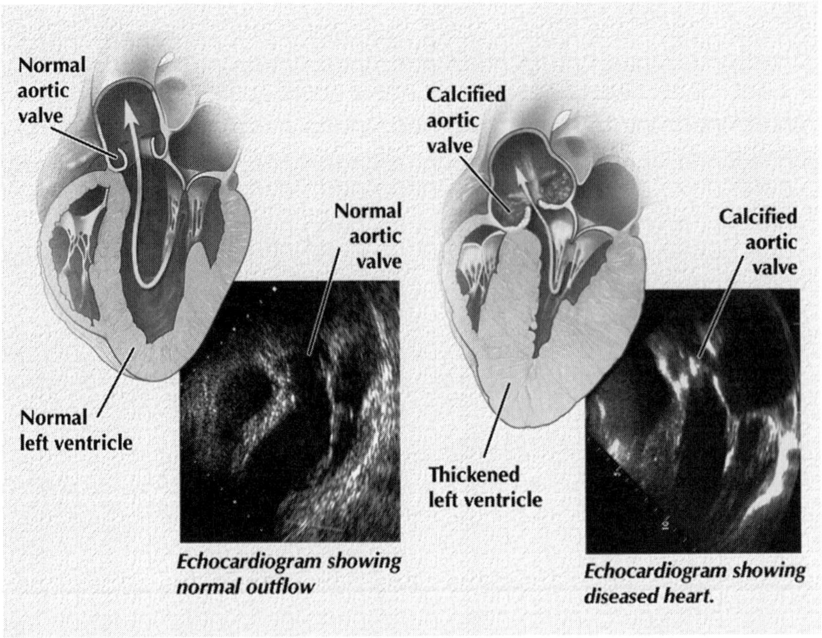

Fig. 8. Normal and calcific aortic valves. Normal aortic valve and ventricle on the left upper diagram, with normal aortic valve appearance and ventricle (*bottom left*). Top right (diagram) and bottom right (echocardiogram) showing a calcified aortic valve that leads to aortic stenosis, increased resistance to outflow, and resultant thickening of the ventricular wall. (*Courtesy of* the Mayo Clinic and Foundation for Medical Education and Research, Rochester, MN; with permission.)

Antiplatelet therapy may be initiated in patients who have TIA and bicuspid calcific aortic stenosis, but anticoagulation is generally not recommended unless atrial fibrillation or another high-risk factor for embolism echocardiographic abnormality is detected [99–102].

Mitral Valve Stenosis

Mitral valve stenosis from rheumatic heart disease with or without atrial fibrillation is an indication for warfarin anticoagulation, with INR ranging between 2.0 and 3.0, to prevent thromboembolic events (cerebral and systemic) [106,107]. Anticoagulation is recommended in some patients who have mitral valve stenosis without atrial fibrillation and have evidence of spontaneous echo contrast ("smoke") within a large left atrium (>5.5 cm). In these patients, valvuloplasty may be attempted after an adequate period of anticoagulation.

Mitral Annular Calcification

Mitral annular calcification (MAC) does not denote simply calcification of the mitral annulus, but rather a syndrome characterized in elderly patients by a calcified mitral annulus, mitral stenosis or regurgitation, aortic stenosis, conduction disturbances, embolic phenomenon, and even endocarditis [102]. Antiplatelet agents are reasonable first-line therapy, but if recurrent embolic events occur or atrial fibrillation develops, anticoagulation or valvular repair (Fig. 9) should be considered [101].

Mitral Valve Prolapse

Mitral valve prolapse (MVP) is the most common echocardiographic finding in normal individuals (4 to 6%) [102]. If symptomatic, palpitations or chest pain may be present. MVP is typically a benign echocardiographic finding and not associated with increased stroke risk unless it occurs in combination with mitral annular calcification, mitral regurgitation, or atrial fibrillation. MVP is being studied in cerebrovascular disease, with some studies showing denudation of the mitral endothelium and platelet-fibrin thrombi, which may embolize. Antiplatelet agents remain first-line therapy, but anticoagulation is considered for recurrent cerebral ischemic events or MVP associated with atrial fibrillation or another embolic risk factor [101].

Prosthetic Cardiac Valves

Antithrombotic therapy depends on the type and location of the prosthetic valve (Fig. 10) and the presence of atrial fibrillation [101]. For metallic valves ("ball in cage" and "caged-disc," see Fig. 10, top right and middle right), warfarin anticoagulation is typically recommended to attain a target INR ranging from 2.5 to 3.5. Prosthetic valves in the mitral position are

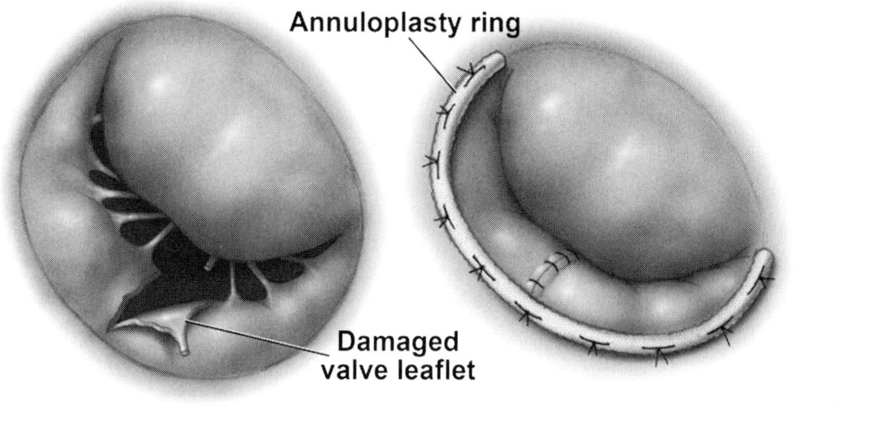

Fig. 9. Mitral valve annuloplasty. Mitral valve annuloplasty (*right*) repairing damaged mitral valve leaflet (*left*). (*Courtesy of* the Mayo Clinic and Foundation for Medical Education and Research, Rochester, MN; with permission.)

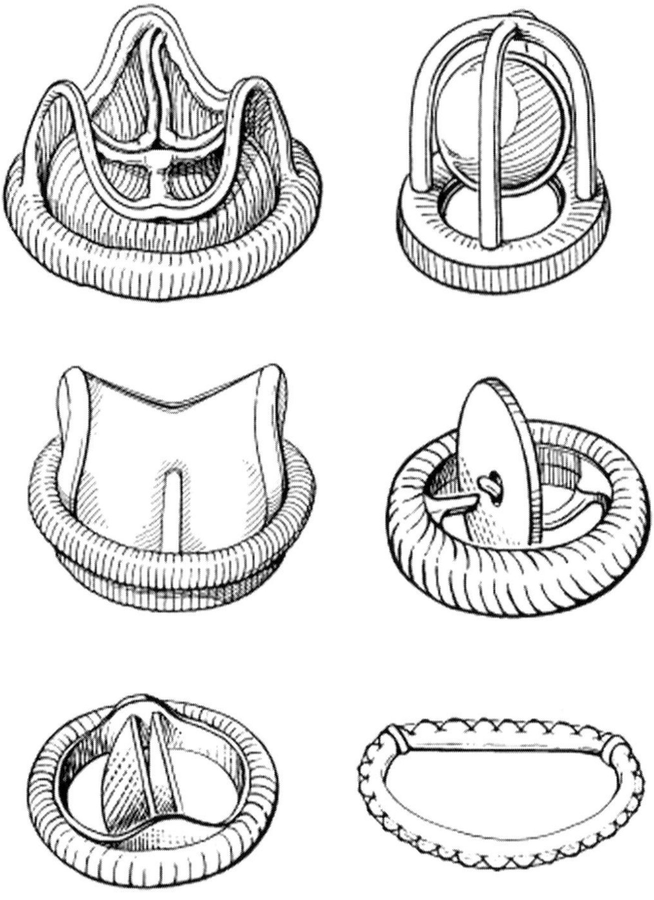

Fig. 10. Different prosthetic heart valves. Bioprosthetic valve (*top left*). Prosthetic bileaflet (*top middle* and *bottom left*). Ball in cage prosthesis (*top right*). Disc in cage prosthesis (*middle right*). Annuloplasty ring (*bottom right*). (*Courtesy of* the Mayo Clinic and Foundation for Medical Education and Research, Rochester, MN; with permission.)

associated with a higher thrombotic risk than those in the aortic position. Patients who have a bileaflet aortic valve (see Fig. 10, middle left and bottom left) without atrial fibrillation or left ventricular dysfunction should receive warfarin to attain a target INR ranging from 2.0 to 3.0 [108]. For high-risk patients, aortic bileaflet valves, mitral bileaflet, or caged disc location with concomitant atrial fibrillation, warfarin with INR intensity of 2.5 to 3.5 and aspirin, 81 to 100 mg/d, may be given [100,108].

Patients who have aortic bioprosthetic valves (eg, porcine) are typically managed with aspirin (325 mg/d) monotherapy, assuming no atrial fibrillation, whereas those who have mitral bioprosthetic valves may require warfarin for the first 3 months before converting to aspirin monotherapy. Bioprosthetic valves complicated by thrombus formation, atrial fibrillation, or thromboembolism failing antiplatelet therapy may require warfarin anticoagulation with an INR ranging from 2.0 to 3.0 [100,108].

Papillary Fibroelastoma (Giant Lambl's Excrescence)

Giant Lambl's excrescence (GLE) are valvular abnormalities that have a frond-like appearance and a stalk-like attachment that arise mostly from left-sided valvular surfaces (aortic more than mitral) and are of unclear cause (neoplastic, hamartomatous, or reparative) [6]. Embolic risk is difficult to quantify for GLE, but seems directly proportional to size and mobility. Initial medical therapy typically involves an antiplatelet agent; if recurrent cerebral ischemic events occur, anticoagulation or surgical resection are considered for large (>1 cm) mobile lesions [6,109,110].

Valvular Strands (Lambl's Excrescences)

Valvular strands [6,111] are common small filiform projections (<1 mm wide and <1 cm long) arising near valve closure lines (mitral more than aortic) that result from traumatic abrasions of the valve surface. Risk factors for valvular strands include age and valvular disease (eg, rheumatic valve disease). Antiplatelet therapy is recommended for patients who have cerebral ischemic events attributable to valvular strands. Whether anticoagulation is superior to antiplatelet therapy for stroke prevention in this condition is unclear [111]; however, administering antiplatelet therapy is reasonable [82].

Nonbacterial Thrombotic Endocarditis

Nonbacterial thrombotic endocarditis (NBTE), or marantic endocarditis, is a noninfectious process affecting normal or degenerative cardiac valves caused by fibrin thrombi deposits in patients who have hypercoaguable states associated with adenocarcinomas of the lung, colon, or pancreas that produce mucin [102]. Patients who have NBTE may present with arterial and venous thromboembolism and disseminated intravascular coagulation. Heparin, but not warfarin, has provided benefit [102] and helped treat the underlying neoplastic disorder.

Libman-Sacks endocarditis is a noninfectious valvular abnormality associated with autoimmune disorders, such as systemic lupus erythematosus and the antiphospholipid antibody syndrome. No large-scale randomized trials exist to provide evidence-based data, but some experts recommend anticoagulation with warfarin as primary treatment to prevent stroke [4].

Infectious Endocarditis

Infectious seeding of heart valves (Fig. 11) or endocarditis before the advent of antibiotics was associated with a very high cerebral embolic rate

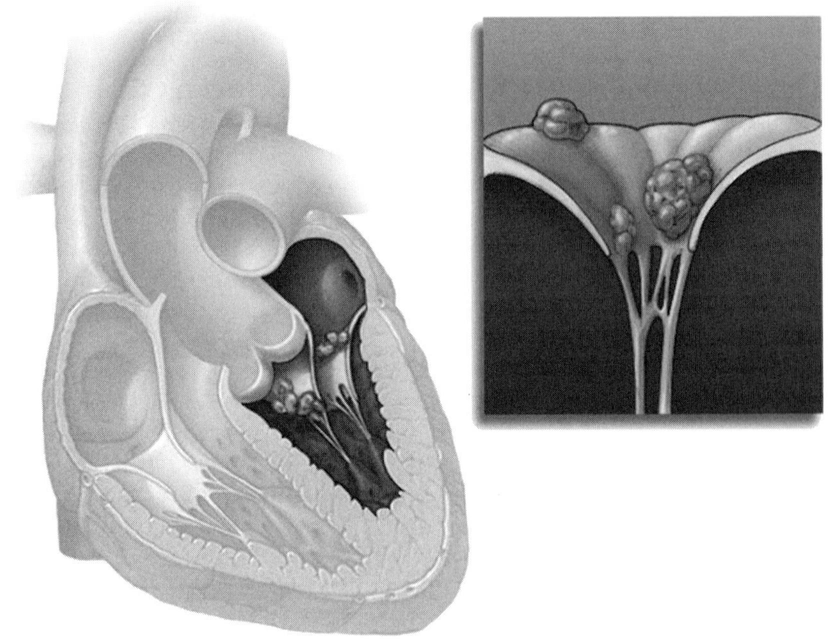

Fig. 11. Mitral valve endocarditis. Mitral valve endocarditis, showing the valvular vegetations on the surface of the mitral valve. (*Courtesy of* the Mayo Clinic and Foundation for Medical Education and Research, Rochester, MN; with permission.)

(70%–90%), which decreased (12%–40%) with the advent of antibiotics [21,23]. Specific antibiotic therapy for endocarditis remains first-line treatment based on blood culture results, whereas anticoagulation remains controversial or contraindicated [102,112–117] given the early rates of cerebral hemorrhage and the fact that anticoagulation does not reduce the incidence of embolism in native valve endocarditis. Patients who have mechanical prosthetic valves, however, may be at higher risk if anticoagulation is discontinued [92]. Exceptions to this rule include patients who have infected aortic bioprosthetic valves and those on antibiotics and in normal sinus rhythm.

Controversy remains about the duration and intensity of anticoagulation in patients who have prosthetic valve endocarditis, given the risk for embolism versus intracranial hemorrhage [102,112–117]. Embolism to the brain may also occur in these patients, and they may develop an infected microscopic nidus (especially in the presence of *Staphylococcus aureus*) or microaneurysm that may be prone to cerebral hemorrhage. Prosthetic valve endocarditis may be considered an anticoagulation dilemma, because patients have equal risks for ischemic stroke and cerebral hemorrhage. The authors recommend carefully considering the patient's valve type, location, and presence of atrial fibrillation in weighing the ischemic and hemorrhagic risks. For example, if the patient had a large ischemic stroke from endocarditis, anticoagulation presents higher risk for brain hemorrhage and may need to be delayed or not administered.

Infective endocarditis of a prosthetic heart valve warrants early surgical consultation. Surgical replacement of an infected prosthetic valve presents a high risk for morbidity and mortality, especially for mitral position valves. Surgical removal or repair is considered for patients who have congestive heart failure, cardiac abscess, or persistently positive blood cultures despite antibiotic treatment. Early surgery is also warranted in fungal endocarditis.

Cardiac Tumors

Primary cardiac tumors are rare (<0.2% in unselected autopsy series), and most are benign (50% myxomas and papillary fibroelastoma) but associated with a high frequency of embolic events. Myxomas commonly occur in the left atrium and arise from the interatrial septum. They may embolize to the systemic circulation, particularly to the brain when tumor pieces break off or secondary thrombus formation occurs. TEE is invaluable in defining tumor location, size, and morphology. Surgical resection of the tumor is recommended in all cases of myxomas to prevent embolization [82,109,110,118].

Papillary fibroelastomas are benign tumors that tend to originate on cardiac valves as single or multiple masses. Embolic events are typically the first clinical manifestation, because they are present on highly mobile valve leaflets. The embolic mechanism is the same as myxomas, caused by tumor fragmentation or secondary thrombus generation. Surgical resection is also indicated for fibroelastomas [82,109,110,118].

Metastatic tumors to the heart are 20 to 40 times more frequent than primary cardiac tumors, which are rare (eg, angiosarcoma, rhabdomyosarcoma) [82,119]. Cerebral embolization can also occur from these tumors. Surgical treatment can be offered but depends on the underlying tumor type and prognosis.

Left Atrial Thrombus

Risk factors for left atrial thrombus formation include atrial fibrillation, mitral stenosis, severe left ventricular dysfunction, left atrial dilatation, or presence of a prosthetic mitral valve. Demonstration of a left atrial appendage thrombus on TEE is associated with a threefold increase in the risk for stroke [120]. Therefore, prophylactic anticoagulation is recommended for at least 3 weeks before electrical cardioversion for atrial fibrillation [82].

Spontaneous Echo Contrast ("Smoke")

Spontaneous echo contrast (SEC) is defined as a smoke-like echo density moving within the cardiac chamber, typically the left atrium, indicating stagnant blood flow. TEE best visualizes SEC in the left atrium. The presence of SEC is a predisposing factor to thrombus formation and risk for ischemic stroke by three- to fourfold [120]. Oral anticoagulation decreases the stroke risk associated with SEC [82,120,121].

References

[1] Asinger RW, Dyken ML, Fisher M, et al. Cardiogenic brain embolism: the second report of Cerebral Embolism Task Force. Arch Neurol 1989;46:723.

[2] Bogousslavsky J, Cachin C, Regli F, et al. Cardiac sources of embolism and crebral infarction–clinical consequences and vascular concomitants: the Lausanne Stroke Registry. Neurology 1991;41:855.

[3] Gage BF, Waterman AD, Shannon W, et al. Validation of clinical classification schemes for predicting stroke: results from the National Registry of Atrial Fibrillation. JAMA 2001; 285:2864.

[4] Sila CA. Neurological therapeutics: principles and practice. In: Noseworthy JH, editor. Cardioembolic Stroke. London: 2003. p. 450–7.

[5] Handke M, Harloff A, Olschewski M, et al. Patent foramen ovale and cryptogenic stroke in older patients. N Engl J Med 2007;357:2262.

[6] Kizer JR, Devereux RB. Clinical practice. Patent foramen ovale in young adults with unexplained stroke. N Engl J Med 2005;353:2361. Erratum appears in N Engl J Med 2006 Jun 1;354(22):2401.

[7] Mas JL, Arquizan C, Lamy C, et al. Recurrent cerebrovascular events associated with patent foramen ovale, atrial septal aneurysm, or both. N Engl J Med 2001;345:1740.

[8] Hendel RC, Patel MR, Kramer CM, et al. ACCF/ACR/SCCT/SCMR/ASNC/NASCI/SCAI/SIR 2006 appropriateness criteria for cardiac computed tomography and cardiac magnetic resonance imaging: a report of the American College of Cardiology Foundation Quality Strategic Directions Committee Appropriateness Criteria Working Group, American College of Radiology, Society of Cardiovascular Computed Tomography, Society for Cardiovascular Magnetic Resonance, American Society of Nuclear Cardiology, North American Society for Cardiac Imaging, Society for Cardiovascular Angiography and Interventions, and Society of Interventional Radiology [see comment]. J Am Coll Cardiol 2006; 48:1475.

[9] Rustemli A, Bhatti TK, Wolff SD. Evaluating cardiac sources of embolic stroke with MRI. Echocardiography 2007;24:301.

[10] Horowitz DR, Tuhrim S, Weinberger JM, et al. Mechanisms in lacunar infarction. Stroke 1992;23:325.

[11] Staaf G, Samuelsson M, Lindgren A, et al. Sensorimotor stroke; clinical features, MRI findings, and cardiac and vascular concomitants in 32 patients. Acta Neurol Scand 1998;97:93.

[12] Hart RG, Pearce LA, Rothbart RM, et al. Stroke with intermittent atrial fibrillation: incidence and predictors during aspirin therapy. Stroke Prevention in Atrial Fibrillation Investigators [see comment]. J Am Coll Cardiol 2000;35:183.

[13] Minematsu K, Yamaguchi T, Omae T. 'Spectacular shrinking deficit': rapid recovery from a major hemispheric syndrome by migration of an embolus. Neurology 1992;42:157.

[14] Caplan LR. Intracranial branch atheromatous disease: a neglected, understudied, and underused concept. Neurology 1989;39:1246–50.

[15] Ramirez-Lassepas M, Cipolle RJ, Bjork RJ, et al. Can embolic stroke be diagnosed on the basis of neurologic clinical criteria? Arch Neurol 1987;44:87.

[16] Caplan LR, Hier DB, D'Cruz I. Cerebral embolism in the Michael Reese Stroke Registry. Stroke 1983;14:530.

[17] Arboix A, Oliveres M, Massons J, et al. Early differentiation of cardioembolic from atherothrombotic cerebral infarction: a multivariate analysis. Eur J Neurol 1999;6:677.

[18] Ferro JM. Cardioembolic stroke: an update. Lancet Neurol 2003;2:177.

[19] Adams HP Jr, del Zoppo G, Alberts MJ, et al. Guidelines for the early management of adults with ischemic stroke: a guideline from the American Heart Association/American Stroke Association Stroke Council, Clinical Cardiology Council, Cardiovascular Radiology and Intervention Council, and the Atherosclerotic Peripheral Vascular Disease and Quality of Care Outcomes in Research Interdisciplinary Working Groups: the American Academy of Neurology affirms the value of this guideline as an educational tool for neurologists. Circulation 2007;115:e478.

[20] Harloff A, Handke M, Reinhard M, et al. Therapeutic strategies after examination by transesophageal echocardiography in 503 patients with ischemic stroke. Stroke 2006;37:859.

[21] Douglas PS, Khandheria B, Stainback RF, et al. ACCF/ASE/ACEP/ASNC/SCAI/SCCT/SCMR 2007 appropriateness criteria for transthoracic and transesophageal echocardiography: a report of the American College of Cardiology Foundation Quality Strategic Directions Committee Appropriateness Criteria Working Group, American Society of Echocardiography, American College of Emergency Physicians, American Society of Nuclear Cardiology, Society for Cardiovascular Angiography and Interventions, Society of Cardiovascular Computed Tomography, and the Society for Cardiovascular Magnetic Resonance endorsed by the American College of Chest Physicians and the Society of Critical Care Medicine. J Am Coll Cardiol 2007;50:187.

[22] Tong DC, Bolger A, Albers GW. Incidence of transcranial Doppler-detected cerebral microemboli in patients referred for echocardiography [see comment]. Stroke 1994;25:2138.

[23] Caplan L. Posterior circulation ischemia: then, now, and tomorrow. The Thomas Willis Lecture-2000. Stroke 2000;31:2011.

[24] Bogousslavsky J, Regli F, Maeder P, et al. The etiology of posterior circulation infarcts: a prospective study using magnetic resonance imaging and magnetic resonance angiography. Neurology 1993;43:1528.

[25] Caplan LR, Wityk RJ, Glass TA, et al. New England Medical Center Posterior Circulation registry. Ann Neurol 2004;56:389.

[26] Glass TA, Hennessey PM, Pazdera L, et al. Outcome at 30 days in the New England Medical Center Posterior Circulation Registry [see comment]. Arch Neurol 2002;59:369.

[27] Schonewille WJ, Wijman CA, Michel P, et al. The Basilar Artery International Cooperative Study (BASICS). Int J Stroke 2007;2:220.

[28] Pessin MS, Lathi ES, Cohen MB, et al. Clinical features and mechanism of occipital infarction. Ann Neurol 1987;21:290.

[29] Yamamoto Y, Georgiadis AL, Chang HM, et al. Posterior cerebral artery territory infarcts in the New England Medical Center Posterior Circulation Registry. Arch Neurol 1999;56:824.

[30] Achenbach S, Sacher D, Ropers D, et al. Electron beam computed tomography for the detection of left atrial thrombi in patients with atrial fibrillation. Heart 2004;90:1477.

[31] Freudenberger RS, Hellkamp AS, Halperin JL, et al. Risk of thromboembolism in heart failure: an analysis from the sudden cardiac death in heart failure trial (SCD-HeFT). Circulation 2007;115:2637.

[32] European Heart Rhythm A, Heart Rhythm S, Fuster V, et al. ACC/AHA/ESC 2006 guidelines for the management of patients with atrial fibrillation–executive summary: a report of the American College of Cardiology/American Heart Association Task Force on Practice Guidelines and the European Society of Cardiology Committee for Practice Guidelines (Writing Committee to Revise the 2001 Guidelines for the Management of Patients With Atrial Fibrillation) [erratum appears in J Am Coll Cardiol 2007 Aug 7;50(6):562]. J Am Coll Cardiol 2006;48:854.

[33] Fuster V, Ryden LE, Cannom DS, et al. ACC/AHA/ESC 2006 guidelines for the management of patients with atrial fibrillation: a report of the American College of Cardiology/

American Heart Association Task Force on Practice Guidelines and the European Society of Cardiology Committee for Practice Guidelines (Writing Committee to Revise the 2001 Guidelines for the Management of Patients With Atrial Fibrillation): developed in collaboration with the European Heart Rhythm Association and the Heart Rhythm Society [erratum appears in Circulation 2007 Aug 7;116(6):e138]. Circulation 2006;114:e257.

[34] Feinberg WM, Blackshear JL, Laupacis A, et al. Prevalence, age distribution, and gender of patients with atrial fibrillation. Analysis and implications. Arch Intern Med 1995;155:469.

[35] Go AS, Hylek EM, Phillips KA, et al. Prevalence of diagnosed atrial fibrillation in adults: national implications for rhythm management and stroke prevention: the AnTicoagulation and Risk Factors in Atrial Fibrillation (ATRIA) Study. JAMA 2001;285:2370.

[36] Frost L, Engholm G, Johnsen S, et al. Incident stroke after discharge from the hospital with a diagnosis of atrial fibrillation. Am J Med 2000;108:36.

[37] Wolf PA, Abbott RD, Kannel WB. Atrial fibrillation as an independent risk factor for stroke: the Framingham Study. Stroke 1991;22:983.

[38] Anonymous. The effect of low-dose warfarin on the risk of stroke in patients with nonrheumatic atrial fibrillation. The Boston area anticoagulation trial for atrial fibrillation investigators [see comment]. N Engl J Med 1990;323:1505.

[39] Ezekowitz MD, Levine JA. Preventing stroke in patients with atrial fibrillation. JAMA 1999;281:1830.

[40] Petersen P, Boysen G, Godtfredsen J, et al. Placebo-controlled, randomised trial of warfarin and aspirin for prevention of thromboembolic complications in chronic atrial fibrillation. The Copenhagen AFASAK study. Lancet 1989;1:175.

[41] Connolly SJ, Laupacis A, Gent M, et al. Canadian Atrial Fibrillation Anticoagulation (CAFA) Study. J Am Coll Cardiol 1991;18:349.

[42] Anonymous. Stroke prevention in Atrial Fibrillation Study. Final results [see comment]. Circulation 1991;84:527.

[43] Pearce LA, Hart RG, Halperin JL. Assessment of three schemes for stratifying stroke risk in patients with nonvalvular atrial fibrillation. Am J Med 2000;109:45.

[44] Anonymous. Risk factors for stroke and efficacy of antithrombotic therapy in atrial fibrillation. Analysis of pooled data from five randomized controlled trials [erratum appears in Arch Intern Med 1994 Oct 10;154(19):2254]. Arch Intern Med 1994;154:1449.

[45] Laupacis A, Albers G, Dalen J, et al. Antithrombotic therapy in atrial fibrillation. Chest 1998;114:579S.

[46] Anonymous. Patients with nonvalvular atrial fibrillation at low risk of stroke during treatment with aspirin: stroke prevention in atrial fibrillation III study. The SPAF III Writing Committee for the stroke prevention in atrial fibrillation investigators [see comment]. JAMA 1998;279:1273.

[47] Hart RG, Pearce LA, Aguilar MI. Meta-analysis: antithrombotic therapy to prevent stroke in patients who have nonvalvular atrial fibrillation. Ann Intern Med 2007;146:857.

[48] Ezekowitz MD, Bridgers SL, James KE, et al. Warfarin in the prevention of stroke associated with nonrheumatic atrial fibrillation. Veterans affairs stroke prevention in nonrheumatic atrial fibrillation investigators [see comment][erratum appears in N Engl J Med 1993 Jan 14;328(2):148]. N Engl J Med 1992;327:1406.

[49] Anonymous. Secondary prevention in non-rheumatic atrial fibrillation after transient ischaemic attack or minor stroke. EAFT (European Atrial Fibrillation Trial) Study Group [see comment]. Lancet 1993;342:1255.

[50] Hart RG, Benavente O, McBride R, et al. Antithrombotic therapy to prevent stroke in patients with atrial fibrillation: a meta-analysis [see comment]. Ann Intern Med 1999; 131:492.

[51] Diener HC, Cunha L, Forbes C, et al. European Stroke Prevention Study. 2. Dipyridamole and acetylsalicylic acid in the secondary prevention of stroke [see comment]. J Neurol Sci 1996;143:1.

[52] Aguilar M, Hart R, Antiplatelet therapy for preventing stroke in patients with non-valvular atrial fibrillation and no previous history of stroke or transient ischemic attacks. [Systematic Review] Cochrane Stroke Group. Cochrane Database of Systematic Reviews 2008.

[53] Posada IS, Barriales V. Alternate-day dosing of aspirin in atrial fibrillation. LASAF Pilot Study Group [see comment]. Am Heart J 1999;138:137.

[54] Sato H, Ishikawa K, Kitabatake A, et al. Low-dose aspirin for prevention of stroke in low-risk patients with atrial fibrillation: Japan Atrial Fibrillation Stroke Trial [see comment]. Stroke 2006;37:447.

[55] Edvardsson N, Juul-Moller S, Omblus R, et al. Effects of low-dose warfarin and aspirin versus no treatment on stroke in a medium-risk patient population with atrial fibrillation. J Intern Med 2003;254:95.

[56] Anonymous. Warfarin versus aspirin for prevention of thromboembolism in atrial fibrillation: stroke prevention in Atrial Fibrillation II Study [see comment]. Lancet 1994;343: 687.

[57] Gullov AL, Koefoed BG, Petersen P, et al. Fixed minidose warfarin and aspirin alone and in combination vs adjusted-dose warfarin for stroke prevention in atrial fibrillation: second Copenhagen atrial fibrillation, aspirin, and anticoagulation study [see comment]. Arch Intern Med 1998;158:1513.

[58] Hellemons BS, Langenberg M, Lodder J, et al. Primary prevention of arterial thromboembolism in non-rheumatic atrial fibrillation in primary care: randomised controlled trial comparing two intensities of coumarin with aspirin [see comment]. BMJ 1999;319:958.

[59] Vemmos KN, Tsivgoulis G, Spengos K, et al. Primary prevention of arterial thromboembolism in the oldest old with atrial fibrillation - a randomized pilot trial comparing adjusted-dose and fixed low-dose coumadin with aspirin. Eur J Intern Med 2006;17:48.

[60] Antithrombotic Therapy in Atrial Fibrillation Study Group. The randomized study of efficacy and safety of antithrombotic therapy in non valvular atrial fibrillation: warfarin compared with aspirin. Zhonghua Xin Xue Guan Bing Za Zhi 2006;34:295.

[61] Rash A, Downes T, Portner R, et al. A randomised controlled trial of warfarin versus aspirin for stroke prevention in octogenarians with atrial fibrillation (WASPO) [see comment]. Age Ageing 2007;36:151.

[62] Morocutti C, Amabile G, Fattapposta F, et al. Indobufen versus warfarin in the secondary prevention of major vascular events in nonrheumatic atrial fibrillation. SIFA (Studio Italiano Fibrillazione Atriale) Investigators. Stroke 1997;28:1015.

[63] Perez-Gomez F, Alegria E, Berjon J, et al. Comparative effects of antiplatelet, anticoagulant, or combined therapy in patients with valvular and nonvalvular atrial fibrillation: a randomized multicenter study [see comment]. J Am Coll Cardiol 2004;44:1557.

[64] Connolly S, Pogue J, Hart R, et al, Active Writing Group on behalf of the ACTIVE Investigators. Clopidogrel plus aspirin versus oral anticoagulation for atrial fibrillation in the Atrial fibrillation Clopidogrel Trial with Irbesartan for prevention of Vascular Events (ACTIVE W): a randomised controlled trial [see comment]. Lancet 2006;367:1903.

[65] Anonymous. Adjusted-dose warfarin versus low-intensity, fixed-dose warfarin plus aspirin for high-risk patients with atrial fibrillation: stroke prevention in atrial fibrillation III randomised clinical trial [see comment]. Lancet 1996;348:633.

[66] Schwedt TJ, Demaerschalk BM, Dodick DW. Patent foramen ovale and migraine: a quantitative systematic review. Cephalalgia 2008;28:531.

[67] Maisel WH, Laskey WK. Patent foramen ovale closure devices: moving beyond equipoise. JAMA 2005;294:366.

[68] Anonymous. Proceedings of the American College of Chest Physicians 5th Consensus on Antithrombotic Therapy. 1998. Chest 1998;114:439S.

[69] Homma S, Sacco RL, Di Tullio MR, et al. Effect of medical treatment in stroke patients with patent foramen ovale: patent foramen ovale in Cryptogenic Stroke Study [see comment]. Circulation 2002;105:2625.

[70] Albers GW, Amarenco P, Easton JD, et al. Antithrombotic and thrombolytic therapy for ischemic stroke: the Seventh ACCP Conference on Antithrombotic and Thrombolytic Therapy. Chest 2004;126:483S.
[71] Messe SR, Silverman IE, Kizer JR, et al. Practice parameter: recurrent stroke with patent foramen ovale and atrial septal aneurysm: report of the Quality Standards Subcommittee of the American Academy of Neurology [see comment]. Neurology 2004;62:1042.
[72] Amarenco P, Cohen A, Tzourio C, et al. Atherosclerotic disease of the aortic arch and the risk of ischemic stroke [see comment]. N Engl J Med 1994;331:1474.
[73] Fujimoto S, Yasaka M, Otsubo R, et al. Aortic arch atherosclerotic lesions and the recurrence of ischemic stroke. Stroke 2004;35:1426.
[74] Tunick PA, Nayar AC, Goodkin GM, et al. Effect of treatment on the incidence of stroke and other emboli in 519 patients with severe thoracic aortic plaque [see comment]. Am J Cardiol 2002;90:1320.
[75] Dressler FA, Craig WR, Castello R, et al. Mobile aortic atheroma and systemic emboli: efficacy of anticoagulation and influence of plaque morphology on recurrent stroke [see comment]. J Am Coll Cardiol 1998;31:134.
[76] Medical Research Council. Assessment of short-term anticoagulant administration after myocardial infarction. BMJ 1969;1:335.
[77] Anonymous. Anticoagulants in acute myocardial infarction. Results of a cooperative clinical trial. JAMA 1973;225:724.
[78] Anonymous. Effect of long-term oral anticoagulant treatment on mortality and cardiovascular morbidity after myocardial infarction. Anticoagulants in the Secondary Prevention of Events in Coronary Thrombosis (ASPECT) Research Group [see comment]. Lancet 1994; 343:499.
[79] Cairns JA, Theroux P, Lewis HD Jr, et al. Antithrombotic agents in coronary artery disease. Chest 1998;114:611S.
[80] Drapkin A, Merskey C. Anticoagulant therapy after acute myocardial infarction. Relation of therapeutic benefit to patient's age, sex, and severity of infarction. JAMA 1972;222:541.
[81] Young JB. Chronic Heart Failure Management. Philadelphia: Lippincott-Raven; 1998.
[82] Di Tullio MR, Homma S. Mechanisms of cardioembolic stroke. Curr Cardiol Rep 2002;4:141.
[83] Mosterd A, Hoes AW, de Bruyne MC, et al. Prevalence of heart failure and left ventricular dysfunction in the general population; the Rotterdam Study. Eur Heart J 1999;20:447.
[84] Witt BJ, Brown RD Jr, Jacobsen SJ, et al. Ischemic stroke after heart failure: a community-based study. Am Heart J 2006;152:102.
[85] Loh E, Sutton MS, Wun CC, et al. Ventricular dysfunction and the risk of stroke after myocardial infarction [see comment]. N Engl J Med 1997;336:251.
[86] Anderson GM, Hull E. The effect of dicumarol upon the mortality and incidence of thromboembolic complications in congestive heart failure. Am Heart J 1950;39:697.
[87] Griffith GC, Stragnell R, Levinson DC, et al. A study of the beneficial effects of anticoagulant therapy in congestive heart failure. Ann Intern Med 1952;37:867.
[88] Harvey WP, Finch CA. Dicumarol prophylaxis of thromboembolic disease in congestive heart failure. N Engl J Med 1950;242:208.
[89] Georgiadis D, Sievert M, Cencetti S, et al. Cerebrovascular reactivity is impaired in patients with cardiac failure [see comment]. Eur Heart J 2000;21:407.
[90] Alves TC, Rays J, Fraguas R Jr, et al. Localized cerebral blood flow reductions in patients with heart failure: a study using 99mTc-HMPAO SPECT. J Neuroimaging 2005;15:150.
[91] Hays AG, Sacco RL, Rundek T, et al. Left ventricular systolic dysfunction and the risk of ischemic stroke in a multiethnic population [see comment]. Stroke 2006;37:1715.
[92] Dries DL, Rosenberg YD, Waclawiw MA, et al. Ejection fraction and risk of thromboembolic events in patients with systolic dysfunction and sinus rhythm: evidence for gender differences in the studies of left ventricular dysfunction trials [erratum appears in J Am Coll Cardiol 1998 Aug;32(2):555]. J Am Coll Cardiol 1997;29:1074.

[93] Koniaris LS, Goldhaber SZ. Anticoagulation in dilated cardiomyopathy [see comment]. J Am Coll Cardiol 1998;31:745.
[94] Dunkman WB, Johnson GR, Carson PE, et al. Incidence of thromboembolic events in congestive heart failure. The V-HeFT VA Cooperative Studies Group. Circulation 1993;87: VI94.
[95] Fuster V, Gersh BJ, Giuliani ER, et al. The natural history of idiopathic dilated cardiomyopathy. Am J Cardiol 1981;47:525.
[96] Kyrle PA, Korninger C, Gossinger H, et al. Prevention of arterial and pulmonary embolism by oral anticoagulants in patients with dilated cardiomyopathy. Thromb Haemost 1985;54: 521.
[97] Massie BM, Krol WF, Ammon SE, et al. The Warfarin and Antiplatelet Therapy in Heart Failure trial (WATCH): rationale, design, and baseline patient characteristics [see comment]. J Card Fail 2004;10:101.
[98] Massie BM, Krol WF, Ammon SE, et al. Final results of the warfarin and antiplatelet trial in chronic heart failure (WATCH): A randomized comparison of warfarin, aspirin, and clopidogrel. Presented at the Annual Scientific Session of the American College of Cardiology: March 9, 2004.
[99] Pullicino P, Thompson JL, Barton B, et al. Warfarin versus aspirin in patients with reduced cardiac ejection fraction (WARCEF): rationale, objectives, and design. J Card Fail 2006;12:39.
[100] ACC/AHA 2006 guidelines for the management of patients with valvular heart disease: a report of the American College of Cardiology/American Heart Association Task Force on Practice Guidelines (writing Committee to Revise the 1998 guidelines for the management of patients with valvular heart disease) developed in collaboration with the Society of Cardiovascular Anesthesiologists endorsed by the Society for Cardiovascular Angiography and Interventions and the Society of Thoracic Surgeons.[erratum] J Am Coll Cardiol 2007;49(9):1014. Journal of the American College of Cardiology 2006;48(3):e1–148
[101] Mills P, Leech G, Davies M, et al. The natural history of a non-stenotic bicuspid aortic valve. Br Heart J 1978;40:951.
[102] Salem DN, Levine HJ, Pauker SG, et al. Antithrombotic therapy in valvular heart disease. Chest 1998;114:590S.
[103] Salgado AV, Furlan A, Salcedo E. Risk of stroke in patients with congenital bicuspid aortic valve. J Stroke Cerebrovasc Dis 1991;1:61.
[104] Stein PD, Dalen JE, Goldman S, et al. Antithrombotic therapy in patients with saphenous vein and internal mammary artery bypass grafts. Chest 1998;114:658S.
[105] Davidson CJ, Skelton TN, Kisslo KB, et al. The risk for systemic embolization associated with percutaneous balloon valvuloplasty in adults. A prospective comprehensive evaluation. Ann Intern Med 1988;108:557.
[106] Petty GW, Orencia AJ, Khandheria BK, et al. A population-based study of stroke in the setting of mitral valve prolapse: risk factors and infarct subtype classification. Mayo Clin Proc 1994;69:632.
[107] Wolf PA, Sila CA. Cerebral ischemia with mitral valve prolapse. Am Heart J 1987;113: 1308.
[108] Stein PD, Alpert JS, Dalen JE, et al. Antithrombotic therapy in patients with mechanical and biological prosthetic heart valves. Chest 1998;114:602S.
[109] Castelman B. Roth S. Tumors of the cardiovascular system, 1st edition. Washington DC: Armed Forces Institute of Pathology; 1978, Vol Fascicle 15.
[110] Reynen K. Frequency of primary tumors of the heart. Am J Cardiol 1996;77:107.
[111] Aziz F, Baciewicz FA Jr. Lambl's excrescences: review and recommendations. Tex Heart Inst J 2007;34:366.
[112] Dismukes WE. Management of infective endocarditis. Cardiovasc Clin 1981;11:189.
[113] Fleming HA. General principles of the treatment of infective endocarditis. J Antimicrob Chemother 1987;(20 Suppl A):143.

[114] Hart RG, Foster JW, Luther MF, et al. Stroke in infective endocarditis. Stroke 1990;21:695.

[115] Prabhakaran S. Neurologic complications of endocarditis. Continuum Lifelong Learning in Neurology 2008;14(1):53–73.

[116] Robbins MJ, Eisenberg ES, Frishman WH. Infective endocarditis: a pathophysiologic approach to therapy. Cardiol Clin 1987;5:545.

[117] Salgado AV, Furlan AJ, Keys TF, et al. Neurologic complications of endocarditis: a 12-year experience. Neurology 1989;39:173.

[118] Reynen K. Cardiac myxomas [see comment]. N Engl J Med 1995;333:1610.

[119] Sastre-Garriga J, Molina C, Montaner J, et al. Mitral papillary fibroelastoma as a cause of cardiogenic embolic stroke: report of two cases and review of the literature. Eur J Neurol 2000;7:449.

[120] Anonymous. Transesophageal echocardiographic correlates of thromboembolism in high-risk patients with nonvalvular atrial fibrillation. The stroke prevention in atrial fibrillation investigators committee on echocardiography [see comment]. Ann Intern Med 1998;128:639.

[121] Leung DY, Black IW, Cranney GB, et al. Prognostic implications of left atrial spontaneous echo contrast in nonvalvular atrial fibrillation. J Am Coll Cardiol 1994;24:755.

[122] Nishimura RA, Holmes DR Jr, Reeder GS. Percutaneous balloon valvuloplasty. Mayo Clin Proc 1990;65:198.

Section IV

Special Populations at Risk for Stroke

ELSEVIER
SAUNDERS

NEUROLOGIC
CLINICS

Neurol Clin 26 (2008) 1161–1176

Stroke in Women: Risk and Prevention Throughout the Lifespan

Cheryl D. Bushnell, MD, MHS

Department of Neurology, Wake Forest University Health Sciences, Medical Center Boulevard, Winston-Salem, NC 27157, USA

About 780,000 people in the United States suffer a stroke each year, and about 15% of these strokes are fatal. Of those who die from stroke, about 60% are women [1]. Women also tend to have worse outcomes (quality of life, depression, disability) than men [2–4]. Although the incidence of stroke is lower in women than men for most of their lifespan, a 65-year-old woman's lifetime risk of stroke is 1 in 5, whereas a 65-year-old man's risk is one in six [5]. There has been an increasing emphasis on gender differences and gender-specific issues in cardiovascular diseases. Therefore, randomized controlled trials and cohort studies limited to women have increased our understanding of the health-related issues that are specific to women. Although the majority of strokes occur in women who are older, it is important to consider the woman's lifespan to best appreciate the impact of stroke in women.

Stroke in girls

Stroke is rare in young children, occurring at a rate of 2.3 to 2.7 per 100,000 children in the United States [6–8]. There have been relatively few studies with adequate numbers of childhood stroke cases to determine differences by gender. However, a large epidemiology study of all children in California found that boys were at higher risk for all stroke types than girls (boys: 2.57/100,000; girls: 2.02/100,000; RR 1.28, 95% CI 1.17–1.39) [8].

This work was supported by Grant No. K02 NS058760 from the National Institutes of Health.

E-mail address: cbushnel@wfubmc.edu

doi:10.1016/j.ncl.2008.05.009 ***neurologic.theclinics.com***

Stroke during child-bearing years

Pregnancy

For women of child-bearing age, the incidence of stroke is low, about 11 per 100,000. During pregnancy, the rate of stroke appears to increase. Reported incidence has ranged from 4 to 34 per 100,000 (Table 1) [9–17]. Three population-based studies have used the Nationwide Inpatient Sample (NIS) to investigate stroke in pregnancy [13,14,18]. The NIS is a 20% stratified sample of all discharges in the United States available for assessments of hospitalization rates using specific ICD-9 codes. This is especially useful for conditions such as pregnancy, because the ICD-9 codes can designate antepartum, delivery, or postpartum hospitalizations. During 1979–1991, the rate of stroke (including intracranial venous thrombosis) was 29.1 per 100,000 deliveries [13], and from 1993 to 1994 the rate was 24.7 per 100,000 [14]. The analysis from 2000 to 2001 [16] reported a slightly higher rate (34.2 per 100,000) than the previous two analyses. This may be related to the use of specific ICD-9 codes for stroke (325, 430, 431, 434, and 436) in addition to the codes for cerebrovascular disorders in the puerperium (674.0) [16]. In addition, it is possible that the incidence of pregnancy-related stroke may be increasing.

The majority of pregnancy-related strokes occur postpartum. For example, of the stroke cases identified by James and colleagues [16], 48% occurred in the postpartum period, versus 41% at delivery, and 11% antepartum. In addition, the Baltimore Washington Cooperative Young Stroke Study found that stroke rate was not increased in pregnant compared with nonpregnant women, but during the postpartum period, there was a fivefold increased risk of ischemic stroke (RR 5.4; 95% CI 2.9–10.0), and an 18-fold increased risk of intracerebral hemorrhage (RR 18.2; 95% CI 8.7–38.1) [11]. In a case series of 20 women with postpartum stroke, eight (40%) occurred within the first 7 days of delivery, seven (35%) between 7 and 14 days, three (15%) between 14 and 21 days, and two (10%) between 28 and 36 days [19]. Although the underlying reason for the increased risk of stroke at delivery and postpartum is not certain, increased risk may be associated with a relative hypercoagulability and the natural selection to protect against fatal hemorrhage at delivery. Others have speculated that the large decrease in blood volume, the rapid fluctuations in hormone levels, or vessel wall changes could profoundly influence cerebral hemodynamics [11].

Pregnancy-related intracerebral hemorrhage (ICH) carries the highest morbidity and mortality of all stroke types [16]. The incidence of pregnancy-related ICH was also studied using the NIS database, and an analysis from 1993 to 2002 showed that the risk of ICH is higher in pregnant (7.1 per 100,000 at-risk person-years) than in nonpregnant women (5.0 per 100,000 person years) [17]. Similar to other stroke types, ICH predominantly occurred postpartum compared with antepartum. In addition, 20% of these women died in the hospital; 18% were discharged to a skilled nursing or other type of facility; and only 44% had routine discharges to home. Factors associated with maternal mortality included advanced maternal age, Hispanic race-ethnicity, and coagulopathy [17].

There are multiple risk factors that have been recognized as risk factors for stroke in pregnancy. One of the most important risks is advanced maternal age. For example, in the NIS analysis from 2000 to 2001, the incidence increased from 35.3 per 100,000 in those aged 30 to 34, to 58.1 per 100,000 in those aged 35 to 39 [16]. In addition, African American women have about a 50% higher risk of stroke than white women (odds ratio [OR] 1.5; 95% CI 1.2–1.9). Novel risk factors that were explored and found to be associated with pregnancy-related stroke in the most recent analysis of the NIS included migraine (OR 16.9; 95% CI 9.7–29.5), thrombophilia (OR 16.0; 95% CI 9.4–27.2), sickle cell disease (OR 9.1; 95% CI 3.7–22.2), and lupus (OR 15.2; 95% CI 7.4–31.2) [16]. Other expected pregnancy-related complications were also identified, such as postpartum infection, postpartum hemorrhage, transfusion, fluid/electrolyte imbalance, and preeclampsia/gestational hypertension [16].

Preeclampsia

One of the hypertensive disorders of pregnancy, preeclampsia occurs in about 5% of pregnancies in the United States; it is an important cause of maternal and infant morbidity and mortality [20,21]. Preeclampsia and gestational hypertension increase the risk of stroke during pregnancy as a result of severe hypertension and disturbed cerebral autoregulation. For example, preeclampsia has been associated with vasculopathies that overlap with hypertensive encephalopathy and lead to cerebral endothelial leakage. This causes an appearance of vasogenic edema on brain imaging, is typically reversible, and rarely associated with ischemic stroke. The other severe consequence of hypertension is the risk of pregnancy-related ICH. As shown in the NIS analysis from 1993 to 2002, preeclampsia/gestational hypertension was associated with a 10-fold risk of pregnancy-related ICH [22]. Preeclampsia can also occur postpartum, and under-recognition of the diagnosis could lead to substantial delays in treatment.

The pathophysiology of preeclampsia is believed to be related to endothelial dysfunction that occurs early during pregnancy [23]. The endothelial dysfunction may also persist following delivery. For example, Chambers and colleagues [24] showed that women with preeclamptic deliveries had poorer endothelial function than women with normal pregnancies, even after adjusting for cardiovascular risk factors. Another case–control study showed that women with a history of preeclampsia evaluated about 15 years after pregnancy had higher glycosylated hemoglobin levels and insulin levels, which were suggestive of metabolic syndrome, as well as an increase

Table 1
Incidence studies of pregnancy-related stroke

Author	Data source	Stroke cases/pregnant population	Incidence (per 100,000 deliveries)	Causes/risk factors
Sharshar et al [9]	Hospital records, France	31/348,295	Non-ICH: 4.3 ICH: 4.6	Eclampsia, AVM, cervical artery dissection, PPA, PS deficiency, DIC
Jaigobin and Silver [10]	Hospital records Toronto, Canada	34/50,711	All: 26 Infarction: 18 ICH: 8	Coagulopathy, preeclampsia, smoking, hypertension, AVM, DIC, aneurysm
Kittner et al [11]	Baltimore-Wash. Cooperative Young Stroke Study Hospital records	31/234,023	All: 8.1	Preeclampsia, CNS vasculopathy, dissection, TTP, cortical vein thrombosis, vasculitis, AVM, cocaine
Ros et al [12]	Inpatient register Sweden, 1987–1995	144/1,003,489 deliveries	Infarction: 4.0 ICH: 3.8 SAH: 2.4	Maternal age > 35, parity ≥ 4, 2 days before to 1 day after delivery
Lanska and Kryscio [13]	National Hospital Discharge Survey (1979–1991)	8,918/50,264,631 deliveries	Stroke: 17.7	Age 35–44, hypertension
Lanska and Kryscio [14]	Nationwide inpatient sample releases 2 and 3	183/1,408,015 deliveries	Stroke: 13	Age 35–44, hypertension, Cesarean delivery, fluid/electrolyte, acid-base disorder, rheumatic fever/valvular heart disease, pneumonia, vomiting
Jeng et al [15]	National Taiwan University Hospital young stroke registry medical records	49/49,796 deliveries	Infarction: 8 ICH: 9 SAH: 1	Hypertension, cardiac disease, hypercholesterolemia, preeclampsia, AVM, aneurysm, coagulopathy

James et al [16]	Nationwide inpatient sample 2000–2001	2,850/8,322,799 deliveries	Stroke: 34	Maternal age >35, African American race, hypertension, heart disease, thrombophilia, sickle cell disease, anemia, thrombocytopenia, lupus, diabetes, migraine headaches, alcohol/substance abuse, smoking, preeclampsia, postpartum hemorrhage, transfusion, postpartum infection, fluid/electrolyte imbalance
Bateman et al [17]	Nationwide inpatient sample 1993–2002	423/6,969,553 deliveries	ICH: 6.1	Maternal age >35, African American race, hypertension, preeclampsia/eclampsia, coagulopathy, tobacco abuse

Abbreviations: AVM, arteriovenous malformation; CNS, central nervous system; DIC, disseminated intravascular coagulation; ICH, intracerebral hemorrhage; PPA, post-partum angiopathy; SAH, subarachnoid hemorrhage; TTP thrombotic thrombocytopenic purpura.

From: Bushnell C. Stroke and the female brain. Nature Clinical Practice Neurology 2007;4:22–33; with permission.

in circulating cellular adhesion molecules (intercellular adhesion molecule [ICAM] and vascular cell adhesion molecule [VCAM]) compared with controls [25]. A separate study demonstrated that women with preeclampsia onset before 34 weeks gestation had elevated carotid intimal medial thickness (ie, a measure of subclinical atherosclerosis), compared with women with normal pregnancies and nulliparous women [26]. These measurements were performed beyond the puerperium, but before lactation had ceased. Although this study was small (only 22 women in each group), it suggests that preeclampsia, in particular the early-onset type, may be associated with accelerated atherosclerosis [26].

The vascular and inflammatory changes in women with a history of preeclampsia may in part explain the observed increased risk of stroke later in life. In a study from Scotland, women with preeclampsia/eclampsia were four times more likely to have hypertension (OR 3.98; 95% CI 2.8–5.6) and three times more likely to have had a self-reported stroke (OR 3.4; 95% CI 0.95–12.2) [27]. The Stroke Prevention in Young Women Study, a case–control study of women with ischemic stroke between ages 15 and 44, showed a 50% higher prevalence of self-reported preeclampsia versus controls, although the association was diminished when adjusted for hypertension [28]. In addition, women with maternal placental syndrome, which includes gestational hypertension, preeclampsia/eclampsia, placental abruption, and placental infarction, have an increased risk of heart disease later in life [29].

Another important consequence of preeclampsia is the risk of infant morbidity and mortality. Preeclampsia was shown to be an independent risk factor for perinatal arterial stroke, increasing the odds by fivefold (OR 5.3: 1.3-22.0) [30]. Therefore, it is important to recognize that preeclampsia is a risk for vasculopathy or stroke during delivery and postpartum (especially ICH), and it poses a risk for stroke later in life as a result of endothelial dysfunction, hypertension, and an increase in cardiovascular risk factors.

Oral contraceptives

The risk of stroke with oral contraceptive pill (OCP) use has been extensively evaluated. The results of three separate meta-analyses summarizing over 30 years of studies have shown that oral contraceptive users have about a twofold increased risk of stroke over non-users [31–33]. Because the incidence of stroke is low in this age group, the absolute risk with oral contraceptive use is also low, at about 8 per 100,000 women [31]. Although most women who use these drugs are healthy, there are some medical conditions that are clearly associated with an accelerated risk. These conditions include hypertension, smoking, migraine headache with aura, thrombophilia, and obesity.

Hypertension is a major risk factor for stroke in women using OCPs [34–37]. When blood pressure is screened before prescribing OCPs–and appropriately managed–the risk of ischemic stroke is reduced [38,39]. It is therefore recommended that blood pressure be screened before prescribing OCPs. The American College of Obstetricians and Gynecologists recommends that if women are under age 35 with well-controlled and monitored hypertension who do not smoke or have evidence of end-organ vascular disease, a trial of low-dose OCPs is acceptable [40].

Like hypertension, cigarette smoking is a well-known risk factor for stroke in women using OCPs. This risk ranges from about twofold to eightfold in OCP users versus nonusers [32,34–36,41,42]. It is recommended that women who plan to use OCPs avoid smoking while on these medications, particularly if the women are over the age of 35.

OCP users who also have migraine headaches have an increased risk of stroke versus women without migraine headaches. The World Health Organization (WHO) Collaborative Study showed that women with migraine headache who used OCPs were roughly eight times more likely to have ischemic stroke than those with either risk factor alone and more than 16 times as likely as those with neither risk factor [43]. When women with both risk factors also smoked, a greater than multiplicative effect was seen on stroke risk, with an OR of 34.4 compared with those with none of the risk factors. Another study found a nearly 14-fold increase in migraineurs who used OCPs compared with those with neither risk factor [44]. A pooled analysis of two studies from the United States found a lower, but still statistically significant, risk of ischemic stroke in migraineurs who used OCPs [45].

Women who have migraines without auras and no other stroke risk factors can safely take OCPs, whereas women with frequent, prolonged, complicated auras should avoid OCPs [46]. The International Headache Society Task Force on Combined Oral Contraceptives and Hormone Replacement Therapy recommends consideration of progestin-only pills in those with stroke risk factors [47]. They also suggest that further evaluation, and possibly cessation of OCPs, may be needed in users who develop new persisting headaches, new-onset migraine with aura, increased headache frequency or intensity, or unusual aura symptoms including prolonged aura [47].

OCP use alters a variety of coagulation factors that may play an important role in the increased risk of stroke in users. There is evidence that women who have underlying thrombophilic disorders are at increased stroke risk when using OCPs. Slooter and colleagues [48] found that OCP users with Factor V Leiden mutation were at a greater than 11-fold increased risk of stroke than nonusers without the mutation. OCP users with the MTHFR 677TT mutation were at a roughly fivefold increased risk compared with those with neither risk factor. The risk of stroke with OCP use and MTHFR mutation is more than double that of either risk factor alone [49].

Obesity, as measured by body mass index and abdominal girth, has also been associated with a small but significant increased risk of stroke [50].

Obesity in combination with OCP use has been demonstrated to further increase the risk of stroke in young women. A large case–control study from the Netherlands noted a fourfold increase in stroke risk in obese OCP users compared with non-obese women who do not use OCPs and a twofold increased risk compared with nonobese women who use OCPs [36]. The best explanation for this synergistic risk is that obese women are at risk for hypercoagulability, insulin-resistance and diabetes, hypertension, and hyperlipidemia, which are all factors that increase the risk of stroke and which are perhaps synergistically increasing the risk in women using OCPs.

Stroke during mid-life

Women under age 50 are generally considered to have a lower incidence and prevalence of stroke than men [1]. However, data from the National Health and Nutrition Examination Survey (NHANES) has shown that women appear to be having a more substantial increase in the prevalence of stroke in midlife versus men. In this analysis, women age 45 to 54 had a significantly higher odds of stroke compared with men the same age (OR 2.39; 95% CI 1.32–4.32) [51]. Consistent with the surge in stroke events, there was a surge in cardiovascular risk in women greater than men, as well. For instance, systolic blood pressure (SBP) increased at a steeper rate in women with each decade from 35 to 44 years (average SBP 113.9 mm Hg), 45 to 54 years (average SBP 123.5 mm Hg), and 55 to 64 years (average SBP 132.0 mm Hg) [51]. Men, however, initially had a higher SBP between ages 35 and 44 (average SBP 120.0 mm Hg) than women, but men showed a more gradual increase to the ages of 55 to 64 (average SBP 128.6 mm Hg). In addition, women had a substantial increase in total cholesterol, triglycerides, waist circumference, homocysteine, glycosylated hemoglobin, and a lowering of the ankle brachial pulsatility index between the ages of 45 to 54 and 55 to 64 [51]. These data suggest that there is an acceleration of multiple risk parameters in women a decade or more before cardiovascular and stroke events traditionally occur in women. Assuming these data are valid, there is a significant opportunity to increase efforts to recognize risk factors in women during midlife and improve prevention strategies.

Menopause

The midlife prevalence of stroke in women has been shown to occur as women would traditionally be experiencing the menopausal transition. Menopause occurs naturally in women with at least one intact and functioning ovary. During perimenopause, estradiol levels decline by about 60% [52]. After menopause, estradiol levels continue to decline but then plateau after one to three years. Overall, there is a sevenfold to 10-fold decrease in estradiol levels from the beginning to the end of the menopausal transition

[53]. In contrast to the rapid decline in estradiol, circulating testosterone levels are decreasing more gradually during this period, [54] leading to a relative androgen excess [54].

The menopausal shifts in hormonal levels and ratios of estrogens to androgens are important because these sex steroids appear to have opposite effects on vascular risk. Estrogens have multiple beneficial effects on the cardiovascular system, including vasodilation and increased cerebral blood flow [55] by decreasing cerebral vascular tone and increasing arterial compliance [56].

In addition to the benefits on vessel function, estrogen may also reduce atherosclerotic risk through its impact on lipids. Exogenous estrogen replacement improves lipid profiles by lowering total and low-density lipoprotein (LDL) cholesterol, lipoprotein (a), and raising high-density lipoprotein (HDL) cholesterol [57,58].

Conversely, androgens have a detrimental effect on cerebral blood vessels by increasing arterial tone. They also lead to a pro-atherogenic profile by decreasing HDL, and by increasing triglycerides, LDL, and total cholesterol [54].

Concurrent with the decline in sex steroids, women develop changes in cardiovascular risk factors during menopause. Lipid measurements in women across the menopausal transition in the Healthy Women Study showed that LDL cholesterol and triglycerides increased and HDL cholesterol decreased during perimenopause, whereas fasting glucose and blood pressure levels increased during postmenopause [59]. Along with a change in body fat distribution leading to abdominal obesity, the lipid, blood pressure, and glucose changes are consistent with metabolic syndrome. In addition to the metabolic changes, estrogen deficiency during menopause also leads to a shift from anti-inflammatory to proinflammatory cytokines such as IL-1β, IL-6, and TNF-α [60]. These cytokines are important because they have been associated with an increased risk of heart disease and stroke [61].

Hormone therapy (including selective estrogen receptor modulators)

Replacing the depletion of endogenous estradiol with replacement hormone therapy was widely believed to be an effective method to reduce cardiovascular disease in women. However, randomized trials of hormone therapy with conjugated equine estrogens (CEE), CEE with medroxyprogesterone acetate (MPA), and 17-beta estradiol showed no benefit for secondary prevention of heart disease [62] and stroke, [63] as well as an increased risk of both types of events in healthy women (ie, the Women's Health Initiative [WHI]) [64]. Multiple analyses of the WHI results have not revealed any particular subgroup of women who are at higher or lower risk of cardiovascular events with hormone therapy (HT). However, a post hoc analysis of events based on the time of initiation following menopause showed that there was a trend for a reduced risk for heart disease for women who initiated HT within 5 years of menopause, but the risk of stroke with HT was elevated regardless of the timing of initiation [65].

Selective estrogen receptor modulators (SERMs) have anti-estrogenic effects in mammary tissues and estrogenic effects on bone and cholesterol levels, making these drugs useful for prevention of breast cancer and osteoporosis. Tamoxifen has been used as adjuvant therapy for surgical resection, radiation and chemotherapy in breast cancer, as well as prevention for high-risk women. Tamoxifen increases the risk of venous thrombosis by twofold to fourfold in users, and it may also be associated with an increased risk of ischemic stroke. A meta-analysis of prevention and adjuvant therapy trials found an 80% increased risk of ischemic stroke (OR 1.82; 95% CI 1.41–2.36), whereas there was a nonsignificant increase in all strokes combined (OR 1.29; 95% CI 0.92–1.81) [66]. A large case–control study, however, found that there was no association between stroke and tamoxifen use in women following breast cancer diagnosis, but that the use of any chemotherapy, regardless of regimen or whether it was combined with tamoxifen, was associated with stroke (OR 2.3; 95% CI 1.4–3.8). Raloxifene, a separate SERM, has been studied in a similar fashion as tamoxifen, but primarily for breast cancer prevention and for osteoporosis. Although an early analysis of cardiovascular events in the Multiple Outcomes of Raloxifene Evaluation suggested protection against cardiovascular events in women at high risk for cardiovascular disease, [67] the Raloxifene Use for the Heart trial showed no protection against heart disease and total strokes, but an increased risk for fatal stroke (OR 1.49; 95% CI 1.00–2.24) [68]. Raloxifene also significantly reduced the risk of invasive breast cancer [68]. Another trial compared the effects of tamoxifen and raloxifene on these same risks in the Study of Tamoxifen and Raloxifene trial [69]. This trial showed no difference in the rates of heart disease or stroke in the two treatment groups, although the risk of venous thromboembolism was lower with raloxifene.

Based on the strong evidence from these trials, the only recommended use for hormone therapy is for treatment of vasomotor symptoms (ie, hot flashes) and osteoporosis [70]. The cardiovascular disease prevention guidelines for women state that neither hormone therapy nor SERMs should be used for primary or secondary prevention (class III, level A) [71].

Stroke in older women

The impending epidemic

The prevalence of stroke is lower in women than men until the ages of 75 [72] to 85 [73]. With the exception of the NHANES analysis suggesting a midlife surge, women appear to be protected from stroke until the oldest age groups. From a population-based perspective, women make up about half of the population at age 50, but the ratio of women to men increases with each decade to a ratio of 2.70 at age 90 [74]. As a result of the larger number of women in older age groups, women comprise an excess of stroke deaths, which will increase as the population ages. Weighing all these factors together, there may be an impending epidemic of women dying from stroke. Health care providers need to be prepared for this by recognizing the risk factors and optimizing prevention in older women. The risk factors for stroke include hypertension, smoking, hyperlipidemia, atrial fibrillation, diabetes mellitus, carotid stenosis, prior stroke or transient ischemic attack, and coronary artery disease.

Guidelines for cardiovascular disease prevention in women

The most recent American Heart Association evidence-based guidelines for Cardiovascular Disease Prevention in Women contains updated clinical information relevant to the care of women at risk of stroke. Although these guidelines are not specific for stroke alone, the majority of the risk factors for stroke and heart disease overlap, and the prevention strategies are relevant for both conditions.

In this update, classification of risk was modified to include high risk, at risk, and optimal risk (Box 1). The rationale for reclassifying women is related to the very high lifetime risk of cardiovascular disease. In fact, the lifetime risk of stroke in women is about 20%, [5] and for all cardiovascular disease, this approaches 40% [75]. The traditional Framingham risk score limits the prediction to 10 years or less, but it may underestimate the future risk of CVD in women who are found to have subclinical disease, measured with coronary artery calcium or carotid intimal-medial thickness [71]. In addition, because women are frequently misclassified as having lower than actual risk by physicians, [76] this redefinition was intended to increase recognition of risk and guide appropriate prevention strategies for women based on a simpler risk classification [71].

The guidelines for women who are not actively being treated for an acute cardiovascular event can be summarized as follows: (1) all women, regardless of risk, should be counseled on class I, level B lifestyle recommendations (smoking cessation, heart-healthy eating patterns, regular physical activity, and weight management); (2) blood pressure control (class I, level A for pharmacotherapy and level B for lifestyle changes), LDL goal < 100 mg/dL (class I, level B), aspirin (class I, level A) or other antiplatelet agents (class I, level B), glycemic control in diabetic women (class I, level B), and aldosterone blocker (class I, level B) in selected women are recommended for high risk women who have not had a recent cardiovascular event and do not meet requirements for acute cardiac or stroke rehabilitation [71]; (3) weight maintenance/reduction be pursued in all women, regardless of risk, to a goal BMI of 18.5 to 24.9 kg/m2 and a waist circumference of ≤ 35 in through a balance of physical activity, caloric intake, and formal

Box 1. Risk classification for cardiovascular disease

High risk
Established coronary heart disease
Cerebrovascular disease
Peripheral arterial disease
Abdominal aortic aneurysm
End-stage or chronic renal disease
Diabetes mellitus
10-year Framingham global risk > 20%

At risk
>1 major risk factor for CVD, including:
- Cigarette smoking
- Poor diet
- Physical inactivity
- Obesity, especially central adiposity
- Family history of premature CVD (CVD at <55 years of age in male relative and <65 years of age in female relative)
- Hypertension
- Dyslipidemia

Evidence of subclinical vascular disease (eg, coronary calcification or carotid intimal–medial thickness)
Metabolic syndrome
Poor exercise capacity on treadmill test and/or abnormal heart rate recovery after stopping exercise

Optimal risk
Framingham global risk <10% and a healthy lifestyle with no risk factors

Adapted from Mosca L, Banka C, Benjamin E, et al. Evidence-based guidelines for cardiovascular disease prevention in women: 2007 update. Circulation 2007;115:1481–501; with permission.

behavioral programs when indicated (class I, level B) [71]. Recommended diets are those rich in fruits and vegetables, whole-grain, high-fiber foods, fish (especially oily fish) at least twice a week, as well as very limited proportions of saturated fats and transfatty acids (class I, level B); (4) physical activity recommendations for women include an accumulated total of at least 30 minutes of moderate-intensity physical exercise (eg, brisk walking) on most days of the week (class I, level B). Women who are working to lose weight or sustain weight should increase to 60 to 90 minutes of moderate-intensity activity on most, if not all, days of the week (class I, level C) [71].

Aspirin for stroke prevention in women

Aspirin has long been the mainstay of secondary prevention of cardiovascular disease. An analysis from the Nurses' Health Study showed that women who used aspirin long-term had significantly lower mortality, especially cardiovascular mortality [77]. The Women's Health Study, a randomized controlled trial of 100 mg of aspirin every other day compared with placebo in healthy women over age 45, is the only study of aspirin for primary prevention in women [78]. The primary result of the trial showed no overall benefit in the composite outcome of first major cardiovascular event (nonfatal myocardial infarction, nonfatal stroke, or death from cardiovascular disease) for the aspirin treated subjects [78]. However, there was a beneficial decrease in ischemic stroke events. The guidelines for cardiovascular prevention in women currently recommend aspirin therapy in doses of 75 to 325 mg per day for high-risk women unless contraindicated (class I, level A), and in women age 65 years or older, aspirin should be considered in doses of 81 mg daily or 100 mg every other day if blood pressure is controlled and the benefit for preventing ischemic stroke or myocardial infarction outweighs the risk of gastrointestinal bleeding and hemorrhagic stroke (class IIa, level B). In women younger than 65 years of age, aspirin should be considered when the benefit for preventing ischemic stroke is likely to outweigh the adverse effects of therapy (class IIb, level B) [71].

References

[1] Rosamund W, Flegal K, Furie K, et al. Heart Disease and Stroke Statistics 2008 Update: A report from the American Heart Association Committee and Stroke Statistics Subcommittee. Circulation 2008;117:e25–146.

[2] Gargano J, Reeves M. Sex differences in stroke recovery and stroke-specific quality of life. Stroke 2007;38:2541–8.

[3] Eriksson M, Asplund K, Glader E-L, et al. Self-reported dperession and the use of antidepressants after stroke: a national survey. Stroke 2004;35:936–41.

[4] Herrmann N, Black S, Lawrence J, et al. The Sunnybrook Stroke Study. A prospective study of depressive symptoms and functional outcome. Stroke 1998;29:618–24.

[5] Seshadri S, Beiser AS, Kelly-Hayes M, et al. The lifetime risk of stroke. Estimates from the framingham study. Stroke 2006;37:345–50.

[6] Broderick J, Talbot G, Prenger E, et al. Stroke in children within a major metropolitan area: the surprising importance of intracerebral hemorrhage. J Child Neurol 1993;8:250–5.

[7] Schoenberg B, Mellinger J, Schoenberg D. Cerebrovascular disease in infants and children: a study of incidence, clinical features, and survival. Neurology 1978;28:763–8.

[8] Fullerton H, Wu Y, Zhao S, et al. Risk of stroke in children. Ethnic and gender disparities. Neurology 2003;61:189–94.

[9] Sharshar T, Lamy C, Mas J. Incidence and causes of strokes associated with pregnancy and puerperium. A study in public hospitals of Ile de France. Stroke 1995;26:930–6.

[10] Jaigobin C, Silver FL. Stroke and pregnancy. Stroke 2000;31:2948–51.

[11] Kittner SJ, Stern BJ, Feeser BR, et al. Pregnancy and the risk of stroke. N Engl J Med 1996; 335:768–74.
[12] Ros HS, Lichtenstein P, Bellocco R, et al. Increased risks of circulatory diseases in late pregnancy and puerperium. Epidemiology 2001;12:456–60.
[13] Lanska DJ, Kryscio RJ. Stroke and intracranial venous thrombosis during pregnancy and puerperium. Neurology 1998;51:1622–8.
[14] Lanska DJ, Kryscio RJ. Risk factors for peripartum and postpartum stroke and intracranial venous thrombosis. Stroke 2000;31:1274–82.
[15] Jeng J-S, Tang S-C, Yip P-K. Stroke in women of reproductive age: comparison between stroke related and unrelated to pregnancy. J Neurol Sci 2004;221:25–9.
[16] James A, Bushnell CD, Jamison M, et al. Incidence and risk factors for stroke in pregnancy and the puerperium. Obstet Gynecol 2005;106:509–16.
[17] Bateman B, Schumacher H, Bushnell CD, et al. Intracerebral hemorrhage in pregnancy. Frequency, risk factors, and outcome. Neurology 2006;67:424–9.
[18] Lanska DJ, Kryscio RJ. Peripartum stroke and intracranial venous thrombosis in the National Hospital Discharge Survey. Obstet Gynecol 1997;89:413–8.
[19] Witlin AG, Mattar F, Sibai BM. Postpartum stroke: a twenty-year experience. Am J Obstet Gynecol 2000;183:83–8.
[20] Kaunitz A, Hughes J, Grimes D, et al. Causes of maternal mortality in the United States. Obstet Gynecol 1985;65:605–12.
[21] Mackay A, Berg C, Atrash H. Pregnancy-related mortality from preeclampsia and eclampsia. Obstet Gynecol 2001;97:533–8.
[22] Bateman B, Schumacher H, Boden-Albala B, et al. Factors associated with in-hospital mortality after administration of thrombolysis in acute ischemic stroke patients. An analysis of the nationwide inpatient sample 1999 to 2002. Stroke 2006;37:440–6.
[23] Roberts JM, Pearson G, Cutler J, et al. Summary of the NHLBI working group on research on hypertension during pregnancy. Hypertension 2003;41:437–45.
[24] Chambers JC, Fusi L, Malik IS, et al. Association of maternal endothelial dysfunction with preeclampsia. JAMA 2001;285:1607–12.
[25] Sattar N, Ramsay J, Crawford L, et al. Classic and novel risk faactor parameters in women with a history of preeclampsia. Hypertension 2003;42:39–42.
[26] Blaauw J, van Pampus M, Van Doormaal J, et al. Increased intima-media thickness after early-onset preeclampsia. Obstet Gynecol 2006;107:1345–51.
[27] Wilson BJ, Watson MS, Prescott GJ, et al. Hypertensive diseases of pregnancy and risk of hypertension and stroke in later life: results from cohort study. BMJ 2003;326:845–52.
[28] Brown DW, Dueker N, Jamieson DJ, et al. Preeclampsia and the risk of ischemic stroke among young women: results from the stroke prevention in young women study. Stroke 2006;37:1055–9.
[29] Ray J, Vermeulen MJ, Schull MJ, et al. Cardiovascular health after maternal placental syndromes (CHAMPS): population-based retrospective cohort study. Lancet 2005;366: 1797–803.
[30] Lee M, Croen L, Backstrand K, et al. Maternal and infant characteristics associated with perinatal arterial stroke in the infant. JAMA 2005;293:723–9.
[31] Gillum LA, Mamidipudi SK, Johnston SC. Ischemic stroke risk with oral contraceptives. A meta-analysis. JAMA 2000;284:72–8.
[32] Chan W-S, Ray J, Wai EK, et al. Risk of stroke in women exposed to low-dose oral contraceptives. A critical evaluation of the evidence. Arch Intern Med 2004;164:741–7.
[33] Baillargeon J, McClish D, Essah P, et al. Association between the current use of low-dose oral contraceptives and cardiovascular arterial disease: a meta-analysis. J Clin Endocrinol Metab 2005;90:3863–70.
[34] WHO Collaborative Study of Cardiovascular Disease and Steroid Hormone Contraception. Ischaemic stroke and combined oral contraceptives: results of an international, multicentre, case-control study. Lancet 1996;348:498–505.

[35] Heinemann L, Lewis M, Spitzer W, et al. Thromboembolic stroke in young women: a European case-control study on oral contraceptives. Contraception 1998;57:29–37.
[36] Kemmeren JM, Tanis BC, van den Bosch MA, et al. Risk of Arterial Thrombosis in Relation to Oral Contraceptives (RATIO) Study. Oral contraceptives and the risk of ischemic stroke. Stroke 2002;33:1202–8.
[37] Lokkegaard E, Jovanovic Z, Heitmann BL, et al. Increased risk of stroke in hypertensive women using hormone therapy. Arch Neurol 2003;60:1379–84.
[38] Curtis K, Mohllajee A, Martins S, et al. Combined oral contraceptive use among women with hypertension: a systematic review. Contraception 2006;73:179–88.
[39] Heinemann LA, Lewis MA, Thorogood M, et al. Case-control study of oral contraceptives and risk of thormboembolic stroke: results from international study on oral contraceptives and health of young women. BMJ 1997;315:1502–4.
[40] American College of Obstetricians and Gynecologists (ACOG). The use of hormonal contraception in women with coexisting medical conditions. ACOG Practice Bulletin 2006;73.
[41] Hannaford P, Croft P, Kay C. Oral contraception and stroke: evidence from the Royal College of General Practitioners' Oral Contraception Study. Stroke 1994;25:935–42.
[42] Siritho S, Thrift AG, McNeil JJ, et al. Risk of ischemic stroke among users of the oral contraceptive pill. The Melbourne Risk Factor Study (MERFS) Group. Stroke 2003;34: 1575–80.
[43] Chang C, Donaghy M, Poulter N. Migraine and stroke in young women: a case-control study. BMJ 1999;318:13–8.
[44] Tzourio C, Tehindrazanarivelo A, Iglesias S, et al. Case-control study of migraine and risk of ischaemic stroke in young women. BMJ 1995;310:803–33.
[45] Schwartz SM, Pettiti DB, Siscovick DS, et al. Stroke and use of low-dose oral contraceptives in young women. A pooled analysis of two US studies. Stroke 1998;29:2277–84.
[46] Allais G, De Lorenzo C, Mana O, et al. Oral contraceptives in women with migraine: balancing risks and benefits. Neurol Sci 2004;25:S211–4.
[47] Bousser M-G, Conrad J, Kittner S, et al. Recommendations on the risk of ischaemic stroke associated with use of combined oral contraceptives and hormone replacement therapy in women with migraine. Cephalalgia 2000;20:155–6.
[48] Slooter AJ, Rosendaal FR, Tanis BC, et al. Prothrombotic conditions, oral contraceptives and the risk of ischemic stroke. J Thrombosis Haemostasis 2005;3:1213–7.
[49] Pezzini A, Grassi M, Iacoviello L, et al. Inherited thrombophilia and stratification of ischaemic stroke risk among users of oral contraceptives. J Neurol Neurosurg Psychiatry 2007;78: 271–6.
[50] Rexrode K, Hennekens C, Willett W, et al. A prospective study of body mass index, weight change, and risk of stroke in women. JAMA 1997;277:1539–45.
[51] Towfighi A, Saver J, Engelhardt R, et al. A midlife stroke surge among women in the United States. Neurology 2007;69:10.1212/1201.wnl.0000268491.0000289956.c0000268492.
[52] Rannevik G, Jeppsson S, Johnell O, et al. A longitudinal study of the perimenopausal transition: altered profiles of steroid and pituitary hormones, SHBG and bone mineral density. Maturitas 1995;21:103–13.
[53] McKinlay SM. The normal menopause transition: an overview. Maturitas 1996;23:137–45.
[54] Liu Y, Ding J, Bush T, et al. Relative androgen excess and increased cardiovascular risk after menopause: a hypothesized relation. Am J Epidemiol 2001;154:489–94.
[55] Rajkumar C, Kingwell BA, Cameron JD, et al. Hormonal therapy increases arterial compliance in postmenopausal women. J Am Coll Cardiol 1997;30:350–6.
[56] Persico N, Mancini F, Artini P, et al. Transdermal HRT and Doppler findings in normotensive and hypertensive postmenopausal patients. Ultrasound Obstet Gynecol 2005;26: 546–51.
[57] The Writing Group for the PEPI Trial. Effects of estrogen or estrogen/progestin regimens on heart disease risk factors in postmenopausal women. The Postmenopausal Estrogen/Progestin Interventions (PEPI) trial. J Am Med Assoc 1995;273:199–208.

[58] Haines C, Chung T, Chang A, et al. Effect of oral estradiol on Lp(a) and other lipoproteins in postmenopausal women. Arch Intern Med 1996;156:866–72.

[59] Matthews KA, Kuller LH, Sutton-Tyrrell K, et al. Changes in cardiovascular risk factors during the perimenopause and postmenopause and carotid artery atherosclerosis in healthy women. Stroke 2001;32:1104–11.

[60] Pfeilschifter J, Koditz R, Pfohl M, et al. Changes in proinflammatory cytokine activity after menopause. Endocr Rev 2002;23:90–119.

[61] Bushnell CD, Hurn PD, Colton C, et al. Advancing the study of stroke in women. Summary and recommendations for future research from an NINDS-sponsored multidisciplinary working group. Stroke 2006;37:2387–99.

[62] Hulley S, Grady D, Bush T, et al. Randomized trial of estrogen plus progestin for secondary prevention of coronary heart disease in postmenopausal women. JAMA 1998;280:605–13.

[63] Viscoli CM, Brass LM, Kernan WN, et al. A clinical trial of estrogen-replacement therapy after ischemic stroke. N Engl J Med 2001;345:1243–9.

[64] Hendrix SL, Wassertheil-Smoller S, Johnson KC, et al. Effects of conjugated equine estrogen on stroke in the women's health initiative. Circulation 2006;113:2425–34.

[65] Rossouw J, Prentice R, Manson J, et al. Postmenopausal hormone therapy and risk of cardiovascular disase by age and years since menopause. JAMA 2007;297:1465–77.

[66] Bushnell CD, Goldstein LB. Risk of ischemic stroke with tamoxifen treatment for breast cancer: a meta-analysis. Neurology 2004;63:1230–3.

[67] Barrett-Connor E, Grady D, Sashegyi A, et al. Raloxifene and cardiovascular events in osteoporotic postmenopausal women. Four-year results from the MORE (Multiple Outcomes of Raloxifene Evaluation) randomized trial. JAMA 2002;287:847–57.

[68] Barrett-Connor E, Mosca L, Collins P, et al. Effects of raloxifene on cardiovascular events and breast cancer in postmenopausal women. N Engl J Med 2006;355:125–37.

[69] Vogel V, Costantino JP, Wickerham DL, et al. Effects of tamoxifen vs. raloxifene on the risk of developing invasive breast cancer and other disease outcomes. The NSABP Study of Tamoxifen and Raloxifene (STAR) P-2 trial. JAMA 2006;295:2727–41.

[70] American College of Obstetrics and Gynecology. Task force on hormone therapy. Obstet Gynecol 2004;104:1S–129S.

[71] Mosca L, Banka C, Benjamin E, et al. Evidence-based guidelines for cardiovascular disease prevention in women: 2007 update. Circulation 2007;115:1481–501.

[72] Lofmark U, Hammarstrom A. Evidence for age-dependent education-related differences in men and women with first-ever stroke. Neuroepidemiology 2007;28:135–41.

[73] Rothwell P, Coull A, Silver L, et al. Population-based study of event-rate, incidence, case fatality, and mortality for all acute vascular events in all arterial territories (Oxford Vascular Study). Lancet 2005;366:1773–83.

[74] U.S. interim projections by age, sex, race, and hispanic origin [Summary Table 1A]. Available at: http://www.census.gov/ipc/www/usinterimproj/. Accessed September 10, 2007.

[75] Lloyd-Jones D, Leip E, Larson M, et al. Prediction of lifetime risk for cardiovascular disease by risk factor burden at 50 years of age. Circulation 2006;113:791–8.

[76] Mosca L, Linfante A, Benjamin E, et al. National study of physician awareness and adherence to cardiovascular disease prevention guidelines. Circulation 2005;111:499–510.

[77] Chan A, Manson J, Feskanich D, et al. Long-term aspirin use and mortality in women. Arch Intern Med 2007;167:562–72.

[78] Ridker PM, Cook NR, Lee I-M, et al. A randomized trial of low-dose aspirin in the primary prevention of cardiovascular disease in women. N Engl J Med 2005;352:1293–304.

ELSEVIER
SAUNDERS

NEUROLOGIC
CLINICS

Neurol Clin 26 (2008) 1177–1190

Stroke in Minorities

Brian Trimble, MD[a,b,*], Lewis B. Morgenstern, MD[c]

[a]*Alaska Native Medical Center, 4315 Diplomacy Dr., Anchorage, AK 99508, USA*
[b]*Department of Neurology, University of Washington, Seattle, WA, USA*
[c]*The University of Michigan Health System, Cardiovascular Center, Room 3194, SPC #5855, Ann Arbor, MI 48109-5855, USA*

There are several reasons why researchers and clinicians should focus on minority health. The first reason is the justice principle [1]. As the authors discuss in this article, minority populations in the United States have an increased stroke burden. The justice principle suggests that the fact that some people within a population suffer more than others is an unfair situation. It is the responsibility of all in the health care system to rectify this disparity.

Another motivation for addressing the problem is cost. Recent studies suggest a large disparity in the cost of stroke among minority populations, notably due to the earlier age of stroke in African Americans and Hispanic Americans [2]. Reducing health disparities could reduce the economic burden.

Finally, understanding why the burden of stroke is different in minorities provides information about the cause and treatment of disease across all populations. For example, clustering of cavernous malformations in Mexican Americans led to the discovery of a genetic locus for cavernous malformations [3]. Physicians now know that a third to a half of cavernous malformations are familial and inherited in an autosomal dominant pattern. Furthermore, the decreased mortality following stroke among Mexican Americans compared with non-Hispanic whites in this decade, holds hope for clues to improved survival in all populations at risk of stroke [4].

This discussion will focus on stroke in African Americans, Hispanic Americans, and American Indian/Alaska Natives. Non-Hispanic whites will serve as the reference group for comparison. The authors discuss the incidence of modifiable risk factors for stroke within these groups, and

Brian Trimble is the principal investigator for the Alaska Native Stroke Registry and is supported in part by the NINDS/NIH (U01 NS048069).

* Corresponding author.
E-mail address: btrimble@anmc.org (B. Trimble).

0733-8619/08/$ - see front matter. Published by Elsevier Inc.
doi:10.1016/j.ncl.2008.05.010

what is being done to reduce the burden of stroke in minorities. The following is an illustrative example of the implications of social factors and cardiovascular risk factors in two African American women.

A tale of two women

Abby and Bea are two African American women in their mid-40s. Both have hypertension; both are overweight; and both have type II diabetes mellitus. Abby is poor, never finished high school, works out of her home providing child care, and does not have health insurance. Bea is part of middle class America; she has a college education and a job that provides her medical insurance. Bea takes medication regularly for her hypertension and diabetes. Because of Abby's limited income, she often has to forgo buying her hypertension and diabetes medications to pay her bills.

Both women are at high risk for stroke, and both illustrate some problems of dealing with stroke in minorities. The burden of stroke may weigh heavier on minorities in the United States because of differences in education, frequency and distribution of risk factors, income, and access to health care rather than to differences in region, race, or ethnic background (Table 1) [5–12]. Minorities are over-represented in groups that are less educated and socioeconomically disadvantaged. In addition, they may face problems with access to care for reasons related to lack of health coverage or because of language and cultural barriers that lead to mistrust (Fig. 1). Consequently, risk factors such as hypertension and diabetes, which are more common in some minorities, go unrecognized or incompletely treated. The consequence of failing to address primary and secondary prevention measures may result in higher incidence of vascular disease, with greater morbidity and mortality [13–20], and seems to affect those in younger age groups [18,19,21]. Socioeconomic status is indelibly interwoven with the concept of race/ethnicity and disease. Understanding the interaction

Table 1
Factors that may be associated with stroke in minorities

Risk factors [5,6,11]:	Patient factors [56]:
Hypertension	Mistrust and misunderstanding of health care system
Type II Diabetes	Greater tendency to refuse recommended treatment
Hyperlipidemia	Provider factors [56]:
Obesity	Bias or prejudice against minorities
Less leisure exercise	Clinical uncertainty about a patient's condition
Tobacco use	Beliefs or stereotypes about minorities
Excessive use of alcohol	Health care systems-level factors [56]:
Socioeconomic factors [8]:	Language barriers
Lower education level	Short appointments
Lower income	Geographic availability of services
Poor perception of health status	

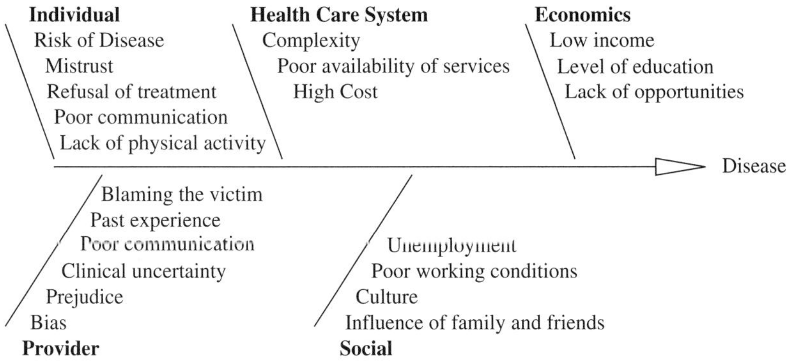

Fig. 1. Cause and effect diagram of factors that contribute to disease in minorities.

between poverty and race/ethnicity may be crucial to understanding health disparities. Although there are reasonable measures of differences in health outcomes in minorities, the measures of socioeconomic status are more challenging, and they may not fully represent the construct of advantage compared with disadvantage. For the purpose of this discussion, race/ethnicity will refer to self-designated social groups sharing similar cultural heritage and ancestry. Race/ethnicity may simply be a proxy for advantage or disadvantage in our society.

Both Abby and Bea are of the same racial background and share similar risk factors for vascular disease. The difference is Abby's lower economic status that may put her at greater risk for vascular disease. This may not only affect her likelihood for access to care, but also the quality of care that she receives.

Health disparities

There are many determinants of inequalities in health. They can be grouped into four broad categories: (1) environment; (2) access and use of services; (3) health status; and (4) difference in health outcomes [22]. In the United States, these inequalities are referred to as health disparities. For the purpose of this discussion, disparity will relate to both unavoidable and avoidable inequalities that lead to stroke. The unavoidable factors such as age, gender, and genetics, give us a better understanding of the causes of stroke. It is the avoidable inequities such as mistrust, refusal of treatment, prejudice, and bias that remind us of the justice principle.

The United States is becoming increasingly diverse. The U.S. Bureau of the Census estimates that by the year 2050, half the United States population will be "minorities." Therefore, a higher burden of disease and mortality among minorities has profound implications for the entire population. For example, there may be higher costs for health due to the loss of productivity of key individuals in the society, and a greater need for health services. The problems racial and ethnic minority groups face accessing high quality care exposes a weakness within our health delivery system. Overall, the United States ranks highly worldwide in the delivery of emergency services, but relatively poorly when it comes to preventive and other services for the population at large [23].

Determining a person's race/ethnicity in epidemiologic studies can be problematic. Since 1960 persons in the United States have specified their own race and ethnicity so that by the 2000 census there were 126 racial and ethnic categories [24]. As mentioned above, the authors define race/ethnicity in terms of history, geography, culture, language, social and economic forces rather than genetics. Actually, genetic research suggests a wide genetic diversity within different racial and ethnic groups [25]. It is likely that a combination of both genetics and environment explain disease states and their outcomes. Consequently, researchers need to understand the contributions and interactions of both. With so many categories of race/ethnicity to choose from, and the complexities of culture and social influence, self-classification may avoid certain potential shortcomings linked to misclassification [26].

An example of how misclassification can skew results can be illustrated in American Indians. For many years it was thought that American Indians had a relatively low incidence of vascular disease. In 1996, a study by the Indian Health Service found large variations in the way race was assigned in American Indians. They found the degree of misreporting race in Native Americans varied from 1.2% in Arizona to 30.4% in California. This resulted in a significant underestimation of coronary artery disease and stroke [27]. Researchers now understand that rates of vascular disease are relatively high in Native Americans, which correlates better with the known high prevalence of risk factors within this group.

The risk and magnitude of stroke in racial and ethnic minorities

Stroke is the third leading cause of death in the United States, and a major cause of disability [28]. However, the burden of fatal and nonfatal stroke is higher and health-related quality of life is lower in racial/ethnic minorities [13,16]. Minority individuals seem to have more hypertension, diabetes, obesity, and less leisure time physical activity than non-Hispanic whites. A higher prevalence of cardiovascular risk factors is further complicated, potentially, by lower education level, poverty, and less access to health care [8,11]. Strokes occur at younger ages and result in greater disability in minority individuals than in non-Hispanic whites [13]. Tables 2–4 lists the findings of age-adjusted stroke incidence for three population-based studies. Non-Hispanic whites were used as the comparison group to calculate rate ratios for each minority group. In Table 2 African Americans between the ages of 35 and 44 years, living in northern Manhattan, New

Table 2
Age and sex adjusted incidence per 100,000 and rate ratios, compared with non-Hispanic whites in four population-based studies of stroke in minorities

Brain attack surveillance in corpus Christy project 2000–2002 [31] (All ischemic strokes)			
Age	Mexican American N = 626	Non-Hispanic White N = 563	Rate ratio
45–59	593	291	2.04
60–74	1875	1187	1.58
≥75	3824	3423	1.12
>45	1375	1137	1.21

York City, NY, have an attack rate ratio for stroke nine times greater than for non-Hispanic whites who are the same age [29]. In Cincinnati, Ohio and northern Kentucky, the incidence rate ratio for stroke was highest for African Americans in the 45 to 55 year age group [30]. Within this age group, the incidence rate ratio for stroke was five times greater than non-Hispanic whites the same age. The attack rate ratio for Hispanics in northern Manhattan was also nearly nine times higher than the non-Hispanic whites in the 35–45 age group. Stroke attack rate ratio was nearly double that of non-Hispanic whites in all age groups in northern Manhattan. In Corpus Christi, Texas, the stroke attack rate ratio in Mexican Americans was higher than non-Hispanic whites but this trend was not as great between Hispanics and non-Hispanic whites in northern Manhattan [31]. Despite the regional and methodology differences, all three studies showed much higher attack rate ratios for stroke in African Americans and Hispanics compared with non-Hispanic whites, particularly in younger age groups.

In the United States, ischemic stroke tends to be more common than hemorrhagic stroke in non-Hispanic whites. This trend is also true for African American, Hispanic, and American Indian/Alaska Native groups. Lacunar strokes are more common in American Indians compared with Hispanics and non-Hispanic whites [32]. Mortality is higher in African Americans compared with non-Hispanic whites for both ischemic and hemorrhagic strokes. In contrast, mortality is lower for American Indian/Alaska

Table 3
Age and sex adjusted incidence per 100,000 and rate ratios, compared with non-Hispanic whites in four population-based studies of stroke in minorities

Greater Cincinnati/Northern Kentucky stroke study 1993 [30] (First ever stroke, including hemorrhagic stroke)			
Age	African American N = 213	Non-Hispanic White[a]	Rate ratio
0–34	7	4	1.75
35–44	121	32	3.78
45–54	320	63	5.08
55–64	637	273	2.33
65–74	972	669	1.45
≥75	1820	736	2.47

[a] Non-Hispanic whites in Rochester, MN 1989 [58].

Table 4
Age and sex adjusted incidence per 100,000 and rate ratios, compared with non-Hispanic whites in four population-based studies of stroke in minorities

Northern Manhattan Stroke Study 1993–1996 [29] (All strokes)

Age	African American N = 148	Hispanic N = 352	Non-Hispanic White N = 162	Rate ratio African American	Rate ratio Hispanic
20–24	19	3	13	1.46	0.23
25–34	0	11	10	0.00	1.10
35–44	54	53	6	9.00	8.83
45–54	184	127	49	3.76	2.59
55–64	366	265	221	1.66	1.20
65–74	636	685	282	2.26	2.43
75–84	1153	804	421	2.74	1.91
≥85	1461	1778	651	2.24	2.73

Natives and Hispanics with ischemic strokes compared with non-Hispanic whites [33]. Some risk factors are more prevalent within a population than others. For example, hypertension is higher in African Americans than any other minority group and diabetes is high in both African Americans and American Indians [7]. This may explain some of the difference in mortality between different minority groups.

Stroke is expensive. The cost was estimated to be $140,000 per patient, for a total cost estimate of $64.7 billion dollars in 2007 [16]. The cost of prevention can pose a challenge as well. There are a growing number of stroke survivors who are unable to afford medications putting them at risk for recurrent stroke. These are mostly African American, poor, female, nonelderly, and ill stroke survivors [34]. Working stroke survivors are unable to afford employer-based health insurance, and disabled stroke survivors age <65 years may not be insured because they do not qualify for Medicare health insurance. Per capita cost of stroke is highest in African Americans at $25,782; followed by Hispanics at $17,201; and non-Hispanic whites at $15,597 [2]. The highest contributor to this cost is loss of earnings. Although the patient and family feel the disability from stroke more acutely, there is also lost productivity, lost wages, and worries about affordability of health care.

To better understand the problem of stroke in minorities in the United States, the authors look at three representative groups: African Americans, Hispanics, and Native Americans. (Although Asian and Pacific Islanders are an important, emerging minority group in the United States with respect to stroke, they are beyond the scope of this review.)

Stroke in African Americans

"African American" refers to a person having origins in a black racial group or Africa [35]. African Americans have approximately double the mortality from stroke compared with other race/ethnic groups [36]. They may achieve less functional improvement after a stroke, though this requires further validation, but despite the higher disability are more likely to be discharged home. Generally, African Americans have a higher prevalence of hypertension, diabetes mellitus, and obesity, and are less likely to report adequate physical activity than non-Hispanics whites. Interestingly, African Americans are more likely to be aware of their hypertension, and they are more often on treatment for their hypertension, but are less likely to have it well controlled [37]. For African Americans, sickle cell anemia is a risk factor for stroke, particularly in children [38]. African American men may use more tobacco and alcohol, whereas African American women may have more hypertension, diabetes, family history of stroke, and less leisure exercise than African American men [39].

Stroke in Hispanics

"Hispanic" refers to a person of Cuban, Mexican, Puerto Rican, South or Central American, or other Spanish culture or origin, regardless of race [35]. Hispanics are the largest minority population in the United States (15%) and Mexican Americans make up the largest subgroup of Hispanics (64%) [31]. Mexican Americans tend to have more diabetes mellitus, and more obesity, lower income, lower education attainment, and report inadequate physical activity compared with non-Hispanic whites [40]. As Table 2 shows, the incidence of stroke in Hispanics is significantly higher than in non-Hispanic whites. Further, the severity and stroke type distributions in Hispanics do not differ from non-Hispanic whites which dispels the myth that stroke in Mexican Americans is predominantly due to small vessel disease [41]. Hispanics are more likely to have a recurrent stroke than African Americans or non-Hispanic whites [42]. Overall stroke mortality is lower in Hispanics except in younger (ages 20–45 years) Hispanics who may have a higher mortality [43]. Hispanics also may have a higher mortality from subarachnoid hemorrhage than other minority groups [31,33].

Stroke in Native Americans

"Native American" refers to a person having origins in any of the original peoples of North, Central, and South America, and who maintains a tribal affiliation or community attachment [35]. Native Americans include both American Indian and Alaska Natives. Native Americans have among the highest rates of risk factors for cardiovascular disease than other race/ethnic groups [44], and the highest prevalence of stroke in non-institutionalized adults [16,28]. Other risk factors include the use of tobacco and alcohol in men. Awareness of diabetes is low, and they report less leisure-time physical activity [45]. Although the prevalence of risk factors is high in this group, they vary by region. Native Americans have more lacunar strokes, and mean age of stroke is generally lower in Native Americans [32].

Little is known about the epidemiology of stroke in Alaska Natives other than the fact that mortality has remained high despite a drop in mortality from stroke nationwide [46]. The Alaska Native Stroke Registry (ANSR) was established in 2005 with funding from the National Institute of Neurological Disorders and Stroke to learn more about stroke in this population [47]. ANSR is a population-based, prospective, surveillance study of stroke in Alaska Natives. The Alaska Native population is well defined and health care is provided through a unique health care delivery system based on a hub and spoke model of care. The aims of the registry are to determine more about the epidemiology of stroke in this population and to monitor the treatment and management of stroke to identify areas where quality of care can be improved. Information from the registry will also help identify critical areas for stroke prevention. Patient entry into ANSR began on October 1, 2005. Information about the frequency of risk factors, stroke type, and stroke incidence rates will be available soon.

Health care to the nearly 20,000 Alaska Native people, many of whom are widely dispersed among more than 200 small communities, is provided largely by the Alaska Tribal Health System. Given the large size of Alaska, the distribution of the population in many small frontier communities, the lack of a comprehensive road system, and the cost and challenges of airplane transportation, health care delivery is organized into a primary, secondary, and tertiary tier system. Primary care is provided in village health clinics staffed by approximately 500 community health aides/practitioners who are community residents trained and certified to provide emergency and primary care in collaboration with physicians based at their regional medical center. Clinics at the farthest reaches of the system feed into 21 tribally-operated health centers and seven tribally-operated hospitals. Regional medical centers are based in the transportation hub of the region and are staffed by physicians who provide primary and secondary care. Patients requiring services not available at the regional centers are referred to the Alaska Native Medical Center in Anchorage, Alaska and, in some cases, tertiary care is provided in other United States cities such as Seattle, Washington, for patients requiring highly specialized services.

Stroke in non-Hispanic whites

Non-Hispanic whites may have higher prevalence of hyperlipidemia, myocardial infarction, and stroke at an older age than other race/ethnic groups. Cardioembolic stroke is more prevalent including atrial fibrillation compared with many minority groups. Mortality from stroke is higher at older age groups than other ethnic groups.

Socioeconomic status also is an important risk factor for stroke. A study in Ontario, Canada, a region with universal health care, found an inverse relationship between income and stroke mortality [48]. Poorer patients were less likely to have access to hospitals and specialty care by neurologists.

They were less likely to have brain imaging with CT and MRI and were less likely to receive rehabilitation services. There was an inverse relation between income and both 30-day and 1-year mortality even after adjustment for age, sex, comorbid conditions, and hospital and physician characteristics.

A recent study in the United States focused on the relationship between wealth, income, and education in relation to risk of stroke [49]. Both wealth and income were independent risk factors for stroke in those 50 to 64 years old; however, wealth was more strongly associated with stroke than other socioeconomic factors. This risk was not found in those over the age of 65, presumably due to a survivor effect. It was concluded that greater wealth is not only a buffer during hard economic times, but wealth also provides the resources that foster a healthy life style. Wealthy people have lower prevalence of smoking, obesity, diabetes, and alcohol consumption.

Reducing disparities in stroke

Healthy People 2010 is a national health promotion and disease prevention initiative instituted by the U. S. Department of Health and Human Services that has a vision for achieving improved health care for all Americans. There are two goals: increase quality and years of healthy life, and eliminate health disparities. With respect to stroke, the goals will focus on both primary and secondary prevention strategies. Especially important is the recognition and treatment of vascular risk factors such as hypertension. An African American community in Maryland demonstrated the effectiveness of using indigenous community health workers to improve control of hypertension [50]. Working in conjunction with an academic health center, local residents were trained to manage, monitor, educate, and counsel people in their community about hypertension. The efforts resulted in a significant reduction in mean blood pressure in the community and an increase in individuals with controlled hypertension. The availability of effective blood pressure lowering drugs may be responsible, at least in part, for the decline in stroke in the United States over the past two decades. In addition, making people aware of stroke symptoms and the need to seek care immediately also may be helpful. The use of thrombolytic therapy is still under-used in the United States. In a study looking at use of recombinant tissue-plasminogen activator (rt-PA) in academic hospitals, researchers found African Americans were one fifth as likely to receive rt-PA than non-Hispanic whites [51].

Children can have a powerful influence on older adults to encourage them to take their medications, have regular check-ups, recognize stroke symptoms, and can alert emergency medical services when those affected are suddenly disabled. In a randomized, controlled trial to teach middle school children about stroke, researchers showed the effectiveness of an educational intervention [52]. The study was done in six middle schools in Corpus Christi, Texas. In three schools, students received 12 hours of classroom instruction on stroke pathophysiology, stroke symptom knowledge, and what to do for witnessed stroke. The other three schools received no instruction. Students were tested about their knowledge in these three areas before and after the intervention. Students in the intervention group showed significant improvement in postintervention testing in all three areas, compared with the students that did not receive the instruction. Children left to the care of older adults can help alert emergency medical services in the event of a stroke.

The American Stroke Association and the National Stroke Association have implemented programs aimed at reaching children, family, and community to heighten awareness of stroke [53,54]. Brainiac Kids and Hip Hop Stroke are both programs for children with ideas for games, plays, and activities to be used at school, home, and in the community, which make learning about stroke fun and easy to remember. Power to End Stroke is a stroke awareness campaign targeting African Americans to heighten awareness of stroke. "Give Me Five for Stroke" (Walk, Talk, Reach, See, Feel) is a joint campaign of the American Academy of Neurology, the American College of Emergency Physicians and the American Heart Association/American Stroke Association to increase awareness among Americans of stroke symptoms and to call 9-1-1 for transport to a nearby hospital emergency department. Another program to help the public recognize the symptoms of stroke and to seek stroke care right away is the "F.A.S.T" campaign (for *F*ace, *A*rm, *S*peech, *T*ime). Studies are needed which can provide scientific evidence that these interventions are effective.

Informal settings such as beauty shops, barbershops, community centers, and churches may be important venues for conducting stroke education. In Atlanta, Georgia and Cincinnati, Ohio, beauticians volunteered to learn about the signs and symptoms and risk factors for stroke. Taking what they learned back to the beauty shop, stroke became a frequent topic in their discussions with customers. As a result, researchers found not only did stroke awareness improve within the community, but this way of educating the community about stroke was also very well received [55]. Blood pressure screenings at community health fairs, grocery stores, and churches can heighten awareness of hypertension. As previously discussed, young people may have an influence on their parents and grandparents by focusing attention on prevention for those at risk. Early intervention to treat or prevent risk factors may lead to lower stroke risk and mortality.

Providers need to do their part to reduce risk factors in minorities. The Institute of Medicine report challenges health care providers and systems to overcome prejudicial attitudes toward minorities and stereotyping which may have a deleterious effect on medical decision-making [56]. To determine the diagnosis and course of treatment, doctors rely on information gained from the patients, coupled with their prior expectations about the patient. If the physician does not accurately understand the symptoms, because of language or cultural barriers, then he or she is more likely to give greater emphasis on predetermined beliefs. These beliefs may be influenced by the age, gender, socioeconomic status, and race/ethnic background of the patient. As a result, patient needs and treatment decisions may not be well matched resulting in mistrust and eventually to refusal of treatment altogether. It is important for all physicians to practice with empathy and cultural sensitivity to build trust and foster a meaningful doctor–patient relationship [57].

Summary

Overall, African Americans, Hispanics, and Native Americans have higher stroke risks, stroke occurrence at an earlier age, and, for some minorities, possibly more severe strokes than non-Hispanic whites. The higher prevalence of risk factors, overall lower socioeconomic status, and health care system challenges for minority patients may contribute to stroke disparities. Stroke is a substantial burden on many minorities in terms of mortality, lost wages, and disability. There are steps, however, that health care providers can take that may reduce this disparity. For example, providers can exhibit sensitivity to the difficulties minority patients may have in negotiating a complicated health care system and attempt to reduce barriers to access to care. Physicians can establish better rapport with patients by better understanding their concerns and the cultural framework that underlie their behaviors and decision-making. Whenever possible, clinicians should use interpreters to facilitate communication when they do not speak the native language of their patients. Being proactive in recognizing vascular risk factors and doing what it takes to reduce them is essential. Health care providers can target populations at risk with programs to heighten awareness of stroke symptoms and risk factors. Informing young people about stroke not only influences the next generation at risk for vascular disease but also helps their parents, other older family members, and friends better understand these disorders, their risk factors, prevention measures, and treatment. By determining what works to change behavior and by breaking down barriers to care, members of the health care system can take critical steps oward reducing stroke disparities.

References

[1] Rawls J. A theory of justice. Cambridge (MA): Belknap Press of Harvard University Press; 1999.
[2] Brown DL, Boden-Albala B, Langa KM, et al. Projected costs of ischemic stroke in the United States. Neurology 2006;67(8):1390–5.
[3] Mindea SA, Yang BP, Shenkar R, et al. Cerebral cavernous malformations: clinical insights from genetic studies. Neurosurg Focus 2006;21(1):e1.
[4] Lisabeth LD, Risser JM, Brown DL, et al. Stroke burden in Mexican Americans: the impact of mortality following stroke. Ann Epidemiol 2006;16(1):33–40.

[5] Richardson A, Yiao Y, Tucker P. Regional and racial differences in prevalence of stroke–23 states and District of Columbia, 2003. MMWR Morb Mortal Wkly Rep 2005;54(19):481–4.

[6] Qureshi AI, Giles WH, Croft JB. Racial differences in the incidence of intracerebral hemorrhage: effects of blood pressure and education. Neurology 1999;52(8):1617–21.

[7] Bolen J, Rhodes L, Powell-Griner E, et al. State-specific prevalence of selected health behaviors, by race and ethnicity–behavioral risk factor surveillance system, 1997. In: U.S. Department of Health and Human Services CfDCap, editor. MMWR CDC surveillance summaries. Vol. 49. March 24, 2000 edition. Washington DC: US Government Printing Office; 2000. p. 1–60.

[8] Bravata DM, Wells CK, Gulanski B, et al. Racial disparities in stroke risk factors: the impact of socioeconomic status. Stroke 2005;36(7):1507–11.

[9] Hayes DK, Greenlund KJ, Denny CH, et al. Racial/ethnic and socioeconomic disparities in multiple risk factors for heart disease and stroke–United States, 2003. MMWR Morb Mortal Wkly Rep 2005;54(5):113–7.

[10] Hayes DK, Greenlund K, Denny C, et al. Racial/ethnic and socioeconomic disparities in multiple risk factors for heart disease and stroke – United States, 2003. MMWR Morb Mortal Wkly Rep 2005;54(05):113–7.

[11] Sacco RL, Boden-Albala B, Abel G, et al. Race-ethnic disparities in the impact of stroke risk factors: the northern Manhattan stroke study. Stroke 2001;32(8):1725–31.

[12] Mensah GA, Mokdad AH, Ford ES, et al. State of disparities in cardiovascular health in the United States. Circulation 2005;111(10):1233–41.

[13] Xie J, Wu EQ, Zheng ZJ, et al. Impact of stroke on health-related quality of life in the noninstitutionalized population in the United States. Stroke 2006;37(10):2567–72.

[14] Shen JJ, Washington EL, Aponte-Soto L. Racial disparities in the pathogenesis and outcomes for patients with ischemic stroke. Manag Care Interface 2004;17(3):28–34.

[15] Kuhlemeier KV, Stiens SA. Racial disparities in severity of cerebrovascular events. Stroke 1994;25(11):2126–31.

[16] Neyer J, Greenlund K, Denny C, et al. Prevalence of stroke – United States, 2005. In: Div for Heart Disease and Stroke Prevention NCfCDPaHP, CDC, editor. MMWR weekly. vol. 56. May 18, 2007 edition. Washington DC: US Government Printing Office; 2007. p. 469–74.

[17] White H, Boden-Albala B, Wang C, et al. Ischemic stroke subtype incidence among Whites, Blacks, and Hispanics: the Northern Manhattan Study. Circulation 2005;111(10):1327–31.

[18] Neyer JR, Greenlund KL, Denny CH, et al. Prevalence of stroke–United States, 2005. MMWR Morb Mortal Wkly Rep 2007;56(19):469–74.

[19] Disparities in deaths from stroke among persons aged <75 years–United States, 2002. In: U.S. Department of Health and Human Services CfDCap, editor. MMWR Morb Mortal Wkly Rep. Vol. 54. 2005/05/20 edition. Washington DC: US Government Printing Office; 2005. p. 477–81.

[20] Liao Y, Tucker P, Giles W. Health status of American Indians compared with other racial/ethnic minority populations – selected states, 2001–2002. In: Div of Adult and Community Health NCfCDPaHP, CDC, editor. MMWR Weekly. vol. 52. Washington DC: US Government Printing Office; 2003. p. 1148–52.

[21] Jacobs BS, Boden-Albala B, Lin IF, et al. Stroke in the young in the northern Manhattan stroke study. Stroke 2002;33(12):2789–93.

[22] Carter-Pokras O, Baquet C. What is a "health disparity"? Public Health Rep 2002;117:426–34.

[23] Holloway RG, Benesch C, Rush SR. Stroke prevention: narrowing the evidence-practice gap. Neurology 2000;54(10):1899–906.

[24] Winker MA. Measuring race and ethnicity: why and how? JAMA 2004;292(13):1612–4.

[25] Burchard EG, Ziv E, Coyle N, et al. The importance of race and ethnic background in biomedical research and clinical practice. N Engl J Med 2003;348(12):1170–5.

[26] Fustinoni O, Biller J. Ethnicity and stroke: beware of the fallacies. Stroke 2000;31(5):1013–5.

[27] Casper M, Denny C, Coolidge J, et al. Atlas of heart disease and stroke among American Indians and Alaska Natives. In: Services DoHaH, editor. Atlanta (GA): US Department of Health and Human Services, Center for Disease Control and Prevention, and Indian Health Service; 2005.

[28] Rosamond W, Flegal K, Furie K, et al. Heart disease and stroke statistics–2008 update: a report from the American Heart Association Statistics Committee and Stroke Statistics Subcommittee. Circulation 2008;117(4):e64.

[29] Sacco RL, Boden-Albala B, Gan R, et al. Stroke incidence among white, black, and Hispanic residents of an urban community: the Northern Manhattan Stroke Study. Am J Epidemiol 1998;147(3):256–68.

[30] Broderick J, Brott T, Kothari R, et al. The Greater Cincinnati/Northern Kentucky Stroke Study: preliminary first-ever and total incidence rates of stroke among Blacks. Stroke 1998;29(2):415–21.

[31] Morgenstern LB, Smith MA, Lisabeth LD, et al. Excess stroke in Mexican Americans compared with Non-Hispanic Whites; The Brain Attack Surveillance in Corpus Christi Project. Am J Epidemiol 2004;160(4):376–83.

[32] Frey JL, Jahnke HK, Bulfinch EW. Differences in stroke between White, Hispanic, and Native American patients: the barrow neurological institute stroke database. Stroke 1998; 29(1):29–33.

[33] Ayala C, Greenlund KJ, Croft JB, et al. Racial/ethnic disparities in mortality by stroke subtype in the United States, 1995–1998. Am J Epidemiol 2001;154(11):1057–63.

[34] Levine DA, Kiefe CI, Howard G, et al. Reduced medication access: a marker for vulnerability in US stroke survivors. Stroke 2007;38(5):1557–64.

[35] Provisional guidance on the implementation of the 1997 standards for federal data on race and ethnicity. In: Budget OoMa, editor. Federal register. vol. 66. Washington DC: US Government Printing Office; 2001. p. 3829–31.

[36] Casper M, Barnett E, Williams GJ, et al. Atlas of stroke mortality: racial, ethnic, and geographic disparites in the United States. In: U.S. Department of Health and Human Services CfDCap, editor. Atlanta (GA): Center for Disease Control and Prevention; 2003. p. 11–2.

[37] Howard G, Prineas R, Moy C, et al. Racial and geographic differences in awareness, treatment, and control of hypertension: the reasons for geographic and racial differences in stroke study. Stroke 2006;37(5):1171–8.

[38] Adams RJ. Big strokes in small persons. Arch Neurol 2007;64(11):1567–74.

[39] Worrall BB, Johnston KC, Kongable G, et al. Stroke risk factor profiles in African American women: an interim report from the African-American Antiplatelet Stroke Prevention Study. Stroke 2002;33(4):913–9.

[40] Smith MA, Risser JMH, Lisabeth LD, et al. Access to care, acculturation, and risk factors for stroke in Mexican Americans: the brain attack surveillance in corpus Christi (BASIC) project. Stroke 2003;34(11):2671–5.

[41] Uchino K, Risser JMH, Smith MA, et al. Ischemic stroke subtypes among Mexican Americans and non-Hispanic whites: the BASIC project. Neurology 2004;63(3): 574–6.

[42] Sheinart K, Tuhrim S, Horowitz DR, et al. Stroke recurrence is more frequent in Blacks and Hispanics. Neuroepidemiology 1998;17(4):188–98.

[43] Karter A, Gazzaniga J, Cohen R, et al. Ischemic heart disease and stroke mortality in African-American, Hispanic, and non-Hispanic white men and women, 1985 to 1991. West J Med 1998;169(3):139–45.

[44] Galloway JM. Cardiovascular health among American Indians and Alaska Natives: successes, challenges, and potentials. Am J Prev Med 2005;29(5 Suppl 1):11–7.

[45] Denny C, Holtzman D, Cobb N. Surveillance for health behaviors of American Indians and Alaska Natives; findings from the behavioral risk factor surveillance system, 1997–2000. MMWR CDC Surveill Summ 2003;52(SS07):1–13.

[46] Day G, Provost E, Lanier A. Alaska native mortality update: 1999–2003. 2006. Available at: www.anthc.org/cs/chs/epi/pubs.cfm. Published Last Modified Date. Accessed July 13, 2008.
[47] Trimble B, Hamel R, Gorelick P, et al. Alaska native stroke registry. International Journal of Stroke 2007;2:60–1.
[48] Kapral MK, Wang H, Mamdani M, et al. Effect of socioeconomic status on treatment and mortality after stroke * editorial comment. Stroke 2002;33(1):268–75.
[49] Avendano M, Glymour MM. Stroke disparities in older Americans. Is wealth a more powerful indicator of risk than income and education? Stroke 2008;39(5):1533–40.
[50] Levine DM, Bone LR, Hill MN, et al. The effectiveness of a community/academic health center partnership in decreasing the level of blood pressure in an urban African-American population. Ethn Dis 2003;13(3):354–61.
[51] Johnston SC, Fung LH, Gillum LA, et al. Utilization of intravenous tissue-type plasminogen activator for ischemic stroke at academic medical centers: the influence of ethnicity editorial comment: it is time to implement stroke practice improvement programs and prevent the racial disparity in stroke care. Stroke 2001;32(5):1061–8.
[52] Morgenstern LB, Gonzales NR, Maddox KE, et al. A randomized, controlled trial to teach middle school children to recognize stroke and call 911: the kids identifying and defeating stroke project. Stroke 2007;38(11):2972–8.
[53] Learn about stroke. Available at: http://www.strokeassociation.org/presenter.jhtml?identifier=3030387. Accessed May 3, 2008, 2008.
[54] Laino C. Hip hop to stroke awareness. Available at: http://www.webmd.com/stroke/news/20070207/hip-hop-to-stroke-awareness. Accessed April 26, 2008.
[55] Smith S, Frankel M, Famikin B, et al. Challenges of community-based research unveiled in the beauty shop stroke education project. Stroke 2007;38(2):612.
[56] Unequal treatment confronting racial and ethnic disparities in health care. In: Smedley BD, Smith AY, Nelson AR, editors. Washington, DC: The National Academies Press; 2003.
[57] LaVeist T, Nickerson K, Bowie J. Attitudes about racism, medial mistrust, and satisfaction with care among African American and white cardiac patients. Med Care Res Rev 2000;57(Suppl 1):146–61.
[58] Brown R, Whisnant JP, Sicks J, et al. Stroke incidence, prevalence, and survival: secular trends in Rochester, Minnesota through 1989. Stroke 1996;27:373–80.

Section V

Prospects for Improving the Quality of Stroke Care

ELSEVIER
SAUNDERS

Neurol Clin 26 (2008) 1191–1207

NEUROLOGIC
CLINICS

National and International Quality Initiatives to Improve Stroke Care

Wende Fedder, RN, MBA

Stroke Center Alexian Brothers Hospital Network, Neuroscience Institute Stroke Center, 800 Biesterfield Road, Elk Grove Village, IL, USA

Stroke is the second leading cause of death worldwide and the third leading cause of death in the United States. Approximately 780,000 new or recurrent strokes occur each year in the United States [1]. It is the leading cause of adult disability and has a significant economic impact. According to Agency for Healthcare Research and Quality, in the United States in 2005 there were an estimated 892,300 hospitalizations for cerebrovascular disease, accounting for 3% of the total costs associated with United States hospital care that year [2]. The Center for Disease Control and Prevention (CDCP) reported that the United States spends $51 billion in lost productivity and health care costs, including $12 billion in nursing home expenditures [3]. Fig. 1 lists present and estimated stroke costs by year in the United States [4]. Because of the major impact and economic burden of stroke around the world, initiatives are underway to improve quality of stroke care that may also reduce cost [1–4]. This article reviews such key national and international quality initiatives.

Prevention initiatives

The United States CDCP sponsors several prevention initiatives designed to improve stroke health. These include Healthy People 2010 and the Paul Coverdell Stroke Registry. Healthy People 2010 is a national prevention statement of health objectives designed to identify the most significant preventable threats to health and to establish national goals to reduce these threats. Overall goals of Healthy People 2010 are to increase the quality and years of healthy life and to eliminate disparities in the burden of disease. The

E-mail address: fedderw@alexian.net

doi:10.1016/j.ncl.2008.06.002

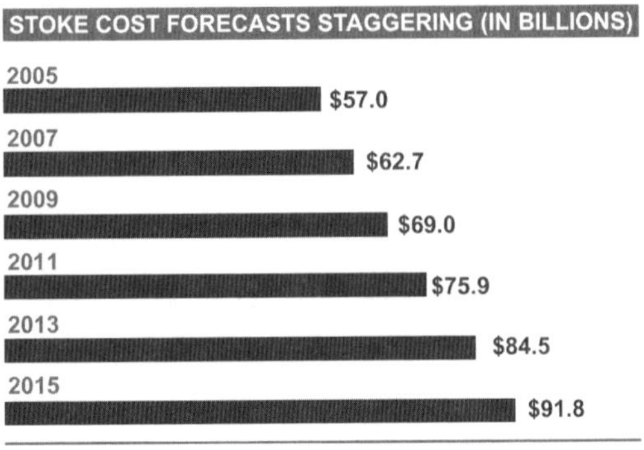

Fig. 1. Stroke cost forecasts in billions of dollars. (*From* Michalke T, Dunne K. The State of Stroke: Organizing for Success. Chicago: NeuStrategy, Inc. 2007; with permission.)

plan has 467 objectives and 16 of those are specifically targeted toward heart disease and stroke [3].

The Paul Coverdell National Acute Stroke Registry [5] was launched in 2001 when Congress requested that the CDCP implement state-based registries to measure and track acute stroke care. Congress named the project after the late United States Senator Paul Coverdell of Georgia, who suffered a fatal stroke in 2000. The long-term goal of this program is to use the registry data to ensure that all Americans receive the highest quality acute stroke care currently available and to prevent deaths attributable to stroke, stroke-related disability, and recurrent stroke. Wave I projects, funded in 2001, were located in Georgia, Massachusetts, Michigan, and Ohio. Wave II projects, funded in 2002, were located in California, Illinois, North Carolina, and Oregon. The project has shown that there are large gaps between generally recommended guidelines for treatment of stroke patients and prevention of subsequent strokes when compared with actual hospital practices [5].

In June 2004, the CDCP provided funds to state health departments of Georgia, Illinois, Massachusetts, and North Carolina to establish statewide Coverdell stroke registries for acute care hospitals. The purpose of these registries was to develop and implement systems for data collection and analysis to guide quality improvement interventions at the hospital level through partnerships with doctors, stroke-care teams, and hospital administrators. By the end of the 2004 to 2007 period, more than 180 hospitals had taken part in a stroke registry program [5].

In June 2007, the CDCP expanded funding to six state health departments in Georgia, Massachusetts, Michigan, Minnesota, Ohio, and North Carolina for the Paul Coverdell National Acute Stroke Registry for a new 5-year funding period. Illinois continues to participate in stroke quality improvement activities and provide information to the CDCP on its progress [5].

Emergency medical service initiatives

In the United States, telephone activation of emergency medical services (EMS) using "911" increases the likelihood that an acute stroke patient will present to the emergency department early enough to be evaluated for acute thrombolytic treatment [6]. Multiple quality initiatives directed at educating potential users of the 911 system have been conducted by the National Stroke Association, the American Stroke Association, and the National Institute of Neurologic Disorders and Stroke. To achieve the goal of accessing 911, the public must be able to recognize the warning signs of stroke and be aware of the need to call the 911 system if symptoms occur. Wein and colleagues [6] have found that education regarding the importance of calling 911 should be directed toward family members, paid caregivers, or coworkers, as those actively experiencing stroke or with a history of stroke may be less likely to access 911.

In addition to the community education challenges, there are challenges associated with integrating the EMS response [7]. For example, state and EMS office personnel and regional and local EMS officials must be educated in relation to the need for pre-hospital notification of stroke patients and development of formal policy for such notification. Additional quality improvements may include transport of patients to the nearest stroke center if a stroke center is located within a reasonable distance, and development of transport or transfer protocols. For EMS rapid transport, it is important to develop quality improvement strategies that address the activation and response by EMS. In addition, these strategies include engaging with pre-hospital and hospital providers in continuous quality improvement processes that comply with protections for the privacy of personal health information. In 1997, the American Heart Association developed a subsidiary called the American Stroke Association (ASA). The first ASA initiatives included the development of a program called Operation Stroke. This was the first program of its type, launched in select cities around the country, to improve the chain of survival for stroke and provide educational campaigns targeted at EMS and community residents. As stroke systems continue to evolve, EMS will have a significant role in stroke quality improvement [7]. It has been said that a good stroke system has a good EMS program as of part of the initiative.

In-hospital stroke center development and designation initiatives

Initial quality improvement

Initial hospital initiatives to improve stroke care were developed for various reasons, including improving fiscal outcomes, creating meaningful evidence-based medicine pertaining to stroke quality, improving overall care. Beginning in the 1970s and 1980s, published articles on stroke quality initiatives began with the focus on stroke rehabilitation program outcomes and development of neurovascular care units, stroke centers, and stroke intensive care units [8–13]. In the 1990s, publications supported designation of stroke units and stroke protocols as ways to reduce length-of-stay for stroke patients and improve quality of care. Wentworth and Atkins [14] published a study showing a reduction in charges and length-of-stay after implementation of a designated stroke unit, medical director, care pathways, and protocols at a community hospital in California. In 1995, Gorelick [15] published an article discussing a strategy to reduce stroke cost called the "Time Zero Plan." He emphasized that hospital length-of-stay was a major variable for inpatient stroke cost. By expediting stroke diagnosis, communicating with the patient and caregiver about the diagnostic and therapeutic plan, and consulting with stroke experts as soon as possible, a high level of quality stroke diagnosis and treatment might be attained. Book and colleagues [16] found that enforcement of care pathway and stroke protocol use had a significant impact on reduction of length-of-stay and improved clinical outcomes in an academic medical center.

In the mid-1990s, the National Stroke Association Stroke Center Network (SCN) [17] hospital stroke program was developed. SCN began in 1996, and helped to establish one of the first National Institutes of Health stroke scale (NIHSS) certification programs and produced several professional, community, and patient education initiatives. SCN contributed data that created Diagnosis Related Group 559, which reimburses hospitals for thrombolytic therapy administration by nearly three times the former amount. SCN developed the National Stroke Association Stroke Center [17] Recommendation Guidelines to build a foundation for stroke center infrastructure. The guidelines were later used by the Brain Attack Coalition (BAC), [18] a group formed in 1996 to improve the understanding of stroke symptoms in the community and improve medical services for stroke. The guidelines served as a foundation to the early draft of Recommendations for the Establishment of Primary Stroke Centers (PSC) in 1998, which were eventually published in the Journal of the American Medicine Association (JAMA) in 2000 [19]. Box 1 provides a list of BAC members [18], which is sponsored by the National Institutes of Health and the National Institute for Neurologic Disorders and Stroke in Bethesda, Maryland. PSCs have specific staffing and infrastructure to first stabilize, then treat acute stroke patients. PSCs are designed to evaluate acute stroke patients for emergent treatment, such as intravenous (IV) thrombolytic therapy, stabilize vital signs, and provide acute brain imaging. Box 2 describes the key components of a PSC [17–19]. A revision of the 2000 publication is underway.

Joint Commission Primary Stroke Center certification

After the PSC guidelines were published, there began a search for a stroke center verification process similar to the American College of Surgeons

Box 1. Brain attack coalition members

American Academy of Neurology
American Association of Neurological Surgeons
American Association of Neuroscience Nurses
American College of Emergency Physicians
American Society of Interventional and Therapeutic Neuroradiology
American Society of Neuroradiology
American Stroke Association
Centers for Disease Control and Prevention
Congress of Neurological Surgeons
National Association of EMS Physicians
National Institute of Neurological Disorders and Stroke
National Stroke Association
Stroke Belt Consortium
Veterans Administration

Data from Brain Attack Coalition. About the Coalition. Available at: http://www.brainattackcoalition.org.

Box 2. Primary Stroke Center components JAMA 2000

Acute Stroke Team (minimum of registered nurse and medical doctor)
Commitment and support of organization and medical director
Continuing medical and allied health education
Emergency departments trained in stroke
EMS education and involvement
Laboratory services, EKG, chest X-ray 24/7
Neuroimaging services 24/7 (CT)
Neurosurgical services within two hours
Outcome and quality improvement
Stroke specific education for stroke team (8 hours)
Stroke Unit designation
Written care protocols

Data from Alberts MJ, Hadaemenos G, Latchaw RE, et al. Recommendations for the establishment of primary stroke centers. JAMA 2000;282:3102–9.

Trauma Center verification process. Kidwell and colleagues [20] published a survey of over 3,000 respondents, including neurosurgeons, neurologists and emergency department physicians who supported the development of stroke centers. In 2003, the ASA, a division of the American Heart Association, and the Joint Commission convened and agreed on a certification process for stroke. Discussions began regarding certification standards for stroke center development. The Joint Commission, founded in 1951, evaluates and accredits approximately 15,000 health care organizations and programs in the United States. As an independent, not-for-profit organization, and the nation's oldest and largest standards setting and accrediting body in health care, the Joint Commission [21,22] was positioned to provide the structure for such a program through their newly developed Disease Specific Certification (DSC) program. DSC was launched as a voluntary program where hospitals could certify a disease management program through an evaluation process. For stroke, the collaboration developed a more consistent approach to clinical outcome measurement and provided a minimum standard for stroke care.

There are three major elements to the Joint Commission's Primary Stroke Center Certification (PSCC). These elements include: compliance with use of evidence-based guidelines, implementation of the Joint Commission standards (Box 3), and measurement of clinical outcomes (Table 1). In addition, receiving the Joint Commission gold seal of approval includes compliance with additional Joint Commission requirements, including The Joint Commission national patient safety goals for disease specific care listed in Box 3 [22,23].

In January 2004, the first hospitals volunteered for PSCC. By April 2005, The Joint Commission reviewed about 15 hospitals each month for PSCC. Out of 4,900 acute hospitals in the United States, 1,200 had reported that they intended to eventually apply for certification [24]. As of May 2008, the Joint Commission had certified over 450 PSCs. In 2007, several states reached greater than 20 Joint Commission certified PSCs. These states include Wisconsin, Texas, Florida, and California [4]. Legislative influences varied among the four states and will be briefly addressed later in subsequent sections (Figs. 2 and 3).

Tracking clinical outcomes

Data collection remains a challenging yet integral component to stroke center quality improvement. Throughout the late 1990s and early 2000s, select stroke registries, including the American Academy of Neurology Stroke Practice Improvement Network Registry, were used to help capture data to improve quality [25]. In 1996, the University Health System Consortium (UHC) conducted their first comprehensive stroke outcome study, reviewing data at member academic medical centers throughout the United States. The UHC conducted subsequent studies over the next 6 years, which

Box 3. The Joint Commission standards and patient safety goals 2008 [16]

The Joint Commission disease specific patient safety goals 2008

Improve the accuracy of patient identification
Improve the effectiveness of communication among caregivers
Reduce the risk of health care-associated infections
Accurately and completely reconcile medications across the continuum of care
Reduce the risk of patient harm resulting from falls
Reduce the risk of influenza and pneumococcal disease in institutionalized older adults
Encourage patients' active involvement in their own care as a patient safety strategy

The Joint Commission disease specific standards

Developing or facilitating care
Program management
Performance measurement
Supporting self management
Clinical information management

From The Joint Commission. Disease specific care certified organizations by disease. Available at: http://www.jointcommission.org/CertificationPrograms/Disease-SpecificCare/DCSPM/. Copyright © The Joint Commission, 2008.

Table 1
Stroke performance measures set following harmonization of measure specifications

No.	Harmonized measure	Ischemic stroke	Hemorrhagic stroke
STK-1	Deep vein thrombosis (DVT) prophylaxis	×	×
STK-2	Discharged on antithrombotic therapy	×	–
STK-3	Patients with atrial fibrillation receiving anticoagulation therapy	×	–
STK-4	Thrombolytic therapy administered	×	–
STK-5	Antithrombotic therapy by end of hospital day two	×	–
STK-6	Discharged on cholesterol reducing medication	×	–
STK-7	Dysphagia screening	×	×
STK-8	Stroke education	×	×
STK-9	Smoking cessation/advice/counseling	×	×
STK-10	Assessed for rehabilitation	×	×

From The Joint Commission. Stroke Performance Measurement Implementation Guide. Available at: http://www.jointcommission.org. (The Joint Commission Web site). January 2008; with permission. Copyright © The Joint Commission, 2008.

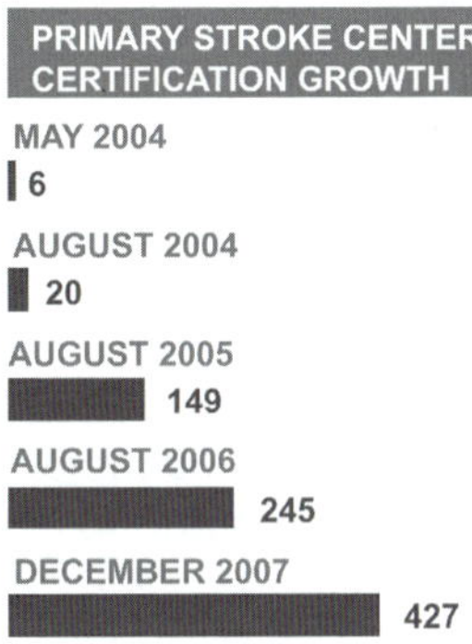

Fig. 2. Primary Stroke Center certification growth in the United States, 2007. (*From* Michalke T, Dunne K. The State of Stroke: Organizing for Success. Chicago: NeuStrategy, Inc. 2007; with permission.)

provided early benchmarking capabilities among academic medical centers. In 2004 to 2005, the ASA began to widely implement the Get With the Guidelines (GWTG)-stroke program, which provided a turnkey approach to continuous quality improvement. The GWTG program provided hospital process and database assistance to meet Joint Commission requirements, including four mandatory preselected clinical outcome measures. As of May 2008, over 1,300 hospitals subscribed to GWTG program [26].

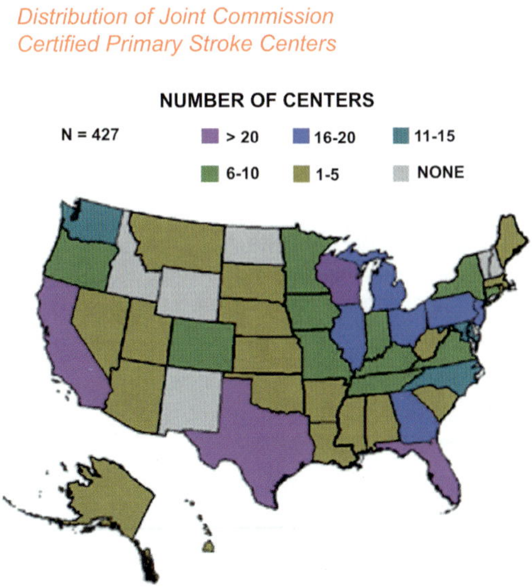

Fig. 3. Primary Stroke Center distribution in the United States, 2007. (*From* Michalke T, Dunne K. The State of Stroke: Organizing for Success. Chicago: NeuStrategy, Inc. 2007; with permission.)

Revisions to clinical measures

In 2008, the Joint Commission introduced new harmonized measures, listed in Table 1. This was accomplished in collaboration with the CDCP and the ASA's GWTG program. By 2008, the Joint Commission certified PSCs were required to collect and electronically report data for all 10 stroke measures. The Joint Commission's [22,23] expert panel recommended, excluding transient ischemic attack patients for reporting purposes based on vagueness or difficulties classifying transient ischemic attack in some cases.

State stroke center designation

In addition to the Joint Commission certification, there are state led designation initiatives. State designation of stroke centers, through state-based public health departments, encourages stroke readiness and requires evaluation for IV thrombolytic therapy. The state of Massachusetts, for example, developed a state-based designation program for stroke centers in 2004. The Massachusetts Department of Health (MDH) statewide stroke prevention and control created a goal to transport stroke patients to an appropriate center within the vital 3-hour treatment window for intravenous tissue-type plasminogen activator or alteplase (tPA) administration. After two years, the MDH drafted an amendment of state regulations creating a license for hospitals with primary stroke services. Massachusetts hospitals able to treat acute stroke within the recommended 3-hour time window for IV tPA are designated by the Department of Public Health as stroke centers [27,28]. Despite several different designation efforts, the impact of these quality initiatives is still being determined.

Does stroke center designation make a difference?

In 2003, Lattimore and colleagues [29] concluded that the establishment of a PSC at a community hospital resulted in a 16% increase in the proportion of patients receiving thrombolytic therapy for ischemic stroke. They concluded that if their experience were generalized, there would be improvements related to reduced cost and clinical outcomes. In 2006, the New York State Stroke Center Designation Project concluded that stroke center designation and selective triage of acute stroke patients improved the quality of care, including access to timely thrombolytic therapy and stroke units. The investigators reported a lack of infrastructure required to treat patients with acute stroke in New York as defined by the BAC guidelines. In 2008, Demaerschalk and colleagues determined it was feasible to develop and operationalize a successful metropolitan-wide matrix of designated stroke centers to accommodate transported patients with acute stroke in a 9,000-square mile region of 3.5 million persons in Arizona. The study showed that after implementation, 18% of the acute stroke population was treated with IV thrombolytic therapy [30,31]. Despite the momentum in favor of stroke center designation, there has been opposition. Concerns surrounding stroke center designation are reviewed elsewhere.

Rehabilitation initiatives

In 2004, the Rehabilitation and Recovery Advisory (RRAB) of the National Stroke Association began to strategically investigate how rehabilitation services could be enhanced so providers who wanted to specialize in stroke rehabilitation could be recognized as leaders in stroke recovery and rehabilitation services. The Commission on Accreditation of Rehabilitation Facilities (CARF) is an international third party accreditation system that currently accredits approximately 5,000 organizations that comprise approximately 38,000 programs. CARF and the National Stroke Association RRAB convened an international standards committee comprised of leading experts in the fields of physical medicine and rehabilitation, reimbursement, allied health and administration. Stroke survivors also played an active role. They produced a set of standards called the Stroke Specialty Program, which was intended for programs seeking accreditation in the United States, Canada, Europe, and South America [32].

These standards can be added to a variety of CARF accreditation programs, such as comprehensive inpatient rehabilitation, outpatient rehabilitation, home and community-based programs, adult day services, assisted living, aging services networks, and long-term care communities. The standards are developed around critical key concepts of rehabilitation, including health, prevention, partnering, life-roles, and supported self-management [32].

Stroke system development and legislation

Quality improvement initiatives reach beyond a single hospital. System-wide approaches have been advocated. For example, in Mississippi this began with a novel statewide approach to care delivery with emphasis on providing various levels of stroke care. In February 2000, the Mississippi Stroke Education Consortium (MSEC), a state-based volunteer advocacy group dedicated to decrease the impact of stroke in Mississippi through continuous education, published a state-based template to promote stroke awareness, prevention, and emergency treatment [33]. The MSEC, which had representation from the state's hospital association, department of health, academic medical centers, and regional affiliate of the American Heart Association proposed five major steps in the development of a statewide emergency stroke network. The steps included: (1) education for professionals and public; (2) stroke care criteria, including acute care availability 24/7, and subacute care with monitoring capability, diagnostic evaluation, and rehabilitation and discharge; (3) medical center designations, including Level I, Level II, and Level III; (4) EMS transport criteria for transporting to Level I, II, or III medical centers; and (5) education with emphasis on public education and continuous education. This template provided a systematic process for educating all the community physicians, allied health, and laypersons about stroke. In addition, it provided a structure for durability, local implementation, comprehensive application, and national reproducibility [33]. David Lee Gordon, MD championed the MSEC.

In 2005, the stroke systems of care related article published in *Stroke* provided a comprehensive approach to building a system of stroke care. The authors were nationally recognized experts in the areas of stroke prevention, emergency medical services, acute stroke treatment, stroke rehabilitation, and health policy development. The article described a stroke system and stated a stroke system should coordinate and promote patient access to the full range of activities and services associated with stroke prevention, treatment, and rehabilitation. The following key components are included in a stroke system of care: primordial and primary prevention, community education, notification and response of emergency medical services, acute stroke treatment, including the hyper-acute and emergency department phases, subacute stroke treatment and secondary prevention, rehabilitation, and continuous quality improvement activities [34].

To support these guidelines, stroke systems of care legislation has occurred on local and national levels. State legislative efforts began in several states, including Georgia, Illinois, Massachusetts, Montana, North Carolina, and Texas. Georgia established the Joint Systems of Care Study Committee designated to examine the stroke systems of care approach. In Illinois, the ASA worked with volunteers and interested groups to introduce the Primary Stroke Center Designation Act. This legislation, which is pending final approval, will allow the director of the Illinois Department of Public Health to designate qualified facilities as stroke ready. In Massachusetts, the state appropriated $500,000 for stroke care to ensure access to quality stroke prevention, treatment, and rehabilitation services. In Montana, the state legislature allocated $1.25 million in funding for the cardiovascular section Public Health and Human Services for stroke awareness and education. Montana is also launching a telemedicine project between a rural hospital and two Montana certified stroke centers. In North Carolina, the General Assembly approved $900,000 in funding to begin efforts to establish a stroke system of care. Texas secured $1.5 million in funding for its previously enacted Stroke Act Texas Legislation. The Texas bill authorizes the Health and Human Services Commission executive commissioner to designate a hospital as a PSC if the hospital is certified by a national medical certification organization such as the Joint Commission [35,36]. No formal state-wide stroke center legislation has been passed in Wisconsin or California. Both states had more than 20 primary stroke centers certified by the Joint Commission, amongst the highest in the Unites States in 2007.

National legislative efforts include the STOP Stroke Act. In March 2007, STOP Stroke Act (H.R. 477) was passed by the full House of Representatives, and in March 2008 the STOP Stroke Act (S.999) was approved by the United States Senate Health, Education, Labor and Pensions Committee. The bipartisan STOP Stroke Act supports stroke recognition and awareness efforts, and encourage medical education and best practice care delivery [37].

In addition to legislative efforts, quality measures are also being evaluated across the acute care continuum. In 2008, the National Quality Forum (NQF) led an effort to evaluate national voluntary consensus standards for prevention and management of stroke across the continuum of care. In this project, NQF identified and endorsed 18 measures that addressed the clinical, system and care coordination aspects involved in effective stroke care across the continuum of care. A steering committee assisted NQF staff in evaluating the candidate measures against the NQF-endorsed measure evaluation criteria of importance, scientific acceptability, usability, and feasibility, as well as standard measure specifications identified by the committee to achieve harmonization [38].

International stroke initiatives

Quality stroke initiatives are increasing among countries around the world, in part because of medical tourism. After the successful launch of domestic DSC primary stroke center certification, Joint Commission International (JCI) began a process of certifying hospitals that met international standards. Approximately 2 years after the launch of their domestic program, the JCI, a division of Joint Commission Resources, the not-for-profit affiliate of The Joint Commission, began development of International Standards for Disease Specific Care. Stroke was included in these standards, and the first health care organizations outside of the United States were certified in stroke in 2006 [21]. Select international programs are in the following sections.

North America

Canada

Each year more than 50,000 Canadians experience a stroke and more than 300,000 currently live with its effects. In 2000, John Manley, Minister of Industry and Minister responsible for the Natural Sciences and Engineering Research Council of Canada and the Social Sciences and Humanities and Research Council, launched the Canadian Stroke Network (CSN), a federal Network of Centers of Excellence. Nearly 20 million dollars was given to develop innovative stroke prevention and recovery strategies. In partnership with the Heart and Stroke Foundation of Canada, in 2006 the CSN developed the Canadian Stroke Strategy. The strategy promoted education and awareness about stroke, the need to use effective treatments, best practices in providing coordinated care in integrated stroke programs, the importance of delivering rehabilitation at the right time and in the right intensity, and the need to support stroke patients and their families in the community [39,40].

In 2008, Lindsay and colleagues [41] identified that despite the evidence supporting best practices in stroke care, significant gaps in translating best practice knowledge into action remain in Canada. An interdisciplinary working group developed best practice recommendations called *Canadian Best Practice Recommendations for Stroke Care*. The best practices consisted of 24 recommendations based on the strongest evidence, and addressed topics across the continuum of stroke care [40]. Recommendations included patient and family education, identification and treatment of depression after stroke, and early assessment of rehabilitation. Implementation and dissemination of these recommendations is in progress [41].

Asia

India, Thailand

In Asia, quality improvement initiatives include programs in India and Thailand. Quality improvement efforts in India include certification by the JCI [40]. Apollo Hospitals, Hyderabad was the first hospital in Asia Pacific to be accredited by the JCI. In addition, Apollo Hospitals, Hyderabad, was the first disease-specific program acute stroke program in the world certified by the JCI [42].

In Thailand, only a few organized stroke units have been established in tertiary medical centers [42]. Thailand, like many countries, faces a major imbalance between the shortage of resources and the large number of patients. However, there are successful quality initiatives. In October 2006, Bumrungrad International in Bangkok, Thailand received disease-specific certification in stroke from the JCI [40]. The hospital's emergency measures, rapid imaging and diagnosis, and effective long-term treatment were reviewed. Bumrungrad International is an internationally accredited, multispecialty hospital, founded in 1980. It is the largest private hospital in Southeast Asia, with 554 beds and over 30 specialty centers. Bumrungrad serves over a million patients annually. Over 400,000 are internationals; they include expatriates who live in Bangkok and nearby countries, plus visitors from 190 countries around the world who come for treatment [42].

South America

Brazil

Stroke quality improvement initiatives are continuing to advance in Brazil. In 2001, the Ministry of Health approved thrombolytic therapy in Brazil for acute ischemic stroke treatment. The health ministry is discussing the possibility of creating a National Stroke Network similar to the CSN.

One of the Brazilian States, Ceará, structured a collaborative network among the institutions involved in acute care and stroke prevention. The majority of stroke patients are treated in public hospitals in Brazil through the Sistema Único de Saúde (SUS; Unified Health System). To improve stroke care in this large health system, there is less need to improve imaging capability; rather, the larger challenge may be to organize an integrated system that improves hospital reimbursement for stroke patients. Hospital Israelita Albert Einstein Stroke Program in São Paulo, Brazil is certified by the JCI [43].

Europe

Norway, United Kingdom, Germany

Stroke is an important cause of morbidity and long-term disability in Europe and imposes a substantial economic burden. In 1998, Ronning and Guldvog [44] published a study that included 802 patients admitted with a stroke diagnosis to a hospital in Norway. During the first few weeks of the study, the case-fatality rate was higher among subjects treated in the general medical ward compared with a stroke unit, especially for subjects with intracerebral hemorrhage. In 2006, the national stroke audit was completed in the United Kingdom and showed differences in stroke care across geographic regions and across hospitals on several similar stroke indicators [41]. A year later, the European Stroke Organization (ESO) founded as a new European society against stroke. The ESO was created from a merger between the European Stroke Council and the European Stroke Initiative. Key objectives of the organization included the development of public policies to reduce the number of stroke-associated deaths [45]. In Germany, a team of stroke specialists standardized the process to develop and implement evidence-based indicators for the measurement of quality of acute hospital stroke care. The development of indicators to measure hospital performance in stroke care is an important step toward improving stroke care on a national level. The chosen standardized evidence-based approaches better ensure maximal transparency, acceptance, and sustainability of the indicators [46].

Australia

Stroke is the second leading cause of death after heart disease in Australia. Every year approximately 53,000 Australians experience stroke. In 2007, the National Stroke Foundation of Australia published an Australian National Stroke Audit (ANSA). The ANSA was the first of its type to represent such a large cross section of hospitals. It examined how often evidence-based recommendations were used in clinical practice and what resources were available to support evidence-based care. The results of the audit were fed back to providers at a local level so that informed decisions to improve stroke care quality could be made. The goals of the ANSA were to provide an overview of the quality of care provided to stroke patients, monitor if clinical guidelines for acute stroke management were being implemented, and describe the variations in stroke services in different parts of Australia and in different hospitals. The results of the ANSA provided a comprehensive overview of the quality of stroke care in Australia and assisted in identifying areas on which to focus ongoing quality improvement activities [47,48].

Summary

Major strides have been made to improve quality of stroke care. The development of stroke units and care pathways has led to improvements in the organization of stroke care. In parallel, there has been the establishment of PSCs and state level programs to improve stroke care. In the future, we may be formally certifying comprehensive stroke centers [49]. Furthermore, the use of quality tools borrowed from other industries may better identify areas for quality improvement in stroke. Finally, as available litigation involving stroke therapy with tPA indicates liability is predominantly associated with failure to provide therapy, quality of care will most certainly remain an important component in the foundation of our medical system [50].

References

[1] American Heart Association. Heart disease and stroke statistics—2008 update. Dallas, (TX): American Heart Association; 2008. Available at: http://www.americanheart.org/downloadable/heart/1200082005246HS_Stats%202008.final.pdf. Accessed April 20, 2008.
[2] Russo CA, Andrews R. Hospital stays for stroke and other cerebrovascular diseases, 2005 Agency for Healthcare Research and Quality (AHRQ) healthcare cost and utilization project. Statistical Brief 51. 2008 May.
[3] Centers for Disease Control. About Healthy People 2010, Hyattsville (MD): CDC, National Center for Health Statistics. Available at: http://www.cdc.gov/DHDSP/stroke_registry.htm. Accessed March 12, 2008.
[4] Michalke T, Dunne K. The state of stroke—organizing for success. 2007.
[5] Centers for Disease Control. The Paul Coverdell National Acute Stroke Registry, Atlanta, GA, CDC, Division of Heart Disease and Stroke Prevention Paul Coverdell National Acute Stroke Registry. Available at: http://www.cdc.gov/DHDSP/stroke_registry.htm. Accessed April 20, 2008.
[6] Wein T, Straub L, Felberg R, et al. Activation of emergency medical services for acute stroke in a nonurban population: the T.L.L. Temple Foundation Stroke Project. Stroke 2000;31:1925–8.
[7] Acker J, Pancioli P, Crocco T, et al. Implementation strategies for emergency medical services within stroke systems of care: a policy statement from the American Heart Association/American Stroke Association Expert Panel on Emergency Medical Services Systems and the Stroke Council. Stroke 2007;38:3097–115.
[8] Kennedy F, Pozen T, Gabelman E. Stroke intensive care: an appraisal. Am Heart J 1970;80:188–96.
[9] Drake W, Hamiltosn M, Carlsson M, et al. Acute stroke management and patient outcome: the value of neurovascular care units (NCU). Stroke 1973;4:933–45.

[10] Millikan C. Stroke intensive care units. Stroke 1979;10:235–7.
[11] Wood-Dauphinee S, Shapiro S, Bass E, et al. A randomized trial of team care following stroke. Stroke 1984;15:864–72.
[12] Norris J, Hachinski V. Stroke units or stroke centers? Stroke 1986;17:360–2.
[13] Reding M, McDowell F. Focused stroke rehabilitation programs improve outcome. Arch Neurol 1989;46:700–1.
[14] Wentworth D, Atkinson R. Implementation of an acute stroke program decreases hospitalization costs and length of stay. Stroke 1996;27:1040–3.
[15] Gorelick P. Acute ischemic stroke and transient ischemic attack: a costly business and strategy to reduce costs: the time zero plan. Journal of Stroke and Cerebrovascular Disease 1995; 5(1):1–5.
[16] Book D, Fedder W, Sunstrom C. Can ischemic stroke clinical outcome tools really improve clinical outcomes? J Stroke Cerebrovasc Dis. 2001;10(4):195, W.B. Saunders Company.
[17] National Stroke Association. For medical professionals. 2006. Available at: http://info.stroke.org. Accessed April 25, 2008.
[18] Brain Attack Coalition. About the Coalition. Available at: http://www.brainattackcoalition.org. Accessed March 20, 2008.
[19] Alberts MJ, Hadaemenos G, Latchaw RE, et al, For the Brain Attack Coalition. Recommendations for the establishment of primary stroke centers. JAMA 2000;282:3102–9.
[20] Kidwell C, Shepherd T, Tonn S, et al. Establishment of primary stroke centers: survey of physician attitudes and hospital resources. Neurology 2003;60:1452–6.
[21] Potter M. Executive Director Disease Specific Care, The Joint Commission 2003–2005. Interview April 2008.
[22] The Joint Commission. Disease specific care certified organizations—by disease Available at: http://www.jointcommission.org/CertificationPrograms/Disease-SpecificCare/DCSPM/. Accessed January 24, 2008.
[23] The Joint Commission. Stroke performance measurement implementation guide (The Joint Commission Web site). Available at: http://www.jointcommission.org/certificationprograms/primarystrokecenters/stroke_pm_edition2.htm. Accessed May 28, 2008.
[24] Zoler M. Rapid growth of organized acute stroke care continues. Family Practice News. Philadelphia Bureau 2005. Volume 35. No (9).
[25] State of New Jersey Department of Health and Senior Services. Development in Stroke Registries. Available at: http://www.state.nj.us/health/healthcarequality/stroke/initiatives.shtml. Accessed May 15, 2008.
[26] American Stroke Association. Get with the guidelines. Available at: http://www.strokeassociation.org/presenter.jhtml?identifier=3002728. Accessed May 5, 2008.
[27] Bettger J. Massachusetts Department of Health. National Association of Chronic Disease Directors. Available at: http://www.chronicdisease.org/files/public/SSS_MA_Stroke_WEB.pdf. Accessed May 5, 2008.
[28] Centers for Medicare and Medicaid. MS-DRG Summary Table. Available at: http://www.cms.hhs.gov/AcuteInpatientPPS/downloads/MSDRGSummaryTable.pdf. Accessed May 5, 2008.
[29] Lattimore SU, Chalela J, Davis L, et al. Impact of establishing a primary stroke center at a community hospital on the use of thrombolytic therapy: the NINDS suburban hospital stroke center experience. Stroke 2003;34:e55–7.
[30] Gropen TI, Gagliano PJ, Blake CA, et al, NYSDOH Stroke Center Designation Project Workgroup. Quality improvement in acute stroke: the New York State Stroke Center Designation Project. Neurology 2006;67(1):88–93.
[31] Demaerschalk B, Bobrow B, Paulseon M. Development of a metropolitan matrix of primary stroke centers: the Phoenix experience. Stroke 2008;39:1246–53.
[32] National Stroke Association. CARF stoke specialty program standards stroke clinical updates for SCN members. Vol. XVII. Issue 1. Summer 2007.

[33] Gordon D. The Mississippi Stroke Education Consortium: a state-based template to promote stroke awareness, prevention and emergency treatment. Neuroepidemiology 2000;19:1–12.
[34] Schwamm L, Pancioli A, Acker J, et al. Recommendations for the establishment of stroke systems of care recommendations from the American Stroke Association's task force on the development of stroke systems. Stroke 2005;36:690–703.
[35] American Heart Association. Heart and Stroke News. Summer 2008.
[36] Texas State Legislature. Emergency Health Care Act; SB No.330. 2006. Available at: http://www.capitol.state.tx.us/tio/79R/billtext/SB00330.HTM. Accessed March 22, 2008.
[37] American Stroke Association. STOP stroke facts bill summary: HR 477/S999 Stroke Treatment and Ongoing Prevention Act (STOP Stroke Act): a bill to improve the prevention, diagnosis, and treatment of stroke. Available at: http://www.heart.org/downloadable/heart/1205765220696STOP%20Stroke%20Fact%20Sheet%2003-14-08.pdf. Accessed May 28, 2008.
[38] National voluntary consensus standards for prevention and management of stroke across the continuum of care. National Quality Forum. 601 13th Street NW, Suite 500 North, Washington, DC 20005. Available at: http://www.qualityforum.org/projects/ongoing/stroke/comments/index.asp. Accessed May 24, 2008.
[39] Canadian Stroke Network and the Heart Foundation of Canada. Canadian stroke strategy, Canadian best practice recommendations for stroke care 2006. National Stroke Nursing Council. Ottowa 2006. p. 43–5.
[40] The Joint Commission International. Joint Commission accredited organizations. Available at: http://www.jointcommissioninternational.org/23218/iortiz/. Accessed May 15, 2008.
[41] Lindsay P, Bayley M, McDonald A, et al. Toward a more effective approach to stroke: Canadian best practice recommendations for stroke care. CMAJ 2008;178(11):1418–25.
[42] Suwanwela NC, Eusattasak N, Phanthumchinda K, et al. Combination of acute stroke unit and short-term stroke ward with early supported discharge decreases mortality and complications after acute ischemic stroke. J Med Assoc Thai 2007;90(6):1089–96.
[43] Massaro Ayrton R. Stroke in Brazil: a South America perspective. International Journal of Stroke 2006;1:113–5.
[44] Ronning OM, Guldvog B. Stroke unit versus general medical wards, II: neurological deficits and activities of daily living. Stroke 1998;29:586–90.
[45] Brainin M, Olsen T, Chamorro A, et al. Organization of stroke care: education, referral, emergency management and imaging, stroke units and rehabilitation. For the EUSI executive committee and the EUSI writing committee. Cerebrovasc Dis 2004;17(Suppl 2):1–14.
[46] Heuschmann P, Biegler M, Busse O, et al. Development and implementation of evidence-based indicators for measuring quality of acute stroke care: The Quality Indicator Board of the German Stroke Registers Study Group (ADSR). Stroke 2006;37(10):2573–8.
[47] National Stroke Foundation 2007. National stroke audit organisational report acute services. Available at: www.strokefoundation.com.au. Accessed May 28, 2008.
[48] National Stroke Foundation 2007. National stroke audit clinical report acute services. Available at: www.strokefoundation.com.au. Accessed May 28, 2008.
[49] Alberts MJ, Latchaw RE, Selman WR, et al, For Brain Attack Coalition. Recommendations for comprehensive stroke centers; a consensus statement from the Brain Attack Coalition. Stroke 2005;36:1597–618.
[50] Liang BA, Zivin JA. Empirical characteristics of litigation involving tissue plasminogen activator and ischemic stroke. Ann Emerg Med 2008;52(2):160–4.

ELSEVIER
SAUNDERS

NEUROLOGIC
CLINICS

Neurol Clin 26 (2008) 1209–1225

Index

Note: Page numbers of article titles are in **boldface** type.

A

doi:10.1016/S0733-8619(08)00130-8
neurologic.theclinics.com

B

C

D

E

N

O

P

Q

R

S

T

United States Postal Service

Statement of Ownership, Management, and Circulation
(All Periodicals Publications Except Requestor Publications)

1. Publication Title: Neurologic Clinics
2. Publication Number: 0 0 0 - 7 1 2
3. Filing Date: 9/15/08
4. Issue Frequency: Feb, May, Aug, Nov
5. Number of Issues Published Annually: 4
6. Annual Subscription Price: $218.00
7. Complete Mailing Address of Known Office of Publication (*Not printer*) (*Street, city, county, state, and ZIP+4*)
Elsevier Inc.
360 Park Avenue South
New York, NY 10010-1710
Contact Person: Stephen Bushing
Telephone (Include area code): 215-239-3688
8. Complete Mailing Address of Headquarters or General Business Office of Publisher (*Not printer*)
Elsevier Inc., 360 Park Avenue South, New York, NY 10010-1710
9. Full Names and Complete Mailing Addresses of Publisher, Editor, and Managing Editor (*Do not leave blank*)

Publisher (*Name and complete mailing address*)
John Schrefer , Elsevier, Inc., 1600 John F. Kennedy Blvd. Suite 1800, Philadelphia, PA 19103-2899

Editor (*Name and complete mailing address*)
Donald Mumford, Elsevier, Inc., 1600 John F. Kennedy Blvd. Suite 1800, Philadelphia, PA 19103-2899

Managing Editor (*Name and complete mailing address*)
Catherine Bewick, Elsevier, Inc., 1600 John F. Kennedy Blvd. Suite 1800, Philadelphia, PA 19103-2899

10. Owner (*Do not leave blank. If the publication is owned by a corporation, give the name and address of the corporation immediately followed by the names and addresses of all stockholders owning or holding 1 percent or more of the total amount of stock. If not owned by a corporation, give the names and addresses of the individual owners. If owned by a partnership or other unincorporated firm, give its name and address as well as those of each individual owner. If the publication is published by a nonprofit organization, give its name and address.*)

Full Name	Complete Mailing Address
Wholly owned subsidiary of	4520 East-West Highway
Reed/Elsevier, US holdings	Bethesda, MD 20814

11. Known Bondholders, Mortgagees, and Other Security Holders Owning or Holding 1 Percent or More of Total Amount of Bonds, Mortgages, or Other Securities. If none, check box → ☐ None

Full Name	Complete Mailing Address
N/A	

12. Tax Status (*For completion by nonprofit organizations authorized to mail at nonprofit rates*) (*Check one*)
The purpose, function, and nonprofit status of this organization and the exempt status for federal income tax purposes:
☐ Has Not Changed During Preceding 12 Months
☐ Has Changed During Preceding 12 Months (*Publisher must submit explanation of change with this statement*)

13. Publication Title: Neurologic Clinics
14. Issue Date for Circulation Data Below: August 2008

15. Extent and Nature of Circulation			Average No. Copies Each Issue During Preceding 12 Months	No. Copies of Single Issue Published Nearest to Filing Date
a. Total Number of Copies (*Net press run*)			2300	2200
b. Paid Circulation (By Mail and Outside the Mail)	(1)	Mailed Outside-County Paid Subscriptions Stated on PS Form 3541. (*Include paid distribution above nominal rate, advertiser's proof copies, and exchange copies*)	1074	996
	(2)	Mailed In-County Paid Subscriptions Stated on PS Form 3541 (*Include paid distribution above nominal rate, advertiser's proof copies, and exchange copies*)		
	(3)	Paid Distribution Outside the Mails Including Sales Through Dealers and Carriers, Street Vendors, Counter Sales, and Other Paid Distribution Outside USPS®	607	585
	(4)	Paid Distribution by Other Classes Mailed Through the USPS (e.g. First-Class Mail®)		
c. Total Paid Distribution (*Sum of 15b (1), (2), (3), and (4)*) ▶			1681	1581
d. Free or Nominal Rate Distribution (By Mail and Outside the Mail)	(1)	Free or Nominal Rate Outside-County Copies Included on PS Form 3541	78	93
	(2)	Free or Nominal Rate In-County Copies Included on PS Form 3541		
	(3)	Free or Nominal Rate Copies Mailed at Other Classes Mailed Through the USPS (e.g. First-Class Mail)		
	(4)	Free or Nominal Rate Distribution Outside the Mail (Carriers or other means)		
e. Total Free or Nominal Rate Distribution (Sum of 15d (1), (2), (3) and (4)			78	93
f. Total Distribution (Sum of 15c and 15e) ▶			1759	1674
g. Copies not Distributed (See instructions to publishers #4 (page #3)) ▶			541	526
h. Total (Sum of 15f and g)			2300	2200
i. Percent Paid (15c divided by 15f times 100) ▶			95.57%	94.44%

16. Publication of Statement of Ownership
☐ If the publication is a general publication, publication of this statement is required. Will be printed in the **November 2008** issue of this publication. ☐ Publication not required

17. Signature and Title of Editor, Publisher, Business Manager, or Owner

Jean Fanucci – Executive Director of Subscription Services — Date: September 15, 2008

I certify that all information furnished on this form is true and complete. I understand that anyone who furnishes false or misleading information on this form or who omits material or information requested on the form may be subject to criminal sanctions (including fines and imprisonment) and/or civil sanctions (including civil penalties).